Radiologic Science

Workbook and Laboratory Manual

Sixth Edition

Stewart C. Bushong, Sc.D., FACR, FACMP
Professor, Department of Radiology
Baylor College of Medicine
Houston, Texas

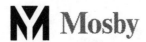 Mosby

St. Louis Baltimore Boston Carlsbad Chicago Naples New York Philadelphia Portland
London Madrid Mexico City Singapore Sydney Tokyo Toronto Wiesbaden

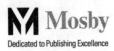
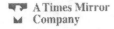

Vice President and Publisher: Don Ladig
Senior Editor: Jeanne Rowland
Senior Developmental Editor: Lisa Potts
Project Manager: Mark Spann
Production Editor: Gina Keckritz, Wordbench
Design and Layout: Ken Wendling, Wordbench
Designer: Judi Lang
Manufacturing Supervisor: Karen Boehme

Cover Photos: Custom Medical Stock Photos, Inc.

Sixth Edition

Printed in the United States of America
Composition by Wordbench
Printed by Plus Communications

Mosby-Year Book, Inc.
11830 Westline Industrial Drive
St. Louis, Missouri 63146

ISBN:0-8151-1580-6

97 98 99 00 01/9 8 7 6 5 4 3 2 1

Consultants

Linda Wendling, MA
Learning Theory Consultant
University of Missouri—St. Louis
St. Louis, Missouri

Joanna Bligh, MEd, RT(R)
Medical Division
Northeast Career Schools
Manchester, New Hampshire

Introduction

The new edition of Bushong's *Radiologic Science* brings with it a completely updated *Workbook and Laboratory Manual*. Questions have been revised, of course, to match the revised text, reflecting new information in the field and applying it in clinical and academic problems. However, some things remain the same: we have retained the popular Experiment and Math Tutor Sections and have updated the Crossword Puzzles, integrating them, this time around, within specific chapters to correspond more directly to the student's text materials. Finally, we have added opportunities for some critical thinking and more project- or action-oriented problems than were in past editions.

We have added a new section to each chapter called "Challenge Questions." These challenge sections offer three kinds of questions:
- The Extended Examination of a topic based completely on text content but more extensive in terms of application and integration than the typical workbook question can afford time for;
- Increased Research Opportunities;
- Occasional Critical Thinking questions that are truly more challenging or difficult. Critical thinking exercises differ from typical objective questions in that they demand (1) integration of information from more than one place or context, (2) sorting and analysis, and/or (3) incorporation of stored knowledge into encountered situations.

To increase student study and interaction opportunities, we strongly suggest that instructors allow students to read and correct each other's worksheets, particularly the essay portions. Although reading essay answers for an entire class is time-consuming for instructors, it can be a valuable review for students. The purpose of the worksheets is to provide for review and test preparation. What better way to prepare than to be challenged repeatedly to ensure that competing answers to a single essay question are all thorough and accurate? We see two ways to use the worksheets to maximum advantage:

- Establish student teams that will take turns reviewing the class's worksheet answers for a specific chapter. Students almost universally find that they perform well above their normal range of test scores on chapters in which they have had the opportunity to do this kind of comparison work. When that realization sets in, they regard the exercise of checking essay and calculation problems for what it is—an excellent study opportunity, one that affords more insights than studying in isolation. (Evaluating multiple-choice questions is not as educational, but fortunately, it only takes minutes to perform!)

- An excellent alternative, and a better one, if time allows, is for each student to check his or her own work in class, as the class is challenged to compare their results in small groups, coming back together for ultimate discussion and confirmation of their conclusions. Students will remember discussions, debates, and verbal challenging of one another's choices more thoroughly than they will remember what they have learned alone with a book, a felt-tip, and a box of Junior Mints—although we continue to support the use of Junior Mints.

The following reviewers provided valuable input that helped in revising the workbook:
Alberto Bello, MEd, RT, Oregon Institute of Technology; Joseph Bittengle, MEd, RT(R), ARRT, University of Arkansas for Medical Sciences; Nadia Bugg, PhD, RT, Midwestern State University; John Clouse, BS, RT, Owensboro Community College; Joseph Dielman, BS, RT(R), ARRT, Triton College; Deborah Edney, BSRT, South Arkansas Community College; Christopher Gould, MS, RT(R), San Jacinto College Central; Wynn J. Harrison, MEd, RT(R)(N), Weber State University; Darrell Hinger, RT(R), Northwest Technical College; John T. Leesburg, RT(R), Jefferson State Community College; Robert Luke, PhD, Boise State University; C. William Mulkey, EdD, RT(R), FASRT, FAERS, Midlands Technical College; Robert J. Parelli, MA, RT(R), Cypress College; Kevin Seisler, BA, RT(R), Mayo Clinic Foundation; Gloria Strickland, MHS, RT(R), Armstrong Atlantic State University; and Natalie Wagner, MS, RT(R)(M), Swedish American Hospital.

A final word for students—we encourage you to form a study group to discuss and review homework and test review materials together. Remember: You are more likely to retain knowledge gained in interaction than that gained in isolation.

As always, Mosby welcomes your comments on this and all our publications in the imaging sciences.

Table of Contents

Worksheets

PART ONE: Radiologic Physics

1   Basic Concepts of Radiation Science, 1
2   Radiographic Definitions and Mathematics Review, 5
3   Fundamentals of the Physics of Radiation Science, 13
4   The Atom, 19
5   Electromagnetic Radiation, 23
6   Electricity, 27
7   Magnetism, 31
8   Electromagnetism, 35

PART TWO: The X-ray Beam

9   The X-ray Unit, 41
10   The X-ray Tube, 47
11   X-ray Production, 51
12   X-ray Emission, 57
13   X-ray Interaction with Matter, 61

PART THREE: The Radiographic Image

14   Radiographic Film, 65
15   Processing the Latent Image, 69
16   Intensifying Screens, 73
17   Scatter Radiation and Beam-Restricting Devices, 79
18   The Grid, 83
19   Radiographic Quality, 87
20   Radiographic Exposure, 91
21   Radiographic Technique, 95

PART FOUR: Special X-ray Imaging

22   Alternative Film Procedures, 101
23   Mammography, 107
24   Mammography Quality Control, 113
25   Fluoroscopy, 117
26   Introduction to Angiography and Interventional Radiology, 123
27   Computer Science, 127
28   Digital X-ray Imaging, 135
29   Computed Tomography, 139

30   Spiral Computed Tomography, 143
31   Quality Assurance and Quality Control, 145
32   Film Artifacts, 149
33   Human Biology, 153

PART FIVE: Radiation Protection

34   Fundamental Principles of Radiobiology, 159
35   Molecular and Cellular Radiobiology, 161
36   Early Effects of Radiation, 165
37   Late Effects of Radiation, 171
38   Health Physics, 175
39   Designing for Radiation Protection, 179
40   Radiation Protection Procedures, 183

Math Tutor by Quinn B. Carroll, MEd, RT, 187

Experiment Section, 217

Worksheet Answers, 295

Math Tutor Answers, 347

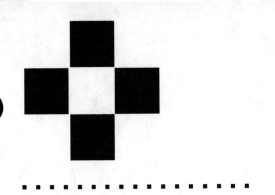

Worksheets

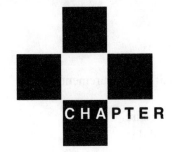

CHAPTER 1   Basic Concepts of
Radiation Science

Match each of the following.

1. _____ Roentgen

2. _____ Einstein

3. _____ Edison

4. _____ Rollins

a. discovered x-rays

b. invented the fluoroscope

c. first used collimation and filtration

d. developed the theory of relativity

Circle the correct answer to each of the following.

5. Matter is defined as:
   a. a gravitational force.
   b. mutual attraction between the earth's mass and the mass of a person.
   c. anything that occupies space.
   d. a force exerted by a body.

6. The principal difference between mass and weight is:
   a. there is no difference; mass and weight are always the same.
   b. when matter changes state (i.e. from solid to liquid), it changes mass.
   c. weight does not change with position, but mass does.
   d. mass is the quantity of matter in an object, and weight is the force exerted by gravity.

7. Geoffrey is the first radiography student to be sent to the moon. He is worried about any physical changes to his body. You assure him that while he is on the moon, his _____ will be the same, even though his _____ will be less.
   a. weight; mass
   b. mass; tissue (matter) distribution
   c. mass; weight
   d. energy; weight

8. Energy is defined as:
   a. a force exerted by a body.
   b. anything that occupies space and has shape.
   c. the ability to do work.
   d. the quantity of matter.

9. Thermal energy is the energy of motion _____; nuclear energy is the energy contained _____.
   a. below ground level; in the air
   b. at the molecular level; in the nucleus of an atom
   c. in volcanic rocks and springs; in the nuclei of molecules
   d. wherever there is heat; wherever there is more than one nucleus

10. Which of the following is an example of kinetic energy?
    a. an unused x-ray machine
    b. a portable x-ray machine in motion
    c. a portable unit parked at a patient's bedside
    d. a and c.

11. An example of chemical energy is that of _____; an example of electrical energy is _____.
    a. a humidifier; a refrigerator
    b. a kiss; making sulphur matches
    c. dynamite; a refrigerator
    d. boiling water; lighting a stove

1

12. Which of the following is *not* electromagnetic radiation?
    a.   ultraviolet rays from the sun
    b.   gravity
    c.   radio waves from a radio tower
    d.   heat from a stove

13. In Einstein's famous $E = mc^2$ equation, c stands for
    a.   mass-energy equivalence.
    b.   the speed of light.
    c.   the theory of relativity.

14. An example of electromagnetic radiation that ionizes matter is:
    a.   slow-moving beta radiation.
    b.   x-rays.
    c.   sound.
    d.   heat.

15. Ionization occurs when:
    a.   an ion pair is converted to gamma rays.
    b.   an orbital electron is released from an atom.
    c.   x-rays and gamma rays interact.
    d.   matter ionizes natural sources of radiation.

16. X-rays and _____ produce enough energy to ionize matter.
    a.   alpha rays
    b.   beta rays
    c.   gamma rays
    d.   ultrasound

17. Examples of the various types of natural environmental radiation include:
    a.   cosmic rays, thorium, and radon.
    b.   increases in altitude; local geology; concrete and gypsum.
    c.   the stars, uranium, and potassium-40.
    d.   the sun, radon, and alpha particles.

18. Which of the following is the largest source of human exposure to man-made radiation?
    a.   nuclear power generating stations
    b.   medical x-rays
    c.   radioactive materials in consumer products
    d.   radioactive fallout

19. The mrad (mGy) unit of measurement relates to:
    a.   radiation overexposure.
    b.   radiation absorbed dose.
    c.   scatter radiation.
    d.   nonionizing radiation.

20. The rad has been changed to the international unit, the:
    a.   gray (Gy).
    b.   sievert (Sv).
    c.   more measurable mrad.
    d.   roentgen.

21. What type of tube was Roentgen using when he discovered x-rays?
    a.   Coolidge tube.
    b.   Crookes' tube.
    c.   anode tube.
    d.   Snook interrupterless transformer.

22. The phosphor that Roentgen employed in his early experiments with x-rays was:
    a.   calcium tungstate.
    b.   rare earth.
    c.   barium platinocyanide.
    d.   zinc cadmium sulfide.

23. The risk of radiation exposure in radiology and diagnostic imaging departments is:
    a.   minimal and thus considered safe.
    b.   high in all radiation areas.
    c.   uncontrolled through collimation, filters, and use of the Bucky grid.
    d.   minimal when patients are held during procedures.

24. Early effects of radiation overdose include _____; latent or late effects include _____.
    a.   decreased sperm count; genetic effects to offspring
    b.   skin cancer; deep tissue cancer
    c.   itching and purpura; blood and chromosomal changes
    d.   birth defects; spontaneous abortion

25. The acronym ALARA:
    a. stands for "Avoiding Low Achievement Radiation Allowance."
    b. suggests that radiographers become as familiar as possible so that they can ignore safety procedures.
    c. suggests that all exposure be kept as low as reasonably achievable.
    d. stands for "American Low-level Radiation Association."

26. The cardinal principles of radiation protection are:
    a. exposure time, badges, and the overhead tube.
    b. protective barrier, monitor, and avoiding unnecessary x-ray exams.
    c. exposure time minimization, yearly mammograms, and fetal monitors.
    d. time, distance, and shielding.

27. The main reason for using aluminum filters in x-ray imaging is to:
    a. reduce low-energy x-rays.
    b. sharpen the image.
    c. absorb penetrating radiation.
    d. absorb heat.

28. Use of collimation:
    a. degrades image quality.
    b. improves image visibility.
    c. increases exposure time.
    d. results in patient discomfort.

29. All of the following help to reduce patient exposure except the use of:
    a. cones.
    b. filtration.
    c. intensifying screens.
    d. fixed protective barriers.

30. Which of the following is *not* one of the 10 basic radiation control principles in diagnostic radiology?
    a. Wear protective apparel during fluoroscopy.
    b. Use gonad shields for every procedure.
    c. Always wear a radiation monitor while at work.
    d. Collimate the x-ray beam to the smallest appropriate field size.

31. During fluoroscopy, a radiographer should always:
    a. remain as close to the patient as possible.
    b. leave the radiation monitor behind the fixed protective barrier.
    c. wear a radiation monitor under the lead apron.
    d. wear protective apparel.

32. The base for a radiographic emulsion prior to World War I was:
    a. cellulose nitrate.
    b. cellulose acetate.
    c. calcium tungstate.
    d. glass.

33. The Coolidge x-ray tube:
    a. was a type of transformer.
    b. has a hot cathode vacuum tube.
    c. did not allow energy and intensity to be accurately selected.
    d. is a series of induction coils for a high-voltage power supply.

34. The Potter-Bucky grid, introduced in 1921:
    a. reduced patient exposure.
    b. increased visibility of the image on film.
    c. reduced examination time.
    d. provided x-ray collimation

CHALLENGE QUESTIONS

■ ■ ■ ■ ■ ■ ■ ■ ■ ■ ■ ■ ■ ■ ■ ■ ■ ■

1. Complete the following statement: "In general, x-ray examinations should be limited to . . ."

2. Discuss ways in which physicians, radiologists, and radiographers at a large medical center can help reduce unnecessary patient exposure to radiation.

3. How many kinds of energy are used during an x-ray examination?

4. List important contributions (include dates) made by Roentgen.

5. What are the NCRP and the ICRP?

6. Explain the concepts of time, distance, and shielding.

7. What were the three most common radiation injuries seen in the early years? Briefly define each.

8. What was Michael Pupin's most significant contribution?

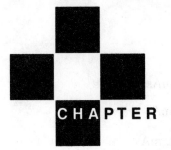

. . . .

Match the following scientific notations to their prefixes and symbols.

1. _____ 10^{12}	a. centi-	i. M
2. _____ 10^{-9}	b. deka-	ii. μ
3. _____ 10^{-2}	c. tera-	iii. m
4. _____ 10^{-6}	d. giga-	iv. k
5. _____ 10^{6}	e. kilo-	v. da
6. _____ 10^{3}	f. nano-	vi. T
7. _____ 10^{-3}	g. micro-	vii. G
8. _____ 10^{9}	h. mega-	viii. n
9. _____ 10	j. milli-	ix. c

. . . .

Circle the correct answer to each of the following.

10. The unit of radiation intensity in air is:
    a. equal to the radiation intensity that will create 2.58×10^{-4} ion pairs in a cubic centimeter of air.
    b. traditionally known as the roengten (R).
    c. in terms of electric charge per unit mass of air.
    d. b and c.
    e. all of the above.

11. In diagnostic radiology, it is acceptable to assume that 1R is equal to:
    a. 1 rem.
    b. 1 Ci.
    c. 1 erg.
    d. 1 J.

12. The formula 1×10^{-2} Gy represents:
    a. one rem or sievert.
    b. the radiation absorbed dose.
    c. the quantity of radiation received by a patient.
    d. the quantity of radioactive material.
    e. b and c.
    f. a and c.

13. A film badge report would express a radiographer's dose equivalent in:
    a. roentgens.
    b. rad.
    c. rem.
    d. curies.

14. Which of the following units expresses the quantity of radioactive material?
    a. becquerel
    b. seivert
    c. Ci
    d. a and c
    e. none of the above

15. In the SI system:
    a.   1 J is approximately equal to 1 MeV.
    b.   the dose equivalent is expressed in units of Gy.
    c.   a dose of 1000 rad is equivalent to 100 Gy.
    d.   a dose of 1000 rad is equivalent to 10 Gy.

Use Tables 2-1 and 2-3 as aids in solving the following problems.

16. Ten kilometers (km) is equivalent to _____ meters (m).

17. 10 μA = _____ mA.

18. If your mass is 70 kg, it is also _____ Mg.

19. 1 nm = _____ m.

20. The normal source-to-image receptor distance (SID) for an upright chest radiograph is 180 cm. This is equivalent to _____ mm.

REVIEW OF MATHEMATICS

Solve the following fraction, decimal, or algebraic equations.

21.   2/4 + 2/12 =

22.   3/8 – 3/16 =

23.   1/2 x 1/4 =

24.   6 7/8 x 2 11/16 =

25.   1/2 ÷ 1/3 =

26.   What is the ratio of 100 mAs to 400 mAs?

27.   8.05 x .693 =

28.   6.02 ÷ 2.567 =

29.   13a = 126; a =

30.   168 + b = 42; b =

31. $\dfrac{x}{8 \text{ mR}} = \dfrac{300 \text{ mAs}}{400 \text{ mAs}}$; x =

32. $\dfrac{75 \text{ kVp}}{80 \text{ kVp}} = \dfrac{210 \text{ mAs}}{x}$; x =

33.   Given that a = bc, if a = 189 and b = 27, then c = ?

Convert each to power-of-ten notation and then perform the indicated operations.

34.   37,000 + 617 =

35. $3.2 \times 48.6 \times 10^{-5}$ =

36. $(10^5)^4$ =

37. $\dfrac{10 \times 10^3 \times 10^{-2} \times 10^5}{10^2 \times 10^{-4}}$

38.   An iodine atom has a diameter of about 4×10^{-10} m. A 60 keV x-ray has a wavelength of 2×10^{-11} m. What is the ratio of the atomic diameter to the x-ray wavelength?

	Fraction	Decimal
39.	1/8 =	_____
40.	1/60 =	_____

	Decimal	Fraction
41.	0.05 =	_____
42.	0.333 =	_____

Solve for x in the following proportions.

43.   x / 7 = 5 / 10

44.   125 / 0.6 = 50 / x

MILLIAMPERE-SECOND CONVERSIONS

Compute the following total mAs values. To benefit from this exercise, do not figure your calculations on paper—do them mentally, then write your answer.

	mA	x	time(s) =	mAs
45.	100	@	0.07 =	_____
46.	500	@	0.004 =	_____
47.	600	@	0.125 =	_____

GRAPHS

Locate the number indicated to the left of each adjacent scale.

48. −0.8

49. 3.6

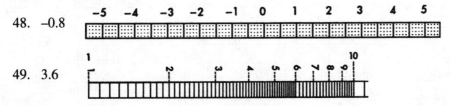

Plot the following set of data on the linear-linear grid and on the linear-log (semilog) graph paper provided.

50. A very small change in filament current results in a very large change in x-ray tube current. A special high-intensity tube design is being tested, and the following data are obtained:

Filament amperes	Tube milliamperes
5.2	25
5.7	50
6.2	100
6.7	200
7.1	300
7.6	500
7.9	700
8.1	900
8.4	1200

51. Radioactive ^{131}I has a half-life of 8 days. An unknown quantity is analyzed today (t = 0 days) and results in 9860 counts per minute (c/min). If analysis of this sample continues at 10-day intervals, the dose might appear as follows:

Time (d)	Activity (c/min)
0	9860
10	4146
20	1744
30	733
40	308
50	130
60	55
70	23
80	10

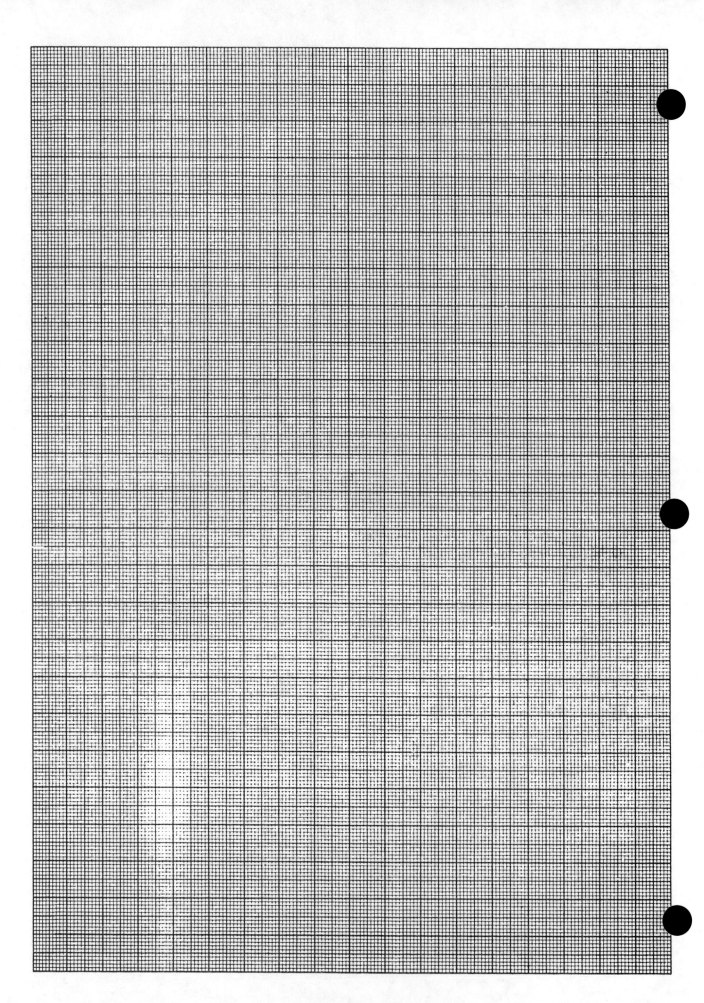

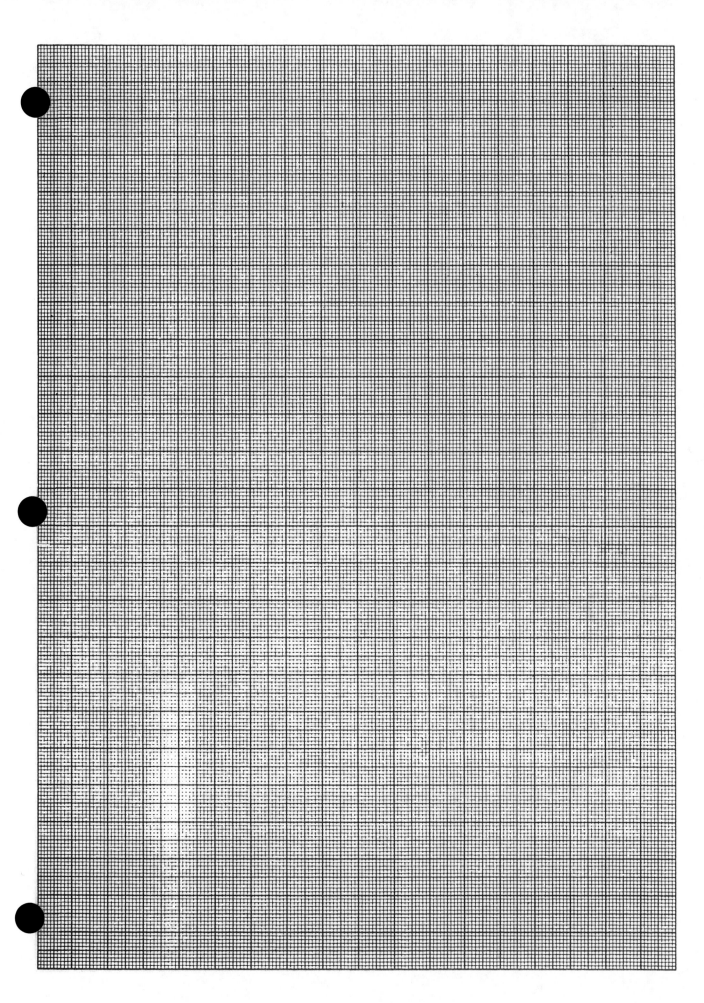

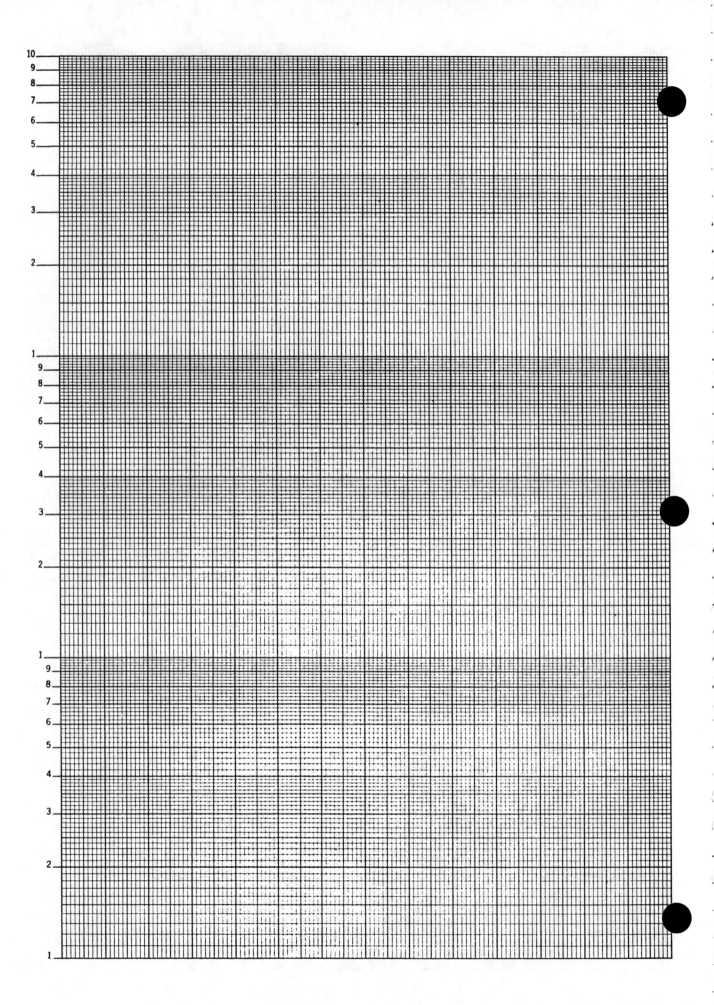

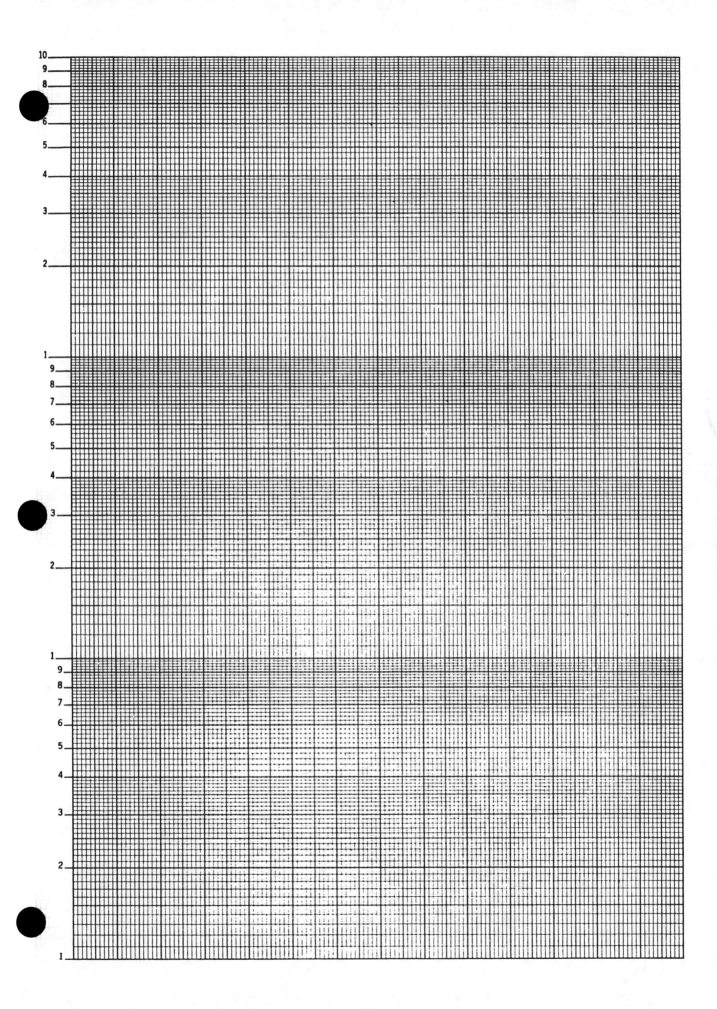

CHALLENGE QUESTIONS

■ ■ ■ ■ ■ ■ ■ ■ ■ ■ ■ ■ ■ ■ ■ ■ ■ ■ ■

1. The number of broken legs is directly proportional to the number of people who fall on the ice skating rink at Rockefeller Plaza. What is the expected number of broken legs for 60 spills on the ice if 20 falls last month resulted in 3 broken legs?

2. A 1/10-second radiographic exposure is equivalent to _____ ms.

3. A PA chest radiograph will expose a patient to approximately 20 mR. This is equivalent to _____ μR.

4. A radiographic unit emits 3.7 mR/mAs (95 μC/kg–mAs). If a given technique requires 120 mAs, what will be the exposure?

5. The radiographic output intensity is 4.3 mR/mAs (111 μC/kg–mAs). If a given technique is 200 mA, 1/60s, what will be the exposure?

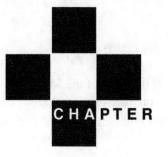

CHAPTER 3

Fundamentals of the Physics of Radiation Science

....

1. Label the figure shown here to illustrate not only the three kinds of quantities measured in physics but examples of each. Naturally, you should not consult your text—except to check your work!

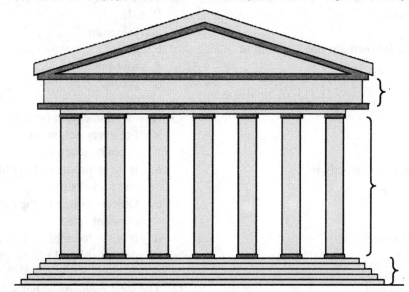

....

2. Complete the following table without consulting your text:

Systems of Units

Unit	British	MKS	_____	SI Units
length	_____	meter	centimeter	_____
mass	_____	_____	_____	_____
time	_____	_____	_____	_____

....

Circle the correct answer to each of the following.

3. The International Bureau of Weights and Measures is located in:
   a. Washington, D.C.
   b. London.
   c. Berlin.
   d. Paris.

4. Which of the following is a base unit in the SI?
   a. coulomb
   b. coulomb/kilogram
   c. kilogram
   d. gray

5. Which of the following standards of measure is correct?
   a. The meter is related to the visible emission from the sun.
   b. The meter is the length of an engraved platinum-iridium bar.
   c. The second is based on the rotation of the earth around the sun.
   d. The second is based on the vibrations of cesium atoms.

6. Which of the following is not a system of units?
   a. SI
   b. CGS
   c. French
   d. British

7. Another name for velocity is:
   a. mass.
   b. speed.
   c. time.
   d. distance/time.

8. Acceleration is also:
   a. a time squared.
   b. a rate of change of velocity with time.
   c. a rate of change of time with velocity.
   d. a rate of change of velocity with distance.

9. The one unit of measure that is the same for all systems is the:
   a. meter.
   b. kilogram.
   c. second.
   d. pound.

10. Which of the following correctly states Newton's first law of motion?
    a. An object with mass (m) and acceleration (a) is acted on by a force given by F = ma.
    b. For every action, there is an opposite and equal reaction.
    c. The total momentum before any interaction is equal to the total momentum after the interaction.
    d. An object at rest will remain at rest unless acted on by an external force.

11. If someone fell off the edge of the south rim of the Grand Canyon, the force exerted would be measured in:
    a. pounds.
    b. kilograms.
    c. newtons.
    d. m/s.

12. The newton is to SI as the _____ is to British.
    a. kilogram
    b. gram
    c. foot-pound
    d. pound

13. How is momentum best described?
    a. For every action, there is an equal and opposite reaction.
    b. It is the product of the mass of an object and its velocity.
    c. Objects falling to the earth accelerate at a constant rate.
    d. It is the force of an object caused by the downward pull of gravity.

14. The total momentum before any interaction is:
    a. decreased by the property of friction, so it is less after the interaction.
    b. an equal and opposite reaction.
    c. equal to the total momentum after the interaction.
    d. greater than the total momentum during the interaction.

15. Which of the following is a unit of work?
    a. rad
    b. joule
    c. gray
    d. newton

16. Which of the following is *not* true?
    a. An object held motionless requires no work applied to it.
    b. The work applied to an object is equal to the force used over a distance.
    c. Power is the product of force and distance.
    d. Power is the rate of work performed over time.

17. A one-bedroom apartment might use 1000 kW-hr of electricity. The kilowatt is a unit of:
    a. power.
    b. energy.
    c. potential energy.
    d. heat.

18. Which of the following statements regarding energy is true?
    a. Energy is the rate of doing work.
    b. Energy is the ability to do work.
    c. Power is a form of energy.
    d. X-rays can be described by their potential energy.

19. Work:
    a. involves the same units as energy.
    b. depends on time.
    c. is performed when a large weight is held motionless.
    d. can be measured in watts.

20. KE is:
    a. directly proportional to velocity.
    b. directly proportional to acceleration.
    c. directly proportional to mass.
    d. a vector quantity.

21. Which of the following is the primary method of heat dissipation from the anode of an x-ray tube?
    a. heat conduction
    b. power reduction
    c. heat convection
    d. thermal radiation

22. Which of the following is the freezing temperature of water?
    a. 0° F
    b. 0° C
    c. 0° K
    d. –273° K

23. In the law of conservation of energy, energy:
    a. can be created or destroyed.
    b. cannot be created or destroyed.
    c. can be transformed from one form to another.
    d. a and c.
    e. b and c.

On a separate sheet of paper, compute the answers for the following questions, using the formulas in your text.

24. A self-propelled, portable x-ray unit can travel the length of a 90 ft (27 m) corridor in 15 s. Express its velocity in ft/s.

25. What is the velocity of a rocket with a mass of 6.1 x 106 kg that develops a takeoff thrust (momentum) of 48.1 x 10^8 N?

26. An automobile is traveling at a velocity of 60 km/hr. It accelerates uniformly to a velocity of 100 km/hr. What was its average velocity during acceleration?

27. Any object dropped near the surface of the earth falls with an acceleration of 9.8 m/s^2. What is its velocity after 2 s if it is released from rest? What is it after 6 s (velocity has units of m/s)?

28. What force is required to move a 68.4 kg portable x-ray machine with an acceleration of 2.31 m/s^2 along a frictionless surface?

29. A radiographer exerts a force of 70 N on a heavy portable x-ray machine and pushes it 40 m in 100 s. What is the work done?

30. What is the power used by the radiographer in the previous problem?

31. Which of the following has more energy?
    a. a 4.5 kg javelin hurled with a velocity of 58 m/s
    b. a 92.5 kg ape in a tree 8.0 m from the ground

Circle the correct answer to each of the following.

32. Which of the following units could be used to express velocity?
    a. m/yr
    b. nm/ns
    c. both of the above
    d. none of the above

33. A stack of x-ray cassettes are sitting on a shelf. In the hallway, a portable x-ray machine is being pushed slowly over the carpet. Which principles have been referred to?
    a. work
    b. power
    c. potential energy
    d. a and b
    e. a and c

34. Kinetic energy is:
    a. mass x gravity x height.
    b. mass x velocity squared.
    c. the energy of motion.
    d. b and c.
    e. a and c.

35. Carole, on assignment in Alaska, is warming her cold hands at a small electric heater in the exam room. As a patient is brought in on a stretcher, she turns toward him, burning her knee on the heater. How has heat been transferred to Carole?
    a. by conduction and thermal radiation first; then by convection
    b. by convection and conduction, initially; then by thermal radiation
    c. by thermal radiation and convection first; then by conduction
    d. by thermal radiation only, although she attempted to use convection

CHALLENGE QUESTIONS
∎ ∎ ∎ ∎ ∎ ∎ ∎ ∎ ∎ ∎ ∎ ∎ ∎ ∎ ∎ ∎

1. Harriet and Jack are going to job interviews at the same hospital in a different city. Harriet knows precisely where to go and how long it will take her to get there. Jack knows how far he has to drive, but has no idea where he's going.
    a. What additional information does Harriet have? What is this called?
    b. What could you call Jack's information (besides "inadequate")?

2. Harriet (from question 1) drives her car 120 miles in 2 hours at a steady rate of 60 mph. Harriet's velocity is _____.
    a. 60 mph
    b. 55 mph
    c. 85 mph
    d. 240 mph

3. Harriet's acceleration was:
    a. 60 mi/hr^2
    b. 0 mi/hr^2
    c. 120 mi/hr^2
    d. not calculable, since not enough data is provided.

4. Jack starts out at a rate of 85 miles per hour, which he cannot maintain for long. As a result, he drops fairly rapidly to 65 miles per hour. He manages to make the trip in 4 hours. What was Jack's average velocity?
    a. 85 mph
    b. 65 mph
    c. 20 mph
    d. 10 mph

5. What was Jack's acceleration?
   a. 5 mi/hr^2
   b. 20 mi/hr^2
   c. 65 mi/hr^2
   d. 85 mi/hr^2

6. Jack drives to another city to apply for another radiographer position. He is late and still has another 150 miles to go to meet his distance goal. Between 1:30 and 2:15, he drives at 85 mph. However, at 2:15 he slows down to 65 mph. He drives at this speed for one hour. At that time, he returns to 85 mph over the next 15 minutes and stays at that speed until his arrival at 4:15. Has Jack's acceleration been positive or negative?

7. What exactly was Jack's acceleration between 2:15 and 3:15? between 3:15 and 4:15?

The Atom

■ ■ ■ ■ ■ ■ ■ ■ ■ ■ ■ ■ ■ ■ ■

CHAPTER 4

1. Identify each of these atom models.

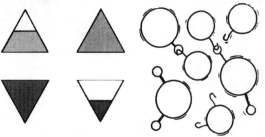

A _____   B _____

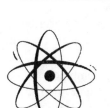

C _____   D _____

■ ■ ■ ■ ■ ■ ■ ■ ■ ■ ■ ■ ■ ■ ■ ■

Circle the correct answer to each of the following.

2. Today, _____ elements have been identified; _____ are naturally occurring, and _____ have been artificially produced.
   a. 104; 52; and 15
   b. 120; 62; and 16
   c. 108; 92; and 16
   d. 104; 92; and 15

3. Particles smaller than the atom:
   a. have never been discovered; the atom is the smallest part of an element.
   b. are quarks.
   c. are called subatomic particles.
   d. were discovered by the Greeks.

4. In developing the term _____, the theorist _____ concluded that each element was composed of identical atoms, each reacting the same way in chemical reactions.
   a. atomic mass; Dalton
   b. identical subparticle; Mendeleev
   c. hook-and-eye elements; Thomson
   d. elemental mass; Rutherford

5. The superscript on a chemical symbol is the:
   a. atomic number.
   b. number of isotopes.
   c. natural occurrence.
   d. atomic charge.

6. Rutherford's model describes the atom as containing a small, dense, _____ center surrounded by _____.
   a. positively charged; a negative cloud of electrons
   b. negative nucleic; a positive cloud of electrons
   c. neutral nucleic; an equally charged layer or "cloud" of electrons
   d. chocolate; a hard candy shell

7. According to _____, in the neutral atom, the number of electrons is equal to the number of _____.
   a. Dalton; positrons
   b. Bohr; positive charges in the nucleus
   c. quantum mechanics; neutrons producing positive ions
   d. Thomson; energy levels or prescribed orbits

8. When two or more atoms combine:
   a. a chemical, ionic bond is formed.
   b. they form molecules, which are also called chemical elements.
   c. they form chemical compounds, called covalent bonds.
   d. they may form molecules, which may join to form larger combinations.

9. Ionic bonding:
   a. is the sharing of electrons.
   b. is the bonding of two atoms with opposite, imbalanced charges.
   c. breaks down the nuclear structures of the atoms involved.
   d. is the attraction of two identical atoms, forming what is called an elemental molecule.

10. The fundamental particles include:
    a. the subatomic mass, the atomic mass unit, and the atomic mass number.
    b. the ion, the valence, and the isotope.
    c. the shell, the nucleus, and the amu.
    d. the electron, proton, and neutron.

11. The atomic mass number of an electron:
    a. is 9.1 x 10-31.
    b. is 0.000549 amu.
    c. equals one-twelfth the mass of a carbon-12 atom.
    d. is 0.

12. The number of protons plus the number of neutrons in the nucleus of an atom is:
    a. called the atomic number.
    b. called the atomic mass number.
    c. represented by A.
    d. a and c.
    e. b and c.

13. The nucleus of the atom:
    a. is mostly empty space, like our solar system.
    b. contains less than 0.001% of the volume of the atom.
    c. contains orbital electrons that can reach orbits thousands of times greater than the diameter of the nucleus.
    d. contains nearly all the mass of the atom.

14. The number of protons:
    a. always determines the number of electrons.
    b. determines the chemical element.
    c. determines the number of isotopes for that atom.
    d. determines an atom's electrical charge.

15. The closer an electron is to the nucleus:
    a. the higher its binding energy.
    b. the more its energy diminishes.
    c. the less accessible it is for binding.
    d. the less it is attracted to electrons in other atoms.

16. An ionized atom:
    a. represents the normal atomic state.
    b. has an electric charge of 0.
    c. occurs by addition or subtraction of protons.
    d. carries a charge equal in magnitude to the difference between the number of electrons and protons.

For each of the following chemical abbreviations, identify the element and its atomic mass.

	Element	Atomic Mass
17. Ag	_____	_____
18. Cu	_____	_____
19. Au	_____	_____
20. C	_____	_____
21. Fe	_____	_____
22. Pb	_____	_____
23. Al	_____	_____
24. Mo	_____	_____
25. W	_____	_____

26. Identify the number of electrons that occupy the outermost shell of the following elements.
    - The number of electrons in the outermost shell of a beryllium atom is _____.
    - The number of electrons in the outermost shell of a calcium atom is _____.
    - The number of electrons in the outermost shell of an iodine atom is _____.
    - The number of electrons in the outermost shell of a barium atom is _____.

27. The maximum number of electrons allowed in any outer shell is ____, which makes the atom _____:
    a. 8; chemically stable
    b. 88; a transitional element
    c. 238; reach maximum atomic mass—in other words, it must be uranium.
    d. 98; in other words, the atom can be determined to have a seventh shell.

Answer each of the following on a separate sheet of paper.

28. What are transitional elements?

29. What is the difference between centripetal force and centrifugal force?

30. What does the symbol E_b stand for?

31. An abnormally excited atom emits particles and energy, transforming itself into another atom in order to reach stability. Is this really possible? If not, describe how such an atom could achieve stability. If it is possible, what is this process called?

32. What is a nuclide, and how can it become a radionuclide?

33. What two things happen at once during beta emission?

34. How does one determine the rate of radioactive decay and the quantity of material present at any given time?

35. What is the half-value layer?

Circle the correct answer to each of the following.

36. Examples of ionizing radiation include:
    a. particulate radiation.
    b. ultrasound.
    c. some electromagnetic radiation.
    d. a and b.
    e. a and c.

37. Which of the following is/are true?
    a. Every subatomic particle is already ionized by virtue of being subatomic.
    b. Electrons are ionized if they are in motion and possess sufficient kinetic energy.
    c. a and b
    d. none of the above

38. Alpha particles:
    a. sustain and transfer kinetic energy for a very long time, once ionized.
    b. easily transfer their kinetic energy to orbital electrons of other atoms.
    c. lose energy quickly.
    d. a and b.
    e. b and c.

39. Beta particles:
    a. are light particles with an atomic mass number of 0.
    b. originate in the nuclei of radioactive atoms.
    c. differ from alpha particles in mass, but not in charge.
    d. a and b.
    e. b and c.

40. Forms of electromagnetic radiation:
    a. are x-rays and gamma rays that have not deteriorated into photons.
    b. differ in their origins and their charges.
    c. include photons that have no mass and no charge.
    d. a and b.
    e. b and c.

41. A beam of photon radiation:
    a. decreases in total intensity as the beam passes through layers of tissue.
    b. is identical in range of motion to a beam of beta radiation.
    c. eventually reaches an intensity of zero.
    d. a and b.
    e. b and c.

CHALLENGE QUESTIONS
■ ■ ■ ■ ■ ■ ■ ■ ■ ■ ■ ■ ■ ■ ■ ■ ■ ■

1. The maximum number of electrons that can exist in each shell is determined by the formula $2n^2$. What does the n stand for?

2. Use only the above formula to answer the following: What is the maximum number of electrons that can exist in (a) the L shell; (b) the N shell; and (c) the Q shell?

3. What is the principal quantum number of the K shell? the M shell? the O shell? How do you know?

4. Describe the relationship between the number of shells in an atom and its position on the periodic table of the elements. Offer three specific examples from the periodic table.

5. What is the number of electrons in the outermost shell called? What does it determine? To what is it numerically equal? How does this differ from period number?

6. Write out the Radioactive Decay Law.

7. Define photons and particulate radiation.

8. Create your own periodic table, using arrows and labels to define and explain (a) period, (b) group, (c) elemental mass number, and (d) atomic number.

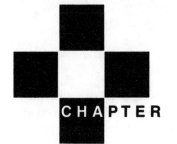

Electromagnetic Radiation

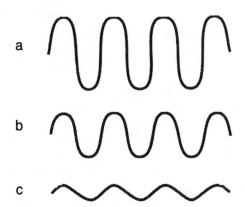

a

b

c

Use the illustration above to answer each of the following questions on a separate sheet of paper.

1. What do these three lines (a, b, and c) represent? What is the most important way these three lines vary? Describe how one would measure these differences.

2. Suppose the lines above represent graphs or models of electromagnetic radiation. (a) What are the most important properties of the sine-wave model? (b) Define each property.

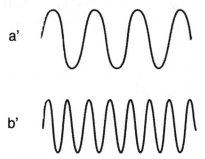

a'

b'

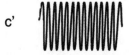

c'

Use the illustration above to answer each of the following questions on a separate sheet of paper.

3. In the illustration above (a', b', and c'), what does the difference in the three lines represent this time?

4. Based on the illustration above, determine the best way to complete this statement: "As _____ is increased, the _____ is decreased."

5. What formula best demonstrates the interrelatedness of the three parameters associated with a wave of the type shown? What is the formula called?

6. Why does the wave equation become simpler whenever one deals with electromagnetic radiation?

Circle the correct answer to each of the following.

7. Photons:
   a. are the smallest quantity of any type of electromagnetic radiation.
   b. are sometimes called quanta.
   c. are energy disturbances that can travel through space at the speed of light.
   d. a and c.
   e. all of the above.

8. James Clerk Maxwell:
   a. showed that visible light has electric properties.
   b. coined the term electromagnetic radiation.
   c. showed that visible light has magnetic properties once it is released, replacing electric properties.
   d. a and c.
   e. a and b.

9. Photons:
   a. have no mass or identifiable form.
   b. have sinusoidal electric fields but not necessarily magnetic fields.
   c. travel through space at 3×10^8 m/s.
   d. a and c.
   e. a and b.

10. The sine-wave model:
    a. describes variations in hertz, wavelength, and frequency of electromagnetic fields as a photon travels.
    b. describes the velocity of a natural phenomenon concerning high-voltage generation.
    c. responds to the properties of frequency, wavelength, and velocity in a moving photon's electromagnetic fields.
    d. none of the above.

11. Frequency:
    a. is the rate of rise and fall of a sine wave.
    b. is measured in wavelengths per second or cycles per second.
    c. is measured as the distance from one crest to another—that is, from any point on the sine wave to the next corresponding point.
    d. none of the above.

12. The wave equation:
    a. is used for sound.
    b. is measured as velocity = frequency **x** sine wave.
    c. is used in electromagnetic radiation.
    d. a and c.
    e. a, b, and c.

13. Sound waves and electromagnetic photons differ in that:
    a. sound wave velocities vary greatly; photons have only one speed.
    b. sources of sound vary.
    c. the velocity of a photon depends on the density of the material it is passing through.
    d. a and b.
    e. all of the above.

14. In electromagnetic radiation:
    a. the product of frequency and wavelength always equals the velocity of light.
    b. as frequency increases, wavelength decreases.
    c. as wavelength increases, frequency increases proportionately.
    d. a and c.
    e. a and b.

15. With electromagnetic radiation:
    a. distance causes the total energy emitted to spread out over an increasingly larger area.
    b. the intensity of light is proportional to the square of the distance of the object from the source.
    c. light intensity increases as velocity and distance increase proportionately.
    d. none of the above.

Fill in the blanks.

16. The intensity of electromagnetic radiation _____ as its distance increases. In other words, the intensity is _____ proportional to the _____ of the distance of an object from the source. This is called the _____ law.

17. In the formula $I_1 / I_2 = (d_2 / d_1)^2$, I_1 is the _____ at distance (d_1) from the source.

18. Visible light photons tend to exhibit more _____ nature than _____ nature. X-ray photons behave more as _____ than as _____. These phenomena illustrate the _____ of radiation.

CHALLENGE QUESTIONS
. . . .

1. If the product of frequency and wavelength always equals the velocity of light for electromagnetic radiation, what does this say about the relationship between frequency and wavelength? Explain your answer.

2. Explain a concrete example that shows the following principle in action: "The intensity of light is inversely proportional to the square of the distance of the object from the source." What is the name of the principle being defined here? Why is this principle true? In other words, what causes this phenomenon to occur?

3. Identify the frequency and wavelength ranges seen in the electromagnetic spectrum.

4. Identify the regions within the known electromagnetic spectrum that have importance to radiography. How does each spectrum differ?

5. What units of measure are used to measure (a) wavelength? (b) frequency? (c) energy? (d) Are these scales of measure related in any way? (c) Why is there no generally accepted, single standard for measuring radiation?

6. Choose which of the statements below is true and then elaborate on it.
   a. The shorter the wavelength of light, the greater the photon of energy.
   b. Light waves behave as though they were circular, like waves in the ocean.
   c. When light waves are absorbed, the energy deposited becomes a reflection.

7. The intensity of an x-ray beam is 400mR (103 μC/kg) at 36 in (90 cm). What will the intensity be at 18 in (45 cm)?

8. What is the energy contained in one photon of radiation from a radio station that has a broadcast frequency of 1260 kHz?

9. Chart five kinds of x-rays and their applications. Choose types that will show the broad variations in applications.

10. Mass and energy are two forms of the same medium. Identify the equivalence of mass to energy for each of the following: (a) 1 meV; (b) 1 keV; (c) 1 eV; (d) a nucleon's mass; and (e) an electron's mass.

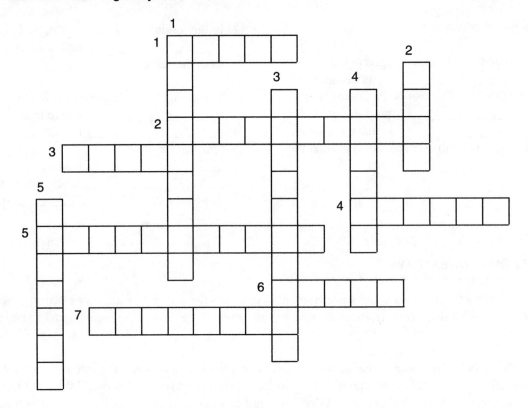

ACROSS

1. Ham operators speak of broadcasting on a 10-_____ or 30-_____.
2. A deviation in the straight line of travel of a photon of visible light is referred to as _____.
3. The abbreviation RF stands for _____ frequency, which comprises a considerble portion of the electromagnetic spectrum.
4. Today, distinguishing between x-rays and gamma rays by_____ is no longer appropriate, thanks to the large particle accelerators now available.
5. _____ light is located in the electromagnetic spectrum between visible light and ionizing radiation.
6. _____ rays come from inside the nucleus of a radioactive atom.
7. Visible light occupies the _____ segment of the electromagnetic spectrum, but it is the only portion that we can sense directly.

DOWN

1. Short wave-length RF is known as _____ radiation.
2. Photons of RF have very low energies and very _____ wavelengths.
3. Photons of visible light are described in physics in terms of _____.
4. In refracted light, the wavelength value of _____ light has a wavelength value of approximately 400 nm.
5. The ability of x-ray and visible light photons to exhibit behaviors of both particles and waves is referred to as wave-particle _____.

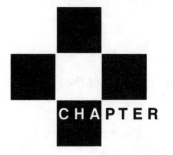

Electricity

CHAPTER 6

Circle the correct answer to each of the following.

1. The smallest units of electric charge are:
   a. mass, form, and energy.
   b. protons and neutrons.
   c. electrons and protons.
   d. positive charges and negative charges.

2. The electric charges associated wtih electrons and protons have the same _____ but opposite _____.
   a. nucleic mass; poles.
   b. magnitude; signs.
   c. form; charges.
   d. velocity; charges.

3. The electron has _____ charge, and the proton has _____ charge.
   a. one unit of negative; one unit of positive
   b. an increased; an inversely proportional decrease of
   c. an ionized; a nonionized
   d. only a negative; either a positive or negative

4. _____ can travel from the outermost shell of one atom to the next, but _____ are fixed inside the nucleus and cannot move.
   a. Ionized particles; nonionized particles
   b. Particles; waves
   c. Electrons; protons
   d. Photons; sine waves

5. _____ occurs when an object becomes charged by the removal or addition of electrons.
   a. Electrification
   b. Electrostatics
   c. Electrolysis
   d. Electrocution

6. _____ refers to electric charges in stationary form.
   a. Electric power
   b. Electric potential
   c. Electrostatics
   d. Neither a, b, nor c

7. An object is said to be electrified when:
   a. it has too few electrons.
   b. it has too many electrons.
   c. its electrons are loosely bound and can easily be removed.
   d. a and c are true.
   e. a, b, and c are true.

8. Electrification can be created:
   a. when a connection causes the flow of electrons.
   b. when electrons are built up as two objects are rubbed together.
   c. when the electrical field of a charged object confers a charge on an uncharged object.
   d. when a, b, or c occur.

9. Friction:
   a. can cause a moving, positive electric charge.
   b. can create the same effect as contact or induction.
   c. creates an electric ground.
   d. is the main cause of lightning.

10. An electric ground:
    a. is a reservoir for stray electric charges.
    b. occurs when an object becomes charged by the addition of electrons.
    c. is an electric charge in stationary form.
    d. is another name for static electricity.

Answer each of the following on a separate sheet of paper.

11. Refer to Figure 6-3 in your textbook. Explain what each illustration signifies.

12. Why is the electron not used as the fundamental unit of electric charge? What is used instead? What is its relationship to the electron?

13. State Coulomb's law, reproducing the equation and identifying what each symbol within that equation stands for.

14. Name and explain the four general laws of electrostatics.

15. Write the equation and explanation of Ohm's law.

Circle the correct answer to each of the following.

16. Under Coulomb's law, the greater the electrostatic charge on either object:
    a. the more directly proportional the electrostatic force is.
    b. the greater its velocity.
    c. the more diminished its electrostatic force (i.e., inverse proportion).
    d. the greater the electrostatic force.

17. Electrostatic forces:
    a. are strong when objects are close but decrease rapidly as objects separate.
    b. have inverse square relationships that are the opposite of that for x-ray intensity.
    c. equation has the same form as that for gravitational force, except that electrostatic forces act only over short distances—the opposite of gravitational forces.
    d. are best described in a and c.
    e. are best described in a and b.

18. Electrostatic forces:
    a. can be attractive or repulsive.
    b. between two charges are unaffected by the presence of a third charge.
    c. between two charges are affected by the presence of a third charge—if it is negative.
    d. are best described in a and c.
    e. are best described in a and b.

Match the following terms and descriptions.

19. __f__   conductor

20. __D__   electric current

21. __A__   electric potential

22. __G__   electrodynamics

23. __C__   electromotive force

24. __h__   insulator

25. __E__   potential energy

26. __J__   semiconductor

27. __I__   superconductivity

28. __B__   volt

a. ability to do work pending release of energy

b. unit of electric potential

c. electric charges positioned close together to make use of electrostatic repulsive force to do work

d. electric charges moving along a wire

e. another word for electric potential or voltage

f. matter through which electrons flow easily

g. electric charges in motion

h. matter that inhibits the flow of electrons

i. limited resistance to electron flow below a critical temperature

j. material that under some conditions behaves as an insulator and under others behaves as a conductor

■ ■ ■ ■ ■ ■ ■ ■ ■ ■ ■ ■ ■ ■ ■ ■ ■

Answer each of the following on a separate sheet of paper.

29. What is the difference between a series circuit and a parallel circuit? How do their "rules" vary? Can you think of an example that would offer a clear visual analogy?

30. Describe some of the differences between direct current and alternating current.

Indicate whether the following statements are true or false.

31. T   F   Electric current consists of electrons flowing in a closed path with controlled resistance.

32. T   F   Electric current is measured in volts; electric potential is measured in amperes, and electric resistance is measured in ohms.

33. T   F   The series circuit has all elements that bridge the conductor.

34. T   F   In direct current, electrons oscillate back and forth along the conductor.

35. T   F   Electric power of 1 watt is equal to 1 A (amp) of current flowing through an electric potential of 1 V (volt).

CHALLENGE QUESTIONS
. . . .

1. Describe the origins of lightning.

2. If a current of 0.75 A flows through a conductor that has a resistance of 8 Ω, what is the voltage across the conductor?

3. An x-ray machine requires 50 kW of electric power and is supplied with 220V. How many amperes of current are drawn?

4. Fill in the table below.

Circuit Element Name	Symbol	Function
resistor		
battery		
capacitor		
ammeter		
voltmeter		
switch		
transformer		
rheostat		
diode		
transistor		

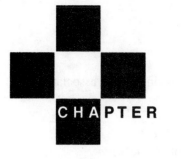

CHAPTER 7

Magnetism

Circle the correct answer to each of the following.

1. Magnetism:
   a. and electrostatics are the same thing; "electrostatics" is simply the older term.
   b. cannot be felt or sensed.
   c. is created in a plane parallel to the field of motion of a moving charged particle.
   d. a and b.

2. A magnetic field:
   a. is the result of electrons circling a nucleus counterclockwise; electrons spinning clockwise cancel each other out.
   b. is created by a pair of electrons circling a nucleus.
   c. exists in atoms with odd numbers of electrons in any shell.
   d. a and b.

3. A magnetic domain is created when:
   a. all domains in an object are aligned, creating a magnet.
   b. a large number of atomic magnets come together with their dipoles aligned.
   c. the proton in a hydrogen nucleus spins on its axis and creates a nuclear magnetic dipole.
   d. electrons circle a nucleus either clockwise or counterclockwise.

4. In ferromagnetic material:
   a. the magnetic dipoles are randomly oriented.
   b. closeness to a bar magnet will cause the magnet's magnetic field lines to be repelled from the ferromagnetic material.
   c. dipoles lose their randomness when exposed to an external magnetic field.
   d. a and c.

5. Permanent magnets:
   a. are artificially produced by charging them in the field of an electromagnet.
   b. are such because their magnetic property cannot be lost—only temporarily disrupted.
   c. are called such because, unlike other magnets, their magnetism is not destroyed by heat or strong percussion.
   d. all of the above.

6. Dimagnetic materials:
   a. have a north and south pole.
   b. cannot be broken down into smallest units.
   c. are unaffected by a magnetic field.
   d. b and c.

7. Examples of dimagnetic materials include:
   a. wood, glass, and plastic.
   b. alnico and gadolinium.
   c. plastic, non-ore glass, and gadolinium.
   d. aluminum, nickle, and cobalt.

8. Alnico:
   a. is a combination of aluminum, nickel, and cobalt.
   b. is one of the more useful magnets produced from ferromagnetic material.
   c. can be permanently magnetized.
   d. a, b, and c.

Answer each of the following on a separate sheet of paper.

9. How are magnets classified?

10. Explain how hydrogen atoms in the body are the basis of magnetic resonance imaging.

11. Write the chemical symbol for magnetite.

12. Explain the derivation of the word *magnetism* and how ancient people discovered it.

13. Define electromagnet.

14. Name and give the magnetic classification of an MRI contrast agent.

15. Define magnetic susceptibility.

16. Explain the effect of Maxwell's field theory on the relationship between the distance between two magnetic poles and their actual magnetic force.

17. Discuss the properties magnetism holds in common with electrostatics.

18. Where is the earth's magnetic field strongest?

19. Name the SI unit of magnetic field strength.

Circle the correct answer to each of the following.

20. When a charged particle moves, a magnetic field is:
    a. erased.
    b. induced perpendicualr to the particle motion.
    c. induced along the directon of particle motion.
    d. induced having the same sign as the particle.

21. When iron is fabricated into a magnet, magnetic domains:
    a. align.
    b. disappear.
    c. cancel.
    d. magnify.

22. Which of the following has an associated magnetic field?
    a. a neutron
    b. a hydrogen nucleus
    c. a hydrogen molecule
    d. none of the above

23. Which of the following is not a principal classification of magnets?
    a. naturally occurring
    b. electro-
    c. superconducting
    d. artificially induced permanent

24. Magnetism:
    a. requires electricity.
    b. is present in some naturally occurring ores.
    c. is defined as a property that can attract glass, wood, or metal.
    d. depends on monopolar atoms.

25. The physical laws of magnetism are similar to the laws of:
    a. the unified field theory.
    b. relativity.
    c. conservation.
    d. gravity.

26. When iron is brought near a permanent magnet, the lines of the magnetic field are:
    a. attracted to the magnet.
    b. repelled by the magnet.
    c. attracted to the iron.
    d. repelled by the iron.

CHALLENGE QUESTIONS
■ ■ ■ ■ ■ ■ ■ ■ ■ ■ ■ ■ ■ ■ ■ ■ ■

1. Copy the headings in Table 7-1, filling in column 1 only. Then, finish filling in the table to demonstrate three fundamental forces in nature.

2. List and explain the four laws of magnetism.

3. If time allows, help organize this class project: Visit an MRI site and discuss magnetic field safety with MRI personnel.

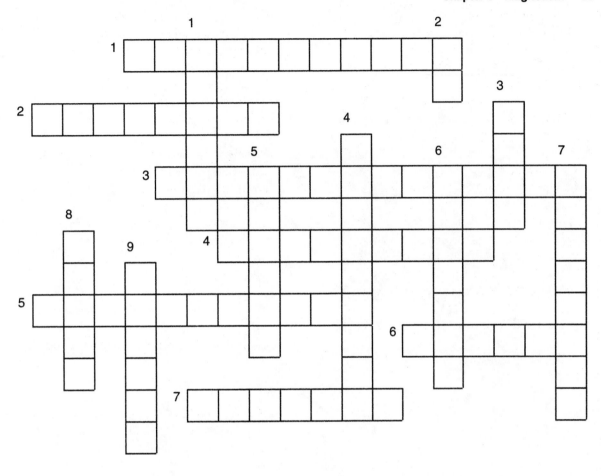

ACROSS

1. Magnetic ores in the earth presumably have strong magnetism in part because they have remained ____ within the earth's magnetic field.
2. An object's magnetic ____-bility refers to the degree to which it can be magnetized.
3. The phenomenon occurring when small objects are attracted to an amber rod rubbed with fur.
4. An oxide of iron that always points toward the North Pole.
5. The imaginary lines of force generated by dipoles in a magnet are deviated by contact with a _____-ic material.
6. When the proton in a hydrogen nucleus spins on its axis, the resultant nuclear magnetic dipole is called a magnetic _____.
7. A magnetic domain is created by an accumulation of many atomic magnets with their dipoles _____.

DOWN

1. The magnet created by an electron orbit is called a magnetic _____.
2. If a material is unaffected when brought into a magnetic field, it is said to be _____-magnetic.
3. Natural magnets generally have an ____ on which they spin.
4. An object that, followed north, was believed to lead to water.
5. A magnetic field is created by an electric _____ spinning on its own axis.
6. When randomly oriented dipoles are _____ by an external magnetic field, they align to that field.
7. Objects that are _____ attracted to a magnet are said to be paramagnetic.
8. Unified _____ theory is concerned with combining gravitational, electric, and magnetic forces with strong nuclear force and weak nuclear interaction.
9. The principle types of magnets are classified by the _____ of each one's magnetic property.

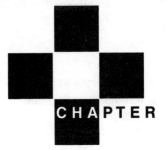

CHAPTER 8

Electromagnetism

Circle the correct answer to each of the following.

1. Electrons in motion are known as:
   a. friction.
   b. electrostatics.
   c. electricity or electromagnetism.
   d. a changing magnetic field.

2. The Voltaic pile:
   a. was invented by Faraday.
   b. is a modern dry cell battery.
   c. consists of zinc and copper plates sand-wiched together.
   d. consists of a magnet and a conductor.

3. EMF:
   a. stands for electrical-mechanical force.
   b. is expressed in units of volts.
   c. is expressed in units of joules per kilo-gram.
   d. was invented by Hans Oersted.

4. The experimental link connecting electric and magnetic forces was discovered by:
   a. Oersted.
   b. Faraday.
   c. Lenz.
   d. Volta.

5. A battery:
   a. converts chemical energy into mechani-cal energy.
   b. is a source of electric resistance.
   c. is a source of electromotive force.
   d. is based on the magnetic property of sim-ilar metals.

6. A modern dry cell battery is a source of:
   a. volts per ohm.
   b. ohms per volt.
   c. coulombs per joule.
   d. joules per coulomb.

7. Which of the following is a symbol for a battery?

   a.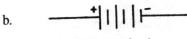
   b.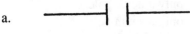
   c.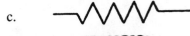
   d.

8. The principal advantage of an electromagnet over a solenoid is magnetic field:
   a. polarity.
   b. variability.
   c. homogeneity.
   d. intensity.

9. Which of the following scientists is *not* asso-ciated with the early development of electro-magnetism?
   a. Volta
   b. Planck
   c. Lenz
   d. Faraday

10. The device designed to measure electron flow in a conductor is known as a (an):
    a. solenoid.
    b. electromagnet.
    c. ammeter.
    d. choke coil.

11. An electric current will flow if the conductor is in a changing magnetic field. This:
    a. is known as Faraday's law.
    b. is the statement of the second law of electromagnetics.
    c. was discovered by Lenz.
    d. was discovered by Volta.

12. The term *electromagnetic induction* refers to the production of:
    a. electromagnetic radiation.
    b. a magnetic field.
    c. an electric current.
    d. a static charge.

13. The magnetic field produced by an electromagnet:
    a. has only a north pole.
    b. has only a south pole.
    c. has neither a north nor a south pole.
    d. is similar to that produced by a bar magnet.

14. Given a closed loop of wire with no electron flow, an electric current can be induced if:
    a. no magnetic field is present.
    b. a constant magnetic field is present.
    c. a changing magnetic field is present.
    d. the loop is opened.

15. Which of the following is based on electromagnetic induction?
    a. radio reception
    b. battery
    c. solenoid
    d. DC current

16. Lenz's Law states that:
    a. an electric current will be induced in a circuit if some part of that circuit is in a magnetic field.
    b. there are two basic types of induction, primary and secondary.
    c. the current induced in a coil by a moving magnet produces a magnetic field opposing the motion of the magnet.
    d. the right-hand rule is used to determine the induced current direction.

17. The principal difference between self-induction and mutual induction is that:
    a. mutual induction is the basis for an electric motor and self-induction is the basis for a transformer.
    b. self-induction requires two coils and mutual induction requires only one.
    c. mutual induction requires two coils and self-induction requires only one.
    d. there is no difference.

18. When an AC source is connected to a coil:
    a. the current flow through the magnetic field changes direction.
    b. electromagnetic radiation will be produced.
    c. mutual induction occurs.
    d. a front EMF will be produced.

19. If two coils are positioned near each other and a varying soucre of EMF is passed through the first coil:
    a. electromagnetic radiation will be produced.
    b. self-induction will occur in the second coil.
    c. mutual induction will occur in the second coil.
    d. such an arrangement is a solenoid.

20. A coil of wire will:
    a. conduct AC relatively unimpeded.
    b. conduct DC relatively unimpeded.
    c. experience mutual induction from a battery.
    d. experience mutual induction from DC.

21. When an electric current is induced by mutual induction, such current flows:
    a. according to Oersted's law.
    b. according to Lenz's law.
    c. in the primary coil.
    d. in the secondary coil.

22. Which of the following is an electromechanical device?
    a. solenoid
    b. battery
    c. generator
    d. transformer

23. The magnetic field produced:
    a. by a solenoid is more intense than that produced by an electromagnet.
    b. in a transformer is based on mutual induction.
    c. in an electromagnet is most intense in the plane perpendicular to its axis.
    d. by an AC source is constant.

Answer each of the following questions on a separate sheet of paper.

24. Tie development of the electric motor with Oersted's experiments.

25. Discuss whose experimenting you believe is most important to the discovery and development of electromechanical devices—Lenz's, Oersted's, or Faraday's.

26. Describe the functioning of an electric generator. How is the coil of wire manipulated to create the desired effect?

27. How many components can you list that are needed to create and run a DC electric motor.

28. Tie development of the electric generator with Faraday's experiments.

29. First, decide which of the following statements is true concerning generators and motors. Then elaborate, explaining your answer:
    a. They convert energy from one form into another.
    b. They have both primary and secondary windings.
    c. They are electromagnets.
    d. They require direct electric contact between primary and secondary coils.

30. Describe the mechanics behind the electric motor.

31. First, decide which of the following would be classified as electromechanical devices. Then, explain why in your own words.
    a. transformers and rectifiers
    b. motors and rectifiers
    c. generators and rectifiers
    d. generators and motors

Circle the correct answer to each of the following.

32. Which of the following is *not* required for an electric generator?
    a. a north pole
    b. source of EMF
    c. magnet
    d. a transformer

33. The main difference between an AC and a DC electric generator is:
    a. the commutator ring.
    b. the source of EMF.
    c. a magnet.
    d. a transformer.

34. Which of the following electric current waveforms is produced by a DC generator?

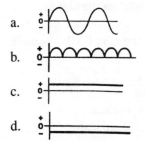

35. The electric current produced by an AC generator has:
    a. constant intensity.
    b. pulsating positive intensity.
    c. pulsating negative intensity.
    d. alternating positive and negative intensity.

36. The electric current intensity produced by a DC generator is:
    a. constant and in one direction.
    b. pulsating and in one direction.
    c. constant and changing direction.
    d. pulsating and changing direction.

37. One difference between an electric generator and an electric motor is the:
    a. types of transformer.
    b. magnetic polarity.
    c. source of EMF.
    d. loop of wire.

38. In electric generators and motors, the commutator ring acts as a:
    a. source of EMF.
    b. converter from DC to AC.
    c. device to vary voltage.
    d. switch.

39. In an induction motor, only the _____ rotates.
    a. rotor
    b. wire loop
    c. stator
    d. electromagnet

40. In an induction motor, an electric current is induced in:
    a. only the rotor.
    b. only the stator.
    c. both the rotor and stator.
    d. neither the rotor nor the stator.

41. In an induction motor, an EMF is supplied to:
    a. only the rotor.
    b. only the stator.
    c. both the rotor and stator.
    d. neither the rotor nor stator.

42. An induction motor is used in an x-ray machine to:
    a. vary voltage.
    b. control current.
    c. rotate the anode.
    d. provide rectification.

Answer each of the following questions on a separate sheet of paper.

43. Explain why the development of the battery led to an increased understanding of electromagnetic phenomena.

44. Explain how to determine the direction of the magnetic field and the electric current in a wire.

45. The magnitude of induced current in Faraday's experiment depends on four factors. Name them.

46. Name and define the two laws of electromagnetics.

47. Name and define the two basic types of electromagnetic induction.

48. Discuss the relationship between primary and secondary voltage in a step-up transformer.

49. Discuss the change in current across a transformer; be sure to address the following issues: (a) Is the change in current in the same direction as the voltage change? (b) What is it proportional to—voltage change or the turns ratio?

50. Discuss the three principle causes for transformer energy losses.

51. Explain the difference between DC and AC systems.

Circle the correct answer to each of the following.

52. Transformers have iron cores in order to intensify the:
    a. magnetic field.
    b. EMF.
    c. electric current.
    d. electric potential.

53. The transformer:
    a. changes electrical potential and current into higher or lower intensities.
    b. can operate on both AC and DC currents.
    c. does not use mutual conduction.
    d. converts one form of energy to another.

54. A transformer "transforms" or changes electric:
    a. impedance.
    b. resistance.
    c. power.
    d. voltage.

55. A transformer with a turns ratio greater than 1 is:
    a. a step-up transformer.
    b. a step-down transformer.
    c. more susceptible to resistance that results in heat generation.
    d. not susceptible to eddy currents that create a loss of transformer efficiency.

56. The transformer that resembles a square donut is called a(n) _____ transformer.
    a. auto
    b. induction
    c. closed-core
    d. shell-type

57. The turns ratio is defined as:
    a. primary voltage + secondary voltage.
    b. secondary amperage + primary amperage.
    c. primary windings ÷ secondary windings.
    d. secondary windings ÷ primary windings.

58. An autotransformer:
    a. is an electromechanical device.
    b. is a shell-type transformer.
    c. contains a single winding to serve as both primary and secondary coils.
    d. is used only to increase voltage.

59. If DC is applied to the primary coil of a transformer:
    a. a secondary voltage will result.
    b. a secondary current will result.
    c. a magnetic field will be produced.
    d. nothing will happen.

60. A rectifier:
    a. refers to a type of electromechanical device.
    b. refers to a type of electromagnetic device.
    c. converts DC to AC.
    d. converts AC to DC.

61. Thermionic emission refers to:
    a. heat conduction.
    b. heat radiation.
    c. electron emission from a heated source.
    d. heat emission from an electric conductor.

62 Which of the following is a component of a tube-type of rectifier?
    a. filament
    b. magnetic core
    c. primary windings
    d. secondary windings

63. In a tube rectifier, or vacuum-tube diode, the electron flow is from:
    a. anode to cathode only when the anode is positive with respect to the cathode.
    b. cathode to anode only when the anode is negative with respect to the cathode.
    c. anode to cathode only when the anode is negative with respect to the cathode.
    d. cathode to anode only when the anode is connected to a positive voltage with respect to the cathode.

64. Near the p-n junction of a semiconductor diode one will find:
    a. p-type material containing excess electrons.
    b. n-type material containing excess electrons.
    c. a heated cathode.
    d. a heated anode.

65. A semiconductor diode:
    a. is also called an electromechanical rectifier.
    b. contains holes also called proton traps.
    c. allows current to flow only from p-type material to n-type.
    d. allows current to flow only from n-type material to p-type.

66. A semiconductor rectifier:
    a. has a heated cathode.
    b. has a heated anode.
    c. is a solid-state device.
    d. is an electromechanical device.

67. In a circuit containing a solid-state diode:
    a. electron flow will be pulsed but uninterrupted.
    b. electrons will be permitted to flow in one direction but not the other.
    c. the result will be contant potential DC.
    d. twice as many electrons will flow in the output coil as in the input coil.

CHALLENGE QUESTIONS
■ ■ ■ ■ ■ ■ ■ ■ ■ ■ ■ ■ ■ ■ ■ ■ ■ ■ ■

1. Describe how you would make an electromagnet. What components would you need?

2. In the following blank p-n junction semiconductor diagram, fill in the holes and electrons and show how electrons are conducted in only one direction.

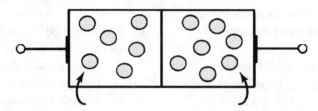

3. Draw the electronic symbol for (a) a vacuum tube; (b) a solid state diode.

4. Draw and label the three types of transformers.

5. Explain the desired effect that all electric generators are expected to produce. Be sure to discuss the efficiency of this process, in terms of percentages of efficacy.

6. A transformer has 10,000 windings on the secondary side and 150 on the primary side. (a) If the primary voltage is 220 V and the primary current is 5 A, what is the turns ratio? Next, calculate (b) the secondary voltage. (c) What is the secondary current?

7. A single rectifier is inserted into a circuit conducting 60 Hz AC so that it suppresses the positive portion of the waveform. Calculate the pulses per second in the output waveform.

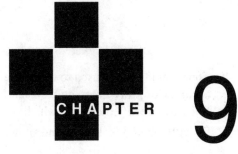

CHAPTER 9

The X-ray Unit

Circle the correct answer to each of the following.

1. Most modern medical x-ray units operate at kilovoltages ranging from _____ and at tube currents ranging from _____ mA.
   a. 25 to 150 kVp; 100 to 1200 mA
   b. 75 to 250 kVp; 1000 to 12000 mA
   c. 50 to 100 kVp; 100 to 500 mA
   d. none of the above.

2. Each x-ray unit, regardless of its design, has the following principal parts:
   a. the operating console, the image intensifier, and the x-ray tube.
   b. the operating console, the x-ray tube, and the fluoroscopic unit.
   c. the x-ray tube, the operating console, and the high-voltage generator.
   d. the x-ray tube, the Bucky tray, and the image intensifier.
   e. the gonad shields, Bucky tray, x-ray tube, and operating console.

3. kVp expresses the:
   a. penetrating quality of x-ray beam.
   b. opposite of half-value layer (HVL).
   c. phototiming.
   d. exposure time.

4. The _____ table is identified by its head and foot tilt.
   a. angiographic
   b. fluoroscopic
   c. radiographic
   d. sinusoidal
   e. floating

5. The line compensator:
   a. measures the voltage provided to the x-ray machine.
   b. adjusts the voltage to precisely 220 volts.
   c. must never be wired to the autotransformer.
   d. is described in a and c.
   e. is described in a and b.

6. The prereading voltmeter:
   a. determines the penetrating quality of the x-ray beam.
   b. actually reads the voltage of the auto-transformer.
   c. registers kilovoltage even when no exposure is being made and no current is flowing in the circuit.
   d. is best described by a and b.
   e. is best described by a, b, and c.

7. The x-ray tube current, the number of electrons crossing from cathode to anode per second, is measured in:
   a. keV.
   b. milliamperes (mA).
   c. kVp.
   d. amperes (A).

8. The timer circuit of an x-ray machine is able to "make" or "break" high voltage across the x-ray tube, nearly always on the _____ side of the high-voltage transformer.
   a. right
   b. zero voltage
   c. filament timer
   d. primary
   e. secondary

9. Electronic timers:
   a. are based on the time required to charge a capacitor through a variable resistance.
   b. must monitor the actual tube current.
   c. automatically terminates the exposure when the required optical density is reached.
   d. incorporates a flat, parallel plate ionization chamber between the patient and the image receptor.

10. X-ray machines with synchronous timers:
    a. have minimum exposure times of as little as 7 milliseconds.
    b. demonstrate timing intervals that increase by multiples.
    c. cannot be used for serial exposures.
    d. are described in a and b.
    e. are described in b and c.

11. A 100-ms image of a spinning top test:
    a. should result in 6 dashes for a half-wave rectified unit.
    b. should result in 6 dashes for a full-wave rectified unit.
    c. is not a reliable way to check exposure times.
    d. none of the above.

12. High-frequency voltage generators:
    a. are responsible for converting low available voltage into a kilovoltage of proper waveform.
    b. do not need rectifiers.
    c. use oil as a heat insulator only.
    d. none of the above.

Indicate whether the following statements are true or false.

13. T F The fluoroscopic x-ray tube is usually attached to an overhead movable crane assembly that permits easy positioning.

14. T F The primary connections conduct the input power to the autotransformer.

15. T F The autotransformer can be designed to increase voltage to approximately three times the input voltage value.

16. T F The spinning top is used to check the accuracy of x-ray timers in half- and full-wave–rectified units in which radiation output is not pulsed.

17. T F When specifying high-voltage generators, the industry standard is to use the maximum tube potential possible at 100 kVp for a 100-millisecond exposure.

18. T F A high-voltage generator for a basic radiographic unit would be rated at 50 to 60 kW.

Calculate the following problems on a separate sheet of paper.

19. A radiograph is made at 350 mA with an exposure time of 85 ms. Express this as mAs.

20. A second radiograph is made at 450 mA with an exposure time of 120 ms. Express this as mAs.

21. A filament transformer with a turns ratio of 1:15 provides 8.3 amperes to the filament. What is the current flowing through the primary coil of the filament transformer?

22. A new filament transformer with a turns ratio of 1:20 provides 7.6 amperes to the filament. What is the current flowing through the primary coil of the filament transformer?

23. An examination calls for 53 kVp and 90 mAs with the 220-mA station. What exposure time should be used?

24. An examination calls for 67 kVp and 85 mAs with the 350-mA station. What exposure time should be used?

25. Before a radiographer can perform a specific procedure, she is asked to determine what secondary voltage will be supplied to the x-ray tube during the procedure. The turns ratio of a high-voltage transformer is 850:1, and the supply voltage is peaked at 230 volts. What is the secondary voltage supplied to the x-ray tube?

26. The turns ratio of a high-voltage transformer is 770:1, and the supply voltage is 180 volts. What is the secondary voltage supplied to the x-ray tube?

27. A low-voltage ripple system is energized at 110 kVp, 100 milliseconds. The maximum tube current possible is 900 mA. What is the power rating?

28. An x-ray machine has a low-voltage ripple system that is energized at 120 kVp, 120 milliseconds. The maximum tube current possible is 950 mA. What is the power rating?

29. A single-phase unit has a maximum capacity of 100 milliseconds of 240 kVp and 600 mA. What is its power rating?

30. A radiographic single-phase unit has a maximum capacity of 100 milliseconds of 200 kVp and 550 mA. What is its power rating?

Answer each of the following on a separate sheet of paper.

31. Describe the functions and principles behind the operations of the autotransformer. How does it relate to the line compensator, and what influences the voltages it receives and sends?

32. What is meant by a prereading voltmeter? What exactly does it do?

33. Explain what is meant by a step-down transformer. Why can a filament transformer be called by that name? What role do precision resistors play?

34. Describe how solid-state radiation detectors work. Who usually uses them?

35. The QC radiographer has been using a full-wave–rectified unit in which radiation output is pulsed. His supervisor asks him one morning to check the accuracy of the x-ray timer. How will he do that?

36. Explain this statement: "X-rays cannot be produced by electrons flowing in reverse direction from anode to cathode."

37. Explain this statement: "The voltage across the x-ray tube during the negative half cycle caused the failure."

38. What is the difference between half-wave and full-wave rectification?

39. What is a shortcoming of half-wave rectification? Why is full-wave rectification preferred?

40. Create a diagram of your own that helps explain how full-wave rectification works. Use details and/or notations to illustrate that the polarity of the x-ray tube remains unchanged, even though the induced secondary voltage alternates between positive and negative.

CHALLENGE QUESTIONS
■ ■ ■ ■ ■ ■ ■ ■ ■ ■ ■ ■ ■ ■ ■ ■

1. List and define the controls on the x-ray machine operating console.

2. Describe, using illustrations, how a phototimer works.

3. Explain, using graphs, how the capacitor discharge generator works in some portable units.

4. Draw the voltage wave forms that illustrate the various power supplies (half-wave, full-wave, etc.).

5. Label the electric circuit diagram for the x-ray unit.

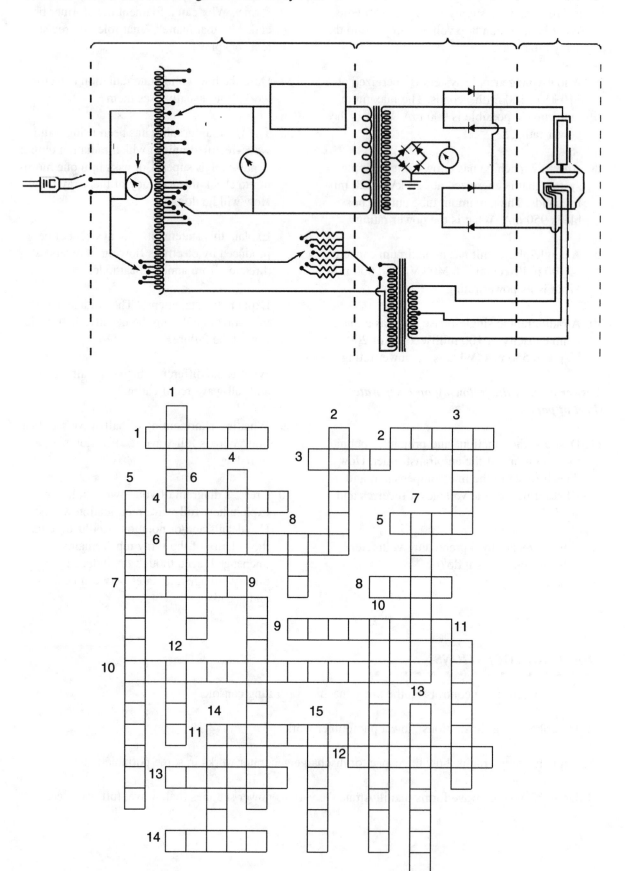

ACROSS

1. Rectification is accomplished through the use of _____.
2. The phototimer used by most manufacturers incorporates a flat, parallel plate _____-ation chamber.
3. One advantage of the high-frequency generator.
4. Inverter circuits convert DC into a series of _____ pulses.
5. For any given radiographic exam, the number of x-rays reaching the image receptor is directly related to current and _____.
6. The penetrating quality of an x-ray beam is expressed by kVp or _____ layer.
7. The incoporation of automatic-exposure control is often referred to as photo _____.
8. A filament transformer is a _____-down transformer.
9. The number of x-rays or the intensity of the beam is usually expressed in mR or mR per mAs and is referred to as the _____ of the x-ray beam.
10. The piece of equipment designed to supply precise voltage to the filament circuit and to the high-voltage circuit of the x-ray machine.
11. In a full-wave–rectified circuit, the negative half cycle corresponding to the inverse voltage is _____-d so that a positive voltage is always directed across the x-ray tube.
12. The continual variation in mAs during an exposure to minimum exposure time is referred to as a _____-load mA.
13. Variation in _____ voltage results in a variation in the x-ray beam.
14. As a filament's current increases, the filament becomes hotter, and electrons are released by _____-ionic emission.

DOWN

1. Since transformers operate only on alternating current, the voltage waveform on both sides of a high-voltage transformer is _____-oidal.
2. One way in which the autotransformer differs from the conventional transformer is that it has a _____ winding.
3. A phototimer measures the quantity of radiation reaching the _____ receptor.
4. A _____-wave–rectified circuit usually contains two diodes, although some contain one or more.
5. The autotransformer works on the principle of _____ induction.
6. The penetrating quality of the x-ray beam, expresed in kVp, refers to the _____ of the x-ray beam.
7. High-frequency voltage generation uses _____ circuits.
8. In controlling the voltage supplied to the high-voltage transformer, it is much safer and easier to vary _____ voltage and then increase it than to increase low voltage to the kilovolt level and then vary its magnitude.
9. Half-wave rectification refers to a condition in which the voltage is not allowed to swing _____ during the negative half of its cycle.
10. The number of electrons emitted by a filament is determined by the filament's _____.
11. Tube _____ is monitored with an mA meter that must be placed in the tube circuit.
12. The voltages an autotransformer receives and provides are in direct relation to the number of _____s of the transformer enclosed by the respective connections.
13. X-ray tube current is controlled through the _____ circuit.
14. Voltage _____ is the variation in peak voltage waveform.
15. Synchronous timers cannot be used for _____ exposures.

The X-ray Tube

Circle the correct answer to each of the following.

1. The most frequently used method for supporting an x-ray tube is:
   a. the ceiling support.
   b. the floor-to-ceiling support.
   c. the image intensifier tower.
   d. none of the above.

2. SID is:
   a. the abbreviation for source-to-image receptor distance.
   b. is the same as FFD.
   c. is said to be standard when the tube is in a detent position.
   d. all of the above.

3. The fluoroscopy tube is mounted:
   a. above the patient.
   b. on a floor-mount system.
   c. without the use of an image intensifier.
   d. underneath the radiographic table.

4. C-arm units:
   a. are also called Crookes' tubes.
   b. are used in portable fluoroscopy.
   c. support x-ray tubes on a support shaped like a C.
   d. none of the above.
   e. b and c.

5. The useful beam is:
   a. only those x-rays emitted through the window.
   b. only those x-rays coming through the protective housing.
   c. only those x-rays moving through the thermal cushion.
   d. a and b.
   e. none of the above.

6. Leakage radiation:
   a. refers to isotropic emissions.
   b. refers to x-rays that escape through the protective housing.
   c. refers only to those x-rays emitted through the window.
   d. a and c.
   e. none of the above.

7. The federal standard for leakage radiation from an x-ray tube is:
   a. less than 80 mR per hour at 1 meter.
   b. less than 100 mR per hour at 1 meter.
   c. less than 1000 mR per hour at 2 meters.
   d. less than 75 mR per hour at 0.5 meter.

8. The protective housing of an x-ray tube:
   a. provides mechanical support for the tube.
   b. protects the tube from damage caused by handling.
   c. protects against electric shock and reduces the level of leakage radiation.
   d. a and c.
   e. all of the above.

9. The oil found in the protective housing around some x-ray tubes:
   a. indicates that the tubes were made before the federal standards for leakage radiation went into effect.
   b. has been found to promote accidental electric shock.
   c. serves as a thermal cushion and electrical insulator.
   d. a and b.

10. An x-ray tube:
    a. has both a cathode and a filament.
    b. has both a cathode and a target anode.
    c. is contained within a glass envelope that can withstand tremendous heat and prevents a vacuum from forming inside the tube.
    d. none of the above.

11. The modern x-ray tube:
    a. is a Coolidge tube.
    b. does away with the need for a vacuum tube.
    c. does not fail if it becomes full of gas molecules.
    d. is a fluorescent tube.

12. Metal envelope tubes:
    a. become coated with vaporized tungsten as they age.
    b. lose their electric potential with aging; the result is arcing.
    c. maintain a constant electric potential between electrons of the tube current and the envelope.
    d. do not have tube windows.

13. The most common cause of tube failure:
    a. is the buildup of tungsten on internal components.
    b. is an open filament.
    c. is a broken or cracked glass envelope.
    d. none of the above.

14. The focal spot is:
    a. the area of the target actually being hit with electrons from which x-rays are emitted.
    b. the actual source of radiation.
    c. the imaginary line generated by the centermost x-ray in the beam.
    d. a and b.
    e. all of the above.

15. The line-focus principle means:
    a. allowing a large area for heating while maintaining a small actual focal spot.
    b. that by angling the target, the effective area of the target is much smaller than the actual area of electron interaction.
    c. a and b.
    d. none of the above.

16. Biangle targets:
    a. have two target angles on the same anode.
    b. have two focal-spot sizes.
    c. cause radiation intensity on the cathode side of the beam to be higher than on the anode side.
    d. are described in a and b.
    e. are described in a and c.

17. The radiographic rating chart:
    a. is the most important.
    b. states which radiographic technical factors are safe.
    c. relates kVp and mAs to other factors in anode cooling.
    d. a and b.
    e. none of the above.

Indicate whether the following statements are true or false.

18. T F The cathode is the negative side of the x-ray tube and has two primary parts—the anode and the focusing cup.

19. T F The x-ray tube current is adjusted by controlling the filament current.

20. T F If the rotor mechanism of a rotating anode fails, the anode may pit or crack because of exposure to heat.

21. T F The effective focal-spot size is the value given when identifying large and small focal spots, which will vary with the target angle.

22. T F The advantage of the line-focus principle is that it simultaneously improves spatial resolution of the x-ray beam as well as the heat capacity of the anode.

23. T F The warm-up procedure used to prevent cracking of an anode from a single excessive exposure will always consist of three exposures 3 seconds apart at 300 mA, 1 second, 80 kVp.

24. T F In x-ray applications, during tube on-time, thermal energy is measured in heat units.

Answer each of the following on a separate sheet of paper.

25. Explain (1) the physics principle behind the need for a focusing cup and (2) specifically how the focusing cup works to condense the electron beam.

26. Describe the three functions of an anode in an x-ray tube.

27. Discuss the use of the two-position exposure switch—in particular, describe its correct use and its effects on tube life.

28. Discuss how a mammography unit might utilize the heel effect to improve image quality.

29. Explain the space-charge effect and saturation current.

30. Describe when the large focal spot should be used. Why?

31. List the common anode materials.

32. Why is tungsten used as the material of choice for the tube target in general rediography?

33. What are the advantages of a rotating target over a stationary target?

34. Label the illustration for the line-focus principle.

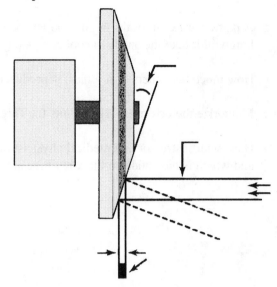

35. Describe the heel effect. How can the heel effect be used advantageously by a radiographer?

36. Explain extrafocal radiation.

37. Name and describe the three major causes of x-ray tube failure.

CHALLENGE QUESTIONS
■ ■ ■ ■ ■ ■ ■ ■ ■ ■ ■ ■ ■ ■ ■ ■ ■

Use the charts and formulas discussed in this chapter to calculate each of the following:

1. Use the charts in Figure 10-26 in your text to determine which of the following exposure factors are safe and which are unsafe:
   a. 98 kVp, 150 mA, 1 second; 3400 rpm; 0.6-millimeter focal spot
   b. 124 kVp, 250 mA, 0.1 second; 3400 rpm; 1-millimeter focal spot
   c. 149 kVp, 400 mA, 0.2 second; 10,000 rpm; 1-millimeter focal spot
   d. 126 kVp, 250 mA, 12 seconds; 10,000 rpm; 1-millimeter focal spot
   e. 75 kVp, 300 mA, 1.7 seconds; 10,000 rpm; 0.6-millimeter focal spot

2. A radiographic exam is done with a tube that has a 1.0-mm focal spot and anode rotation of 3400 rpm. The exam requires technique factors of 100 kVp, 1500 mAs. What is the shortest possible exposure time for this examination?

3. A certain radiographic exam requires 75 kVp at 400 mAs. How many heat units are generated by this exposure?

4. A fluoroscopic exam is performed at 100 kVp and 2.5 mA for 2 minutes. How many heat units are generated?

5. A particular exam results in 200,000 HU being delivered to the anode in a matter of seconds. How long will it take the anode to cool completely if the chart in Figure 10-27 of the text applies?

6. How much heat energy (in joules) is produced during a single exposure of 50 kVp at 400 mAs?

7. Memorize the box titled "Heat Units for Three-Phase Units" on page 123.

8. Have your instructor or a medical physicist or engineer help your class identify which is the cathode and which is the anode on the x-ray tube at your clinical site.

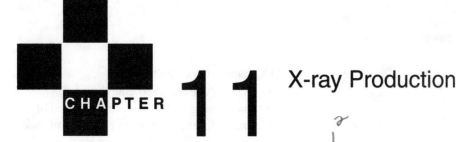

CHAPTER 11 X-ray Production

$KE = \frac{1}{2}mXv^2$

Circle the correct answer to each of the following.

1. A 1200-kilogram Mustang and a 300-kilogram Harley Davidson motorcycle are both traveling at the same speed. The Mustang:
   a. will have the same kinetic energy as the Harley, but only if the Harley doubles its speed.
   b. has four times more kinetic energy than the motorcycle.
   c. has no calculable kinetic energy as long as we do not know its speed.
   d. is accurately discussed in a and b.
   e. is accurately discussed in none of the above.

2. Electron kinetic energy in an x-ray tube is increased by raising:
   a. mass.
   b. acceleration.
   c. kVp.
   d. a and b.
   e. a and c.

3. As electron kinetic energy in an x-ray tube is increased:
   a. mAs of the x-ray beam increases.
   b. kVp of the x-ray beam increases.
   c. kVp of the x-ray beam becomes inversely proportional to the electron kinetic energy.
   d. a and b are true.
   e. a and c are true.

4. The efficiency of x-ray production:
   a. is dependent on the tube current.
   b. increases with increasing kVp.
   c. is dependent on what mA station is selected.
   d. is such that 99% of the kinetic energy of projectile electrons is used in the production of radiation.

5. Characteristic x-rays result when a projectile electron:
   a. violently interacts with an outer-shell electron.
   b. ionizes the target atom by removing an inner shell electron.
   c. interacts violently with a nucleic electron to remove an inner-shell electron.
   d. interacts violently with an outer-shell electron to remove an outer-shell electron.

6. A projectile electron interacts violently with an electron in the K shell of an atom. When the K-shell electron is subsequently ionized, which of the following responses will help in emission of an x-ray?
   a. An outer-shell electron fills the vacancy in the K shell.
   b. An M-shell electron's displacement makes the shell impenetrable by any other projectile electrons.
   c. A low-energy excitation occurs in the nucleus.
   d. Outer-shell electrons are raised to an excited level with the emission of infrared radiation or heat.

7. In characteristic radiation, the x-ray's energy is calculated by:
   a. subtracting the binding energies of the orbital electrons involved.
   b. subtracting the mass of the new electron from the projectile electron's binding energy.
   c. multiplying the masses of the orbital electrons.
   d. squaring the binding energy of the inner-shell electron and multiplying by the binding energy of the projectile electron.

8. An x-ray resulting from an M-to-K electron transition:
   a. is called an M x-ray.
   b. is called a K x-ray.
   c. is more energetic than an L x-ray.
   d. has a lower binding energy than an L x-ray.

9. Characteristic x-rays:
   a. are called thus because they are characteristic of the target element.
   b. are produced by transitions of orbital electrons from inner to outer shells.
   c. show an increase in effective energy that is inversely proportional to an increase in atomic number of the target element.
   d. are described accurately in a and c.
   e. are described accurately in all of the above.

10. Bremsstrahlung radiation:
    a. results when a projectile atom avoids the orbital electrons as it passes through the target atom and penetrates the atom's nucleus instead.
    b. results when a projectile electron loses all kinetic energy and is absorbed into the nucleus of the target atom.
    c. results when a projectile electron slows and changes course as it passes the target atom's nucleus.
    d. results in x-rays that have more specified energies than characteristic x-rays have.

11. The difference in origins of a low-energy bremsstrahlung x-ray and a maximum-energy x-ray is that the maximum-energy x-ray is produced when the projectile electron:
    a. loses all its kinetic energy and drifts away from the nucleus.
    b. is barely influenced by the nucleus, maintaining a maximum level of energy.
    c. requires a specific tube potential of at least 70 kVp.
    d. gains kinetic energy and is violently absorbed by the nucleus.

12. Characteristic x-rays:
    a. have precisely fixed energies.
    b. have energies that are characteristic of the differences between electron-binding energies of a particular element.
    c. have energies that range from the peak electron energy all the way down to zero.
    d. are described in b and c.
    e. are described in a and b.

Indicate whether the following statements are true or false.

13. T F The equation used to calculate kinetic energy is $KE = 1/2 \, (mv)^2$.

14. T F According to the theory of relativity, the mass of the electron increases as it approaches the speed of light.

15. T F X-ray tubes are inefficient because the production of heat in the anode increases directly with increasing tube current and kVp.

16. T F The efficiency of x-ray production is independent of the tube current.

17. T F K-shell electrons have a higher binding energy than outer-shell electrons.

18. T F Low-energy x-rays are more likely to be absorbed in the target.

Calculate the following problems on a separate sheet of paper.

19. A K-shell electron is removed from a tungsten atom and is replaced by an O-shell electron. (a) What is the resultant x-ray called? (b) Why? (c) What is the energy of the characteristic x-ray that is emitted?

20. An O-shell electron is removed from a tungsten atom and is replaced by a P-shell electron. (a) What is the resultant x-ray called? (b) Why? (c) What is the energy of the characteristic x-ray that is emitted?

21. Using data from Figure 11-4 and Table 11-1, calculate the effective level of energy that results when a K-shell electron is removed from a tungsten atom and is replaced by one of the following:
    a. an L-shell electron.
    b. an N-shell electron.
    c. an O-shell electron.

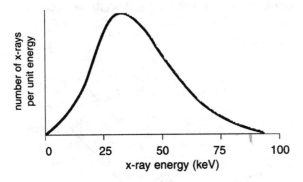

22. If the illustration above shows a bremsstrahlung x-ray spectrum for a specific x-ray machine, do you have enough information to determine at what kVp the machine was operated? If no, what information is missing? If yes, at what kVp was the machine operated, and how can you tell?

23. An x-ray unit is operated at 82 kVp. (a) How much kinetic energy can its projectile electrons have? (b) What will be the range of energy in a bremsstrahlung interaction?

24. Plot the expected emission spectrum for an x-ray machine with a pure molybdenum target (effective energy of the K x-ray equals 17 keV) operated at 87 kVp.

25. Solve the following: What is the minimum wavelength associated with the x-rays emitted from an x-ray machine operated at 100 kVp?

26. Solve the following: What would be the minimum wavelength associated with the x-rays emitted from an x-ray machine if it could be operated at 50 kVp?

Answer each of the following on a separate sheet of paper.

27. Draw and label the x-ray emission spectrum.

28. Describe the differences in a characteristic x-ray emission spectrum and a bremsstrahlung x-ray emission spectrum.

29. The electrons accelerated from cathode to anode do not all have the peak kinetic energy. Why?

30. Why is external filtration so frequently added to the x-ray tube assembly?

31. What is the relationship between x-ray energy and x-ray wavelength?

32. (a) Describe how the relative position of an emission spectrum along the energy axis reflects the quality of the x-ray beam and the quantity of photons in the beam. (b) Next, predict what will happen if the mA station is changed to a lower mA.

33. (a) How is the x-ray emission spectrum affected by a change in kVp? What happens when kVp is raised? (b) What rule does this partially explain? (c) How is this rule used?

34. Describe the effect of hardening the x-ray beam on (a) the characteristic spectrum; (b) bremsstrahlung x-ray emission; (c) the maximum energy of x-ray emission; and (d) low- and high-energy x-rays.

35. Describe the effect of an increase in the atomic number of the target material on the following: (a) bremsstrahlung radiation; (b) the characteristic spectrum.

CHALLENGE QUESTIONS
. . . .

1. In order to perform specific procedures, two x-ray students are both instructed to increase the kVp by 15%. One machine has been operating at 50 kVp, while the other has been operating at 110 kVp. (a) How much kVp will be used by each at the new levels? (b) One student predicts that the 15% increase will double the output intensity from his machine to obtain an optimum optical density on the radiograph, but the other student says it will be equivalent to doubling the mAs. Who, if either, is right? If both are partially right, explain. (c) Is only a 15% increase necessary?

2. Label the illustrations below, and then explain the formation of characteristic and bremsstrahlung x-ray production.

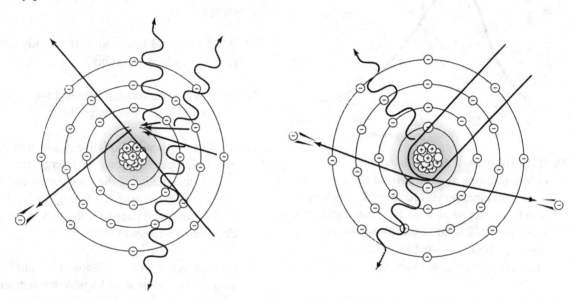

3. What are the four principle factors influencing the shape of an x-ray emission spectrum?

4. Discuss the effect of each of the following five factors on the x-ray emission spectrum: mA, kVp, filtration, target material, and voltage waveform.

5. Calculate a 15% increase in the following kVp levels.

	15% increase
a. 55 kVp	_____
b. 60 kVp	_____
c. 72 kVp	_____
d. 80 kVp	_____
e. 90 kVp	_____
f. 120 kVp	_____

6. Fill in both tables below.

Changes in X-ray Beam Quality and Quantity by Factors That Influence the Emission Spectrum

Increased	Results
mAs	
kVp	
Added mm Al	
Target material	
Voltage ripple	

Factors Affecting the Size and Position of X-ray Emission Spectra

Factor	Effect
Tube current	
Tube voltage	
Added filtration	
Target material (Z)	
Voltage waveform	

CHAPTER 12 X-ray Emission

Circle the correct answer to each of the following.

1. The roentgen is a measure of the:
   a. number of ion pairs produced in air by a quantity of x-rays.
   b. quality of the x-ray beam.
   c. number of coulombs of charge per kilogram in an x-ray.
   d. a and b.
   e. a and c.

2. The radiation quantity is:
   a. the number of x-rays in the useful beam.
   b. the number of x-rays emitted from the x-ray tube.
   c. the number of electrons hitting the target.
   d. a and b.
   e. all of the above.

3. X-ray quantity is:
   a. directly proportional to the penetrability of the x-rays in tissue.
   b. doubled every time the number of electrons striking the tube target is increased by 15%.
   c. directly proportional to the mAs.
   d. inversely proportional to the square of the distance from the target.

4. To maintain a constant exposure of the film, an increase of 15% in kVp should be accompanied by:
   a. a one-quarter increase in mAs as well.
   b. a constant mAs level.
   c. a one-half reduction in mAs.
   d. a squaring of the difference between the two mR levels.
   e. none of the above.

5. The primary purpose of metal filters in x-ray units is to:
   a. absorb all x-rays that have no diagnostic value.
   b. reduce the number of low-energy x-rays that reach the patient.
   c. use their metallic surfaces to intensify the diagnostic value of the half-value layer.
   d. serve none of the above functions.

6. Radiation intensity from an x-ray tube:
   a. varies inversely with the square of the distance from the target.
   b. varies inversely with the square root of the distance from the target.
   c. varies in direct proportion to the product of kVp and mAs squared.
   d. is not calculated by any of the above formulas.

7. As mAs is increased:
   a. optical density decreases proportionately.
   b. x-ray quantity increases proportionately.
   c. x-ray quantity is reduced.
   d. optical density decreases.

8. The half-value layer:
   a. is affected by the kVp and amount of filtration.
   b. refers to the thickness of absorbing material necessary to reduce the x-ray intensity to half of its original value.
   c. is the numerical expression of x-ray quality.
   d. is described in a and c only.
   e. is described in a, b, and c.

9. High-energy x-rays:
   a. are more penetrating than low-energy x-rays.
   b. are attenuated at a higher rate than low-energy x-rays.
   c. are absorbed at a higher rate than low-energy x-rays.
   d. are described in a and b.
   e. are described in b and c.

10. A diagnostic x-ray beam:
    a. has a half-value layer in the range of 3 to 5 millimeters of soft tissue.
    b. is characterized by the half-value layer.
    c. has a half-value layer in the range of 4 to 6 centimeters of aluminum.
    d. is described in a and b only.
    e. is described in b and c only.

11. Hard x-rays:
    a. are those with low penetrability.
    b. are identical numerically to the HVl value.
    c. are those with high penetrability.
    d. are inversely proportional to the half-value layer.

Indicate whether the following statements are true or false.

12. T F The mAs is a measure of the total number of electrons that travel from cathode to anode to produce x-rays.

13. T F The thickness of filtration that increases x-ray intensity to one and a half times its original value is the half-value layer.

14. T F The ideally filtered x-ray beam would be monoenergetic.

15. T F The purpose of the thinness of the window through which x-rays are emitted from the glass envelope is to provide high inherent filtration.

Calculate the following problems on a separate sheet of paper.

16. A specific radiographic technique calls for 120 kVp at 15 mAs, which results in an x-ray intensity of 40 mR to the patient. If the mAs is increased to 30 mAs, what will the x-ray intensity be?

17. A radiographic technique calls for 115 kVp at 12 mAs, which results in an x-ray intensity of 37 mR to the patient. If the mAs is increased to 36 mAs, what will the x-ray intensity be?

18. The radiographic technical factor for a procedure is 65 kVp at 60 mAs. The result is a patient exposure of 200 mR. What will be the potential exposure if the mAs can be reduced to 30 mAs?

19. A procedure calls for 75 kVp at 50 mAs. The result is a patient exposure of 220 mR. What will be the potential exposure (in mR) if the mAs can be reduced to 40 mAs?

20. A technique using 100 kVp at 20 mAs results in an x-ray intensity of 36 mR. Using the first kVp formula on page 141, what will be the intensity if the radiographer retakes the image with the kVp increased to 150 but using the same mAs?

21. A technique using 100 kVp at 10 mAs results in an x-ray intensity of 40 mR. Using the first kVp formula, what will be the intensity if the radiographer retakes the image with the kVp increased to 180 but using the same mAs?

22. Instead of increasing the kVp, as in problem 21, the radiographer decides to decrease it from its original 100 kVp to 85 kVp. What will be the intensity, provided the same mAs is used?

23. An exam at 80 kVp and 50 mAs produces an intensity of 150 mR. However, it will now be necessary to increase the kVp by 15%. How can the radiographer maintain a constant density on the film? What will be the expected intensity as a result?

24. Use the inverse square law to solve the following problem: A radiographer will take a portable x-ray unit to several inpatients. The first exam is normally conducted at 100 cm SID and results in an intensity of 15 mR at the film. If 80 cm is the maximum SID that can be obtained for a specific patient's situation, what will be the radiation intensity at the film?

25. A particular exam is usually taken at 130 kVp at 4 mAs taken at an SID of 200 centimeters. The intensity at the image receptor is 14 mR. If the same technique is performed at an SID of 100 centimeters, what will be the x-ray intensity?

26. An exam is usually taken at 124 kVp at 6 mAs taken at an SID of 240 centimeters. The intensity at the image receptor is 17 mR. If the same technique is performed at an SID of 80 centimeters, what will be the x-ray intensity?

27. An x-ray tube has a half-value layer of 2.7 millimeters of aluminum. The exposure from this machine is 3 mR/mAs at 150 centimeters SID. If 2.7 millimeters of aluminum is added to the beam, what will be the x-ray intensity?

Answer each of the following on a separate sheet of paper.

28. Describe the steps in determining the half-value layer of an x-ray beam.

29. Describe the differences between inherent filtration and added filtration in terms of tube parts involved, effectiveness, and extent of filtration of each.

30. Why does added filtration result in a harder x-ray beam?

31. Name four factors that affect x-ray quantity and describe their effect on radiographic optical density.

32. X-ray quantity (mR) is _____ _____ to the mAs.

33. IR = _____ _____ c/kg.

    IC = _____ _____ electrons.

34. Write and explain the inverse square law.

35. Define *penetrability* of the x-ray beam.

36. List and explain the factors that affect x-ray quality and the effect on optical density.

37. Define light-localizing variable-aperature collimation.

CHALLENGE QUESTIONS
. . . .

1. You are assigned to spend two hours observing an experienced radiographer in a large metropolitan hospital. This radiographer's role is to demonstrate a variety of radiographic techniques. The first patient this afternoon is Mr. Henson, who has severe pneumonia and fluid in one of his lungs. The radiographer tells you she is going to need to use a compensating filter. What is the purpose of a compensating filter? Give an example of how it will help obtain an effective image of Mr. Henson's chest.

2. Next, the radiographer from the previous question is about to take a chest radiograph for Mr. Gibson, who is in excellent health but is receiving a chest radiograph as part of a medical exam needed for an overseas job assignment. But even though you know that Mr. Gibson's physician reports his health as excellent, the radiographer still uses a special filter? What kind will she use? Why?

3. Finally, the last patient needs an anterior-posterior (AP) radiograph of his foot. Describe how you would ensure uniformity in such an image.

4. Explain the compensating filter used in Figure 12-9.

5. Use the nomogram in Figure 12-1 to determine the appropriate x-ray beam intensity for each of the following situations:

   a. a total filtration of 2 mm Al with 70 kVp

   b. a total filtration of 2 mm Al with 80 kVp

   c. a total filtration of 1 mm Al with 40 kVp

   d. a total filtration of 4 mm Al with 40 kVp

   e. a total filtration of 4 mm Al with 80 kVp

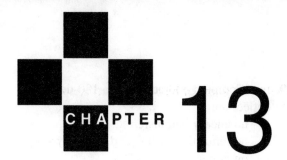

CHAPTER 13

X-ray Interaction with Matter

Match each term to its description or function.

1. _____ classical scattering

2. _____ Rayleigh scattering

3. _____ Compton effect

4. _____ secondary electron

5. _____ backscatter radiation

6. _____ photoelectric effect

7. _____ secondary radiation

8. _____ pair production

9. _____ photodisintegration

10. _____ radiopaque

11. _____ radiolucent

12. _____ differential absorption

13. _____ attenuation

14. _____ remnant radiation

15. _____ contrast agent

a. x-rays scattered back in the direction of the incident x-ray beam

b. having high x-ray absorption

c. x-ray absorption interaction in which the x-ray is not scattered but is totally absorbed

d. total reduction in x-rays remaining in an x-ray beam after penetration through a given thickness of tissue

e. compound used as an aid in imaging organs.

f. electron that interacts with moderate-energy x-rays in Compton scattering

g. difference between those x-rays absorbed photoelectrically and those not absorbed at all

h. characteristic x-ray emission after a photo-electric interaction; occurs when an outer-shell electron fills a vacancy in the K shell

i. interaction of moderate-energy x-rays with outer-shell electrons; reduces the x-ray's energy and ionizes the atom

j. the interaction of low-energy x-rays with the entire atom

k. direct absorption of very high-energy x-rays by the nucleus of an atom, causing the nucleus to emit a nuclear fragment

l. means by which low-energy incident x-rays interact with matter; also called coherent scattering

m. interaction in which an incident x-ray disappears after interacting with the nucleus of an atom, leaving in its place a positron and a negatively charged electron

n. beam exiting from tissue and hitting the x-ray film emulsion; remains of an x-ray after attenuation by matter

o. property of a structure through which x-rays pass

Circle the correct answer to each of the following.

16. Classical scattering:
    a. is the same thing as coherent scattering.
    b. includes Rayleigh, Thomson, and Compton scattering.
    c. is the interaction of low-energy x-rays with matter.
    d. is accurately described in a and c.
    e. is accurately described in a, b, and c.

17. The Compton effect:
    a. results from moderate-energy x-ray interactions with nuclei of atoms.
    b. not only scatters the x-ray but ionizes it as well.
    c. results in a scattered x-ray whose wavelength is greater than that of the incident x-ray.
    d. is accurately described in a and c.
    e. is accurately described in a, b, and c.

18. The energy of a Compton-scattered x-ray is equal to:
    a. the difference between the energy of the incident x-ray and the energy of the ejected electron.
    b. the binding energy of the ejected electron plus its own kinetic energy.
    c. its own binding energy plus the kinetic energy it has when it leaves the atom.
    d. a and c.
    e. none of the above.

19. In a Compton interaction:
    a. the scattered x-ray usually retains less energy than the secondary electron.
    b. the secondary electron drops into a vacancy in an electron shell previously created by some other ionizing event.
    c. the secondary electron loses all of its kinetic energy and is absorbed.
    d. a and c are true.
    e. a and b are true.

20. In a Compton interaction, at a 180-degree deflection,
    a. no energy is transferred.
    b. no ionization occurs and the x-ray keeps on going.
    c. the least amount of energy is transferred to the secondary electron because of backscatter radiation.
    d. the scattered x-ray retains about two-thirds of its original energy.
    e. none of the above is true.

21. The probability of Compton effect:
    a. depends on the atomic number of the atom involved.
    b. is more likely to occur in an atom of bone than in an atom of soft tissue.
    c. is a function of both the x-ray energy and the atomic number of the atom involved.
    d. decreases as x-ray energy increases.
    e. increases proportionally as x-ray energy increases.

22. In the photoelectric effect:
    a. the x-ray is totally absorbed.
    b. the incident photon does not disappear but is ejected from the atom as a photoelectron.
    c. the electron escapes with kinetic energy equal to the difference between the energy of the incident x-ray and the binding energy of the electron.
    d. a and c are true.
    e. a, b, and c are true.

23. As atomic number of matter increases:
    a. it will have no effect on probability of Compton scattering.
    b. it will proportionately increase the probability of Compton scattering.
    c. it will have an inverse effect on probability of Compton scattering.
    d. it will increase probability of Compton scattering—relative to photoelectric effect.
    e. it will reduce probability of Compton scattering with loosely bound electrons.

24. The probability of photoelectric effect:
    a. increases with the third power of the photon energy.
    b. is inversely proportional to the third power of the x-ray energy and directly proportional to the third power of the atomic number of the absorbing material.
    c. is inversely proportional to the third power of the x-ray energy and to the third power of the atomic number of the absorbing material.
    d. is described in a and b.
    e. is not described here.

25. As x-ray energy increases, there is:
    a. less probability of penetration through tissue without interaction.
    b. more probability of photoelectric effect relative to Compton scattering.
    c. reduced absolute photoelectric effect.
    d. more photoelectric effect.
    e. none of the above.

26. When very high-energy x-rays escape interaction with electrons and the nuclear electrostatic field:
    a. they are more likely to be absorbed directly by the nucleus.
    b. the nucleus instantaneously emits a nucleon or other nuclear fragment.
    c. photodisintegration can occur.
    d. a and b occur.
    e. b and c occur.

27. Basically, an x-ray image results from:
    a. the difference between those x-rays absorbed photoelectrically and those not absorbed at all.
    b. the Compton effect.
    c. the differential absorption.
    d. a and b.
    e. a and c.

28. At low energies, the majority of x-ray interactions:
    a. require a lower mAs.
    b. are predominantly Compton scattering.
    c. show an increased chance of occurring.
    d. demonstrate that more x-rays get to the film.
    e. are photoelectric.

29. Mass density:
    a. is the same as optical density.
    b. is the quantity of matter per unit volume.
    c. when doubled, doubles the chance for x-ray interaction.
    d. is best described in a and b.
    e. is best described in b and c.

Calculate the following problems on a separate sheet of paper.

30. A 40-keV x-ray ionizes an atom of barium by ejecting an O-shell electron with 16 keV of kinetic energy. The O-shell has a binding energy of .04 keV. What is the energy of the scattered x-ray?

31. A 36-keV x-ray ionizes an atom of barium by ejecting an O-shell electron with 14 keV of kinetic energy. What is the energy of the scattered x-ray?

32. A 60-keV x-ray interacts photoelectrically with (a) a carbon atom and (b) a barium atom. What is the kinetic energy of each photoelectron and the energy of each characteristic x-ray if an L-to-K transition occurs?

33. (a) If the relative probability of photoelectric interaction with soft tissue for a 30-keV x-ray is 1, how much less likely will an interaction be for a 60-keV x-ray? (b) How much more likely is interaction with air than with lung tissue for a 70-keV x-ray?

34. A student radiographer is about to take a radiograph of a patient's lower leg after an accident with a nail gun. Some nail fragments are thought to have entered the bone, while some have entered muscle and fat tissue only. How much more likely is an x-ray to interact with the bone than muscle or fat?

35. A student radiographer is taking a series of radiographs that are all photoelectric. What is the differential absorption of x-rays in lung relative to fat?

Answer each of the following on a separate sheet of paper.

36. Using Figure 13-13, at what keV for bone and soft tissue does the chance of photoelectric absorption equal the chance of Compton interaction?

37. Is the photoelectric effect the same thing as absorption? Why or why not?

38. What is attenuation? How would you relate it to absorption and scattering?

39. Create a table that demonstrates the characteristics of differential absorption (a) as x-ray energy increases; (b) as tissue atomic number increases; (c) as tissue mass density increases.

40. Illustrate the following interactions between x-rays and atoms:
    • classical scattering (Figure 13-1)
    • Compton effect (Figure 13-2)
    • photoelectric effect (Figure 13-5)
    • pair production (Figure 13-8)
    • photodisintegration (Figure 13-9)

CHALLENGE QUESTIONS

1. What are the principles for the use of contrast agents? How is this useful in radiography? Give examples.

2. If Compton-scattered x-rays provide no useful information on the radiograph, why are they important to our understanding about dose and image production?

3. Outline the following characteristics of Compton scattering: (a) Where and in what situations are they most likely to occur? (b) How does increased x-ray energy affect Compton scattering? (c) What happens as atomic number of matter increasses? (d) What happens as mass density of matter increases?

4. Describe the process by which characteristic x-rays are produced after a photoelectric interaction. What are these characteristic x-rays called? Describe their behavior.

5. What do we mean, regarding photoelectric effect, when we say, "The probability of interaction proportional to the third power of the atomic number of the absorbing material changes rapidly"?

6. Describe what can happen if an incident x-ray has sufficient energy to escape interaction with the electron shells and instead comes close enough to be influenced by the atom's nucleus. How often does this occur in the diagnostic x-ray range? Is it possible for us to know exactly how much energy an x-ray must have to accomplish this?

7. What percentage of the x-rays emitted by an x-ray unit reach the film or contribute to the radiographic image? What does this suggest is necessary to produce a high-quality of a radiograph?

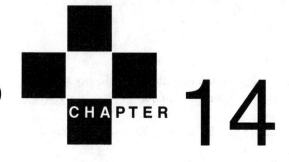

CHAPTER 14

Radiographic Film

Circle the correct answer to each of the following.

1. The remnant beam:
   a. is the portion of the x-ray beam before attenuation by matter.
   b. does not contribute to the diagnostic quality of the image.
   c. activates the phosphor within the intensifying screens, exposing the radiographic film.

2. The primary purpose of the radiographic film base is to:
   a. provide a rigid structure to be coated with emulsion.
   b. provide uniform lucency.
   c. prevent flammability.
   d. interact with x-rays or light photons from screens, transferring information that is exposed by emulsion.

3. Light photons emitted from intensifying screens form an image primarily by interacting with:
   a. the high-Z atoms in the iodine and gelatin mixture.
   b. the high-Z atoms in silver-halide crystals.
   c. dissolved metallic silver (Ag).
   d. the sensitivity speck.
   e. none of the above.

4. The sensitivity speck, thought to be formed by a chemical contaminant:
   a. is primarily responsible for "ghost" images on faulty radiographs.
   b. must be removed during the precipitation process.
   c. is the location where silver atoms are attracted and concentrated during processing.

5. Silver-halide crystals are made by dissolving and mixing:
   a. silver (Ag).
   b. nitric acid (HNO_3).
   c. silver nitrate ($AgNO_3$).
   d. a and b.
   e. b and c.

6. The emulsion consists of a mixture of:
   a. cellulose triacetate.
   b. gelatin.
   c. silver-halide crystals.
   d. b and c.
   e. a, b, and c.

7. Duplitized x-ray film:
   a. can be reproduced using the original film when a copy of a radiograph is necessary.
   b. does not have a supercoating to protect the emulsion.
   c. is coated on both sides with emulsion.

8. Which of the following statements is true?
   a. Green-sensitive film is sensitive to green light only, making it "orthochromatic."
   b. Green-sensitive film is matched to rare-earth screens, although a few rare-earth phosphors emit in the blue-violet area of the spectrum.
   c. If calcium tungstate screens are used, they should be matched with a film that is sensitive not only to blue light but also to green light.
   d. Panchromatic film is sensitive to the entire visible-light spectrum and is thus most appropriate for modern radiographic exposure techniques.
   e. Lanthanum oxybromide screens and green-sensitive films are spectrally matched.

9. What happens if spectral emission of a screen and spectral sensitivity of the film are mismatched?
   a. The image-receptor speed will be too fast, causing underexposure.
   b. The patient dose will be reduced.
   c. The image-receptor speed will be greatly increased.
   d. The light photons from the intensifying screens will be inadequate to create a properly exposed image.
   e. There will be a correct film-screen combination.

10. Reciprocity law failure:
    a. occurs when film is exposed to light from intensifying screens.
    b. is of no concern with long exposure times.
    c. is of no concern with short exposure times.
    d. occurs most often during pediatric examinations.
    e. may be compensated for by reducing technique.

11. Which of the following statements is true?
    a. Processing is the term applied to chemical reactions that transform the latent image into a manifest image.
    b. The principle function of the base is to provide mechanical support for the silver-halide crystals by holding them uniformly in place.
    c. When the remnant radiation deposits energy into the atoms of silver halide, this energy forms a latent image, which can be seen immediately.
    d. Silver-halide crystals are 95% silver iodide and 5% silver bromide.

12. In the formation of a latent image, in what order do the following events occur?
    _____ Light or radiation interaction releases electrons.
    _____ The silver grain results.
    _____ Electrons migrate to the sensitivity speck and are neutralized.
    _____ The buildup of silver atoms and the disappearance of negative surface electrification occur.
    _____ At the sensitivity speck, atomic silver is formed.

Fill in the blanks in the following statements.

13. Radiographic film consists of two basic parts: _____ and _____.

14. The thickest layer of radiographic film is the _____.

15. In forming silver halide, the _____ is precipitated.

16. When photons interact with radiographic film, most of the energy is transferred to the _____, forming the latent image.

17. In the Gurney-Mott theory of photon interaction with silver-halide crystal, both Compton and photoelectric interactions cause the release of _____ with sufficient energy to cross the crystal lattice, releasing more electrons.

18. Silver bromide is formed by mixing _____ with _____.

19. The _____ refers to the formation of the latent image.

Answer each of the following on a separate sheet of paper.

20. Define the following radiographic film characteristics: spectral matching, speed, contrast, latitude.

21. Draw cross-sections of film and intensifying screens that illustrate the following:
    - crossover
    - reduced crossover when an anti-crossover layer is added to the film base

22. What does the Gurney-Mott theory propose?

23. It is the first job in radiography for both you and your colleague in a brand-new hospital in your community. Consequently, every time a different kind of film or screen is required, both you and your colleague in the radiography exam room are thrown into a panic because neither of you knows whether your safelight and filter are adequate. Without consulting your text, create a quick, simple chart or table that can be displayed at all times that will indicate appropriate safelight filters for each major type of film and screen. Research to find out; then incorporate appropriate watt and distance combinations.

24. Why is direct-exposure film rarely used any more? What has replaced it? Give two examples of replacements.

25. What is used to reduce reflection of screen-light that is transmitted through the emulsion and base in mammography, and what is this preventable effect called?

26. Describe the process for creating an image on video film.

27. You are about to participate in your first video imaging procedure. What must you remember about (a) patient dose? (b) film choice?

28. Prepare a brief summary in your own words of each type of specialty film.

29. Develop a chart that could be displayed, offering guidelines for the handling and storage of films, including the following: artifact prevention, heat, humidity, light, and radiation factors. In addition, add a notation about shelf life.

CHALLENGE QUESTIONS
■ ■ ■ ■ ■ ■ ■ ■ ■ ■ ■ ■ ■ ■ ■ ■ ■

1. List a series of events leading from film exposure to production of manifest image, dropping each in random order up and down a sheet of lined paper. Make two photocopies and exchange with two peers. Reorder their list by numbering each step consecutively. By the time you have corrected or reordered two lists made by someone else, you will find you have a much stronger sense of the whole process leading up to a manifest image.

2. This next exercise, which discusses the silver-halide crystal's structure, is accomplished in several steps, outlined below.

    Step 1:   Create a model of the silver-halide crystal and make a photocopy. Exchange with a peer.

    Step 2:   Next, add onto this drawing, inserting labels to add the following information to this model: (a) Silver is a positive ion; bromine and iodine are negative ions. (b) Silver atoms are positiviely charged; bromine and iodine atoms are negatively charged. (c) The halide ions are generally in greatest concentration along the surface of the crystal.

    Step 3:   Next, determine what kind of charge the crystal takes on on its surface, and interstitially. Label it, based on your conclusions.

    Step 4:   Return the drawing to its original creator. Check each other's work, altering each model as necessary. Then, finally, when you get your own drawing back, check your work once again.

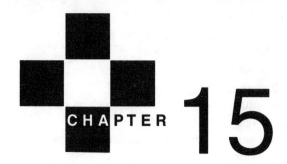

CHAPTER 15

Processing the Latent Image

Match each of the actions or descriptions in the left-hand column to the appropriate term in the right-hand column.

1. _____ development

2. _____ reduction

3. _____ stop bath

4. _____ Pako

5. _____ sequestering agent

6. _____ synergism

7. _____ fixation

8. _____ oxidation

9. _____ Konica

10. _____ solvent

11. _____ aerial oxidation

a. liquid into which chemicals can be dissolved, generally water

b. dissolution and removal from the emulsion of any silver halide not exposed to radiation or light

c. first to produce an automatic film processor with a processing cycle of approximately 45 seconds

d. introduced first automatic x-ray film processor, which could process 120 films per hour

e. neutralization of a positive ion when an electron is given up by the developing agent

f. production of a manifest image from the latent image

g. reaction that produces an electron

h. situation in which the action of two agents working together is greater than the sum of the action of each agent working independently

i. air introduced into the chemistry when it is mixed, handled, and stored

j. substance that forms stable complexes with metallic ions and salts so that they will not accelerate the oxidation of hydroquinone

k. termination of development and removal of excess chemical from emulsion

Circle the correct answer to each of the following.

12. Only silver halide crystals that contain
    _____ are reduced to metallic silver by
    the addition of developer.
    a. surface electrification
    b. chemical ions
    c. the latent image
    d. unexposed areas

13. What is the significance of the development
    of the roller transport system in automatic
    processing?
    a. It was able to handle the workload of
        busy departments more efficiently.
    b. Technical factors were standardized.
    c. Finished radiographs were available in 6
        minutes rather than 40 minutes.
    d. Variations in development and artifacts
        from handling were eliminated.
    e. All of the above.

14. Ammonium thiosulfate:
    a. neutralizes the developer and stops its
        action.
    b. removes undeveloped silver bromine
        from emulsion.
    c. removes aluminum ions.
    d. stiffens and shrinks the emulsion.
    e. maintains proper pH.

15. Mixing developer chemicals requires caution
    because:
    a. the preservative may enhance aerial oxi-
        dation.
    b. alkali compounds used as buffering
        agents are caustic to the skin.
    c. hydroquinone and phenidone may react
        suddenly.

16. An exposed silver-halide crystal:
    a. is permeable to the developing agent
        only in the region of the sensitivity
        speck.
    b. has a negative electrostatic charge dis-
        tributed over its entire surface.
    c. has a positive electrostatic charge distrib-
        uted over its surface except in the region
        of the sensitivity speck.

17. Fixation:
    a. may incorporate the stop bath as part of
        one step.
    b. hardens the gelatin portion of the emul-
        sion.
    c. produces a film of archival quality.
    d. all of the above.

18. Compounds such as hydroquinone, pheni-
    done, and metol:
    a. are oxidation agents.
    b. are composed of ions with electrons near
        their outside surfaces that can neutralize
        positive silver ions.
    c. take electrons from the silver halide crys-
        tals.

19. The wetting agent:
    a. was originally water; it has now been
        replaced by chelates.
    b. is the universal solvent—water.
    c. removes excess chemicals from emul-
        sion.
    d. is a silver halide solution.
    e. is used in a stop bath to remove silver
        halide or other excess chemicals from
        emulsion.

20. In automatic processing:
    a. temperatures are higher than for manual
        processing.
    b. chemical concentrations are higher than
        for manual processing.
    c. the chemicals involved are basically the
        same as for manual processing.
    d. all of the above

Indicate whether the following are true or false.

21. T F In automatic processing, a stop bath
            is not used because the squeegee
            action of the rollers of the transport
            system and the action of acetic acid
            take its place.

22. T F The developer temperature is usually
            maintained within plus or minus 0.5°
            F of the optimal temperature.

23. T F Potassium bromide is an antifog agent that keeps unexposed crystals from being chemically attacked.

24. T F The replenishment system regularly adds to each tank the proper amount of developer and fixer and recirculates wash water.

25. T F Hypo retention improves the archival quality of a radiograph.

Circle the correct answer to each of the following.

26. What is the reason damp films may drop into the receiving bin?
    a. The hardener in the fixer has been depleted.
    b. Failure to add sodium sulfite has caused the developer to oxidise.
    c. Pottasium bromide has been left out, causing a lack of restraining action.
    d. Glutaraldehyde, which controls the swelling and softening of the emulsion, has been depleted.
    e. Silver reduction has swollen the emulsion too much when the chelates were added.

27. What is the reason that developer may oxidize too rapidly?
    a. Impurities were mixed into the developer by error.
    b. Chelates were left out of the developer tank.
    c. Sodium sulfide was not added to the developer solution.
    d. All of the above.

28. What is the difference between the chemicals sodium sulfite and sodium hydroxide used in automatic processing?
    a. Sodium sulfite is a preservative that maintains chemical balance; sodium hydroxide is a buffering agent.
    b. Sodium sulfite controls aerial oxidation; sodium hydroxide is an alkali compound.
    c. Sodium sulfite helps maintain proper development rate; sodium hydroxide controls pH.
    d. All of the above.

29. Archival quality:
    a. refers to the permanence of the radiograph.
    b. implies that an image does not deteriorate with age.
    c. doesn't occur until the fixing stage.
    d. all of the above.

Answer each of the following on a separate sheet of paper.

30. List the three-step process for converting the latent image into a manifest image.

31. Discuss the importance of feeding the film properly into the automatic processor.

32. Explain how a film is transported around the bend in a transport-rack subassembly.

33. What is the optimal temperature for the developer tank in Fahrenheit and Celsius?

34. What is the minimum flow rate for the wash tank in most processors?

35. What are the replenishment rates of developer and fixer for every 14 inches of film?

36. List and describe the three alternative processing methods.

37. What is the purpose of the replenishment system?

38. Discuss the differences in reduction and oxidation.

39. Create an illustrated flow chart of what happens to crystals during development. Add notations to explain what is happening in each diagram you create.

CHALLENGE QUESTIONS
. . . .

1. Create a chart on fairly large paper that lists each step in the sequence of processing steps. Run these steps down the left-hand column. Many students find it helpful to use a horizontal rather than vertical layout. Be sure to leave equal spaces between each item to allow space for "editing" or correcting later. Place four headings across the top of your table so that you can later enter appropriate information under each, adjacent to each appropriate step. The headings you need are as follows: "Manual Time," "Automatic Time," "Purpose," "Processing Chemical Involved," and "Function of Chemical." Now fill in the table.

2. This exercise works well when done either individually or in small teams: Research articles that demonstrate specific problems or solutions labs have sometimes encountered in darkroom and film processing techniques. Use these as a basis for creating your own fictitious "case study." Write specific questions on how to improve or solve these situations. Your instructor or librarian can show you how to use the directories for various radiographic journals. (You don't want to use the same articles as everyone else in class!) Exchange case studies and solve. Sample articles might include: "Reducing the Risks in X-ray Processing," by P. Hewitt in *Occupational Health* 46(7), July 1994, p. 244; "Dry-process Film Eliminates Need for Darkroom and Chemicals," by L.E. Ketchum in *Applied Radiology* 23(5), May 1994, p. 39; "Study Shows Inconsistency in Film Processing Quality," by O.L. Pirtle in *Radiologic Technology* 64(3), Jan.–Feb. 1993, p. 154; or "Solving Your Darkroom Problem," by D. Utt in *Radiologic Technology* 66(1), Sept.–Oct. 1994, p. 65.

   Remember, however, that once you have a directory at hand, you can find more varied and more recent articles than are available at the time of press of this book.

3. On separate index cards, briefly describe a key function of each of the system components that make up an automatic processor (e.g., transport system, replenishment system, etc.). If you prefer, draw a quick, labeled diagram, but *do not identify the system being described.* You should have six cards when you're finished. Exchange two cards, without checking to see that they describe the same systems. Continue to exchange until you no longer have any of your own original cards. Then label each card until you encounter a duplicate. Do not label the duplicate. Instead, exchange cards with another student, again, not looking to see what they're offering you. Continue to exchange until you have a complete set of components for an automatic processor. (This activity also works well as a card game, in which all players in turn "draw" or "discard" until someone wins by collecting a complete set.)

4. This next exercise works well in teams but can be done individually also. Prepare a table and very brief presentation that highlight the differences in rapid processing, extended processing, and daylight processing. Mix some of the most important features among the three; then invite verbal feedback. If students do not catch your "errors," offer to repeat the presentation, offering lead questions or clues, if you like, to guide them in the right direction. Prepare a mini-quiz to follow the presentation.

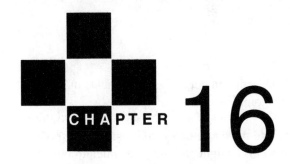

Intensifying Screens

CHAPTER 16

. . . .

Circle the correct answer to each of the following.

1. The use of an intensifying screen:
   a. amplifies the remnant radiation reaching the film.
   b. requires spectral matching with phosphor afterglow.
   c. results in increased patient dose.
   d. generates decreased subject contrast and poorer detail.
   e. eliminates blurring of the image.

2. The phosphor:
   a. is an inactive layer in the intensifying screen.
   b. emits light after stimulation by x-rays.
   c. layer ranges in thickness from 300-400 µm.
   d. has only one purpose—to convert the energy of the x-ray beam to visible light.

3. There is a reflective layer between the phosphor and the base. When x-rays interact with the phosphor:
   a. less than half the light is emitted in the direction of the film.
   b. light is emitted with equal intensity in all directions.
   c. the reflective layer intercepts light headed in other directions and redirects it to the film.
   d. light is emitted isotropically.
   e. all of the above

4. Phosphorescence:
   a. occurs when visible light is emitted during the stimulation of the phosphor.
   b. has occurred if the electron returns to its normal state with the emission of light within one revolution after stimulation.
   c. occurs when phosphor continues to emit light after stimulation of the phosphor.
   d. is desirable.

5. The term *rare earth* describes:
   a. yttrium and barium fluorochloride.
   b. nearly all of the newer phosphors developed since 1972.
   c. those elements of group IIa in the periodic table.
   d. gadolinium, lanthanum, and calcium tungstate.
   e. transitional metals found in abundance in nature.

6. At x-ray energies below the K-shell electron binding energy:
   a. the two K-shell electrons become available for photoelectric interaction.
   b. the incident photon does not have sufficient energy to ionize K-shell electrons.
   c. there is an abrupt increase in the probability of photoelectric absorption.
   d. another rapid reduction in photoelectric absorption occurs with increasing x-ray energy.
   e. all of the above

7. When rare-earth materials are used for radiographic intensifying screens:
   a. all have atomic numbers less than that for tungsten.
   b. all have increased K-shell electron binding energy.
   c. all but one has a lower K-shell electron binding energy.
   d. all have a higher x-ray absorption probability over most of the x-ray absorption spectrum.

8. When a luminescent material is stimulated, the following events happen in what order?
   a. The atom becomes unstable.
   b. The outer shell electrons are raised to an excited energy state.
   c. As the electron returns to its normal state, electromagnetic energy is emitted as visible-light photons.
   d. A hole in the outer electron shell is filled, as the excited electron returns to its normal state.

9. Label the four principle layers of the intensifying screen with micrometer measurements.

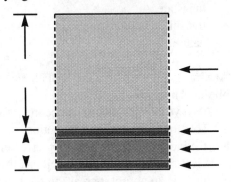

Answer the following on a separate sheet of paper.

10. Give the names and chemical symbols of the materials that have been used as phosphors prior to and since 1972. Refer to the elemental table in your medical dictionary for the chemical symbols.

11. Fill in the blanks to explain the properties of an intensifying screen base.
    It must be _____ and _____. It must not suffer radiation damage nor _____ with age. It must be _____ and not interact with the phosphor layer. It must be _____. It must not contain _____ that would be imaged by x-rays.

12. Name and briefly define the four primary characteristics of intensifying screens.

13. List the six proprietary manufacturer's designs of intensifying screens.

14. Describe in detail the components of a radiographic cassette.

15. Use the figure below to illustrate the spectrums of light emitted from calcium tungstate and rare-earth intensifying screens.

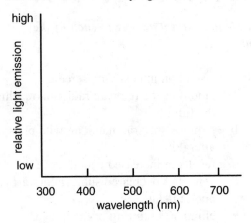

16. What is the DQE? What factors are involved in DQE calculations?

17. An examination using 100-speed screens is taken at 60 kVp, 10 mAs and results in an exposure to the patient of 240 mR. A similar exam taken without screens would result in a patient exposure of 7600 mR. What is the approximate intensification factor?

18. An examination using 300-speed screens is taken at 100 kVp, 5 mAs and results in an exposure to the patient of 180 mR. A similar exam taken without screens would result in a patient exposure of 7200 mR. What is the approximate intensification factor?

19. An examination using 200-speed screens is taken at 80 kVp, 100 mAs and results in an exposure to the patient of 200 mR. A similar exam taken without screens would result in a patient exposure of 6400 mR. What is the approximate intensification factor?

20. List the activator and color associated with the composition and emission of the following phosphors:
    - barum sulfate
    - yttrium tantalate
    - zinc sulfide
    - calcium tungstate
    - gadolinium oxysulfide
    - lanthanum oxysulfide

21. In luminescence, on what sorts of factors do energy states of outer-shell electrons and emitted light wavelengths and colors depend?

22. Describe the purpose, construction, and advantages of asymmetric screens.

23. Using Table 16-4, relate characteristics of calcium tunstate intensifying screens to modern rare-earth intensifying screens.

24. Discuss the use of carbon fiber in radiographic devices.

25. You have noticed that there are areas of blurring on too many of the radiographs your department has produced today. You decide to perform a screen-film contact evaluation. (a) How is this done, and how often? (b) Describe the process.

26. What are the most common causes of poor screen-film contact?

27. (a) Discuss the x-ray absorption below the K-shell absorption edge for the rare-earth elements and above the K-shell absorption edge for tungsten. When is it higher for the rare-earth elements? (b) The absorption curve of the rare-earth screens is characteristic of what factors? (c) Overall, how would you summarize absorption properties of rare-earth screens as opposed to calcium-tungstate screens?

28. Your supervisor notices that the screens used in your department are not being properly taken care of. She asks you to prepare a department handout on when and how to clean screens. What instructions will you include?

CHALLENGE QUESTIONS
■ ■ ■ ■ ■ ■ ■ ■ ■ ■ ■ ■ ■ ■ ■ ■ ■ ■

1. You have been made design coordinator for a brand-new company that will design x-ray machines and apparatus. Because design is your specialty, your first assignment for the company is to call together all engineers and designers who will be working on intensifying screen manufacturing, and to give them a list of design characteristics that will affect x-ray absorption and x-ray-to-light conversion efficiency. What will you include in this list?

2. Howard's office has just switched from direct-exposure film to a film-screen imaging system. Describe how he would determine the amount of dose reduction, if any, the patient would require in moving from nonscreen radiography to intensifying screen radiography.

3. Suppose now that what Howard (from the previous question) knows is this: An exam taken without screen used to result in a patient exposure of 6300 mR. Now, with a 100-speed screen, taken at 80 kVp, 100 mAs, results in a patient exposure of 700 mR. What is the approximate intensification factor of Howard's 100-speed screen-film combination?

4. Prepare a demonstration of the use of a line-pair test pattern. If possible, can you gain access to one to show the class? Discuss measurements you would expect use of this test to produce for an 800 to 1000 class image receptor. What about a 100 class image receptor? To put these numbers in perspective for the rest of the class, give expected scores for the unaided eye; for direct exposure film.

5. Create a model or poster-size diagram of a cross-sectional view of a cassette containing front and back screens and loaded with double-emulsion film. Exchange with a colleague and label.

6. Track the relative number of x-ray and light photons at various stages for radiographs taken with direct-exposure film and with a calcium tungstate screen-film. At what stages might you expect to see major differences? What will these be due to?

7. With a partner, design debate strategies that argue both the pros and cons of using rare-earth screens and their calcium-tungstate screen counterparts. What arguments can you come up with for each side?

8. Prepare audiovisuals or a demonstration that adresses this issue: How can you prevent artifacts and degradation of the radiographic image from poor film-screen contact?

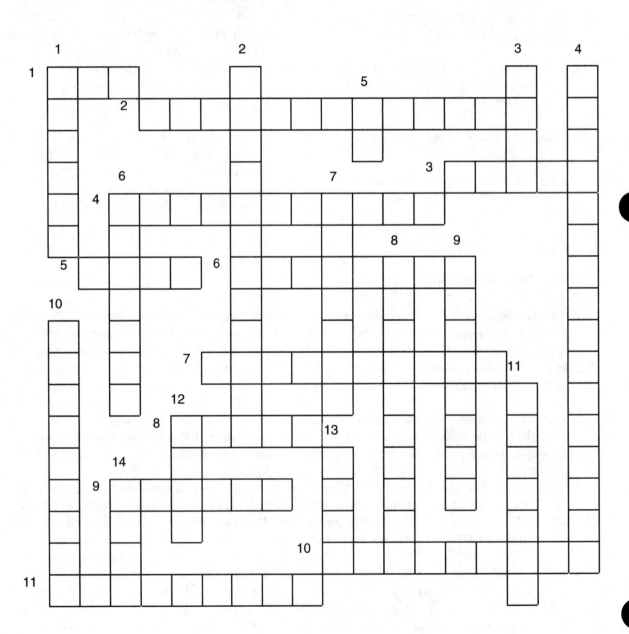

ACROSS

1. Each of the rare-earth screens has an absorption curve characteristic of the phosphor that determines the speed of the screen and how it changes with _____.
2. A disadvantage of some of the fastest rare-earth screens are the noticeable effects of _____ _____.
3. When a luminescent material is stimulated, the ____ -shell electrons are raised to an excited energy state.
4. When an outer-shell electron is raised to an excited state and returns to its _____ _____ with the emission of a light photon, luminescence occurs.
5. An example of a good material for a compression device to be placed between each screen and the cassette to maintain close film-screen contact is _____.
6. An intensifying screen base must not _____ with the phosphor layer; it must be chemically inert.
7. In order for x-ray absorption to be high, the intensifying screen should have a phosphor with a _____ _____ number.
8. If you were to x-ray an intensifying screen in a darkened x-ray room, the luminescence would be visible because there are many _____ photons released with each x-ray interaction.
9. For mammography, a _____ screen is used on the far side of the emulsion to reduce screen blur.
10. In a calcium-tungstate screen, it is the _____ atom that determines its absorption properties.
11. As x-ray energy increases, the probability of absorption _____ rapidly until the x-ray energy is equal to the binding energy of the K-shell electrons.

DOWN

1. When an incident x-ray has energy equal to the _____ electron binding energy, photoelectric absorption is maximum for those electrons.
2. Phosphorescence becomes objectionable, referred to as *afterglow*, when it occurs in an _____ screen.
3. One of the most common causes of poor screen-film contact is _____ latches or hinges.
4. An example of a transitional, rare-earth phosphor found in low abundance in nature is _____ _____.
5. One advantage of screen-film over direct-exposure film use is a decrease in x-ray tube _____.
6. Reduction in spatial resolution is _____ when phosphor layers are thick or when crystal size is large.
7. Use of rare-earth screens results in lower patient dose and less _____ stress on the x-ray tube.
8. Adequate x-ray conversion efficiency requires that the phosphor emit a large amount of light per _____ of x-ray photons.
9. The presence of a reflective layer in an intensifying screen increases x-ray-_____-_____ conversion efficiency but also increases image blur.
10. Rare-earth screens obtain their _____ sensitivity through higher x-ray absorption and more efficient conversion of x-ray energy into light.
11. A disadvangtage of intensifying screens is a lower _____ resolution compared with direct-exposure radiographs.
12. Resolution is usually measured by the _____ pairs per millimeter that can be detected on the radiograph.
13. Carbon fiber was useful in the early days of the space program because of its high strength and _____ resistance.
14. The light emitted by calcium-tungstate screens is readily absorbed if the radiographic film is _____-trally matched.

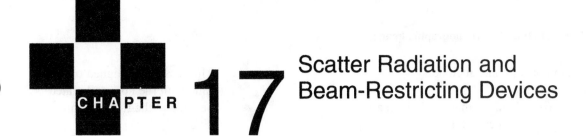

Circle the correct answer to each of the following.

1. The x-rays responsible for the optical density on a radiograph are:
   a. those scattered in the patient as a result of Compton interaction.
   b. only those that make contact with the back intensifying screen.
   c. those that pass through the patient without interacting.
   d. a and c.
   e. a, b, and c.

2. Imaging a wrist:
   a. produces a sharper image than an abdomen or chest radiograph because of reduced scatter radiation.
   b. produces an image with less contrast than an abdominal radiograph because there is less mass to absorb scatter radiation and therefore it escapes.
   c. produces a sharper image than an abdomen or chest radiograph because of increased scatter radiation.
   d. produces a smaller angle of scatter in the remnant beam, resulting in loss of contrast.

3. Factors influencing scatter radiation intensity within the film include:
   a. kilovoltage.
   b. x-ray beam field size.
   c. anatomic part thickness.
   d. all of the above.

4. The relative intensity of scatter radiation:
   a. decreases with a greater field size.
   b. increases with increasing field size.
   c. is not affected by field size.
   d. increases or decreases depending only on collimation, not field size.

5. With increasing x-ray energy:
   a. the number of x-rays that undergo Compton interaction decreases.
   b. the absolute number of Compton interactions decreases.
   c. the number of photoelectric interactions increases.
   d. a and b.
   e. b and c.

6. Joachim prepares to take an abdominal radiograph when he notices a small, bright light is projecting a small cross-hair pattern onto the patient. Which statement or statements best describe what is happening?
   a. Scatter radiation has been detected; Joachim must stop and correct for cone-cutting before taking this radiograph.
   b. The two crossed lines mark the projection of the central ray onto the center of the tissue; Joachim can use this to check alignment and then proceed.
   c. The positive beam limiting device has malfunctioned.
   d. This signals a high mAs and remnant radiation. The patient must have gonad shielding, and a cone collimator must be added.

7. Aperture diaphragms:
   a. in dental radiography use an 18-, 20- or 40-centimeter SID.
   b. in dental radiography must provide an elliptical beam not exceeding 7–9 centimeters in diameter at the skin level.
   c. must have their long axis perpendicular to the long axis of the image receptor.
   d. have a fixed SID and should always project an image 1 centimeter smaller on all sides than the size of the image receptor.

8. Limitations of cones include:
   a. alignment.
   b. fixed openings that make them appropriate for general, but not specific, procedures.
   c. their invariable shape—the cone—which always produces a circular beam only.
   d. cone cutting, a misalignment that damages the cone so that it no longer produces a pervectly circular useful beam.

9. Why are there two sets of shutters in a light-localizing variable-aperture collimator?
   a. They control off-focus radiation.
   b. One set controls longitudinal field changes; the other controls transverse field changes.
   c. They are independently controlled.
   d. all of the above.

10. Gordon is weighing advantages and disadvantages of field-size beam restriction. Several other students willingly offer their "insights." Whose advice should he take?
    a. Wallace says that restriction of field size will improve image quality to a significant degree only during fluoroscopy, rather than radiography.
    b. Henry says field-size beam restriction is not recommended in radiography because of lower radiographic optical density.
    c. Harris says when an x-ray beam is collimated, exposure factors may have to be increased.
    d. Wallace says Harris is right, but this is because reduced scatter radiation results in lower radiographic optical density.

11. Below are steps that take place as a positive beam limiting (PBL) device automatically adjusts collimation. Some may or may not be true. Select those that are true and then assign them their proper sequence in the order of events that occur.
    _____ a. An electric signal is transmitted to the collimator housing.
    _____ b. Sensing devices respond to the electric signal, adjusting the collimator leaves to the correct size.
    _____ c. The cassette is aligned one more time with the now collimated beam, and the radiograph is taken.
    _____ d. Sensing devices identify size and alignment.
    _____ e. The collimator leaves are moved to a precalibrated position to restrict the size of the x-ray beam.

Fill in the blanks in the following.

12. Two kinds of x-rays are responsible for the optical density on a radiograph: (1) those that _____ and (2) those that _____. Together, these two types of x-rays are called _____.

13. Three factors that contribute to an increase in scatter radiation include _____, _____, and _____.

14. Dorothy takes spot films of a test pattern in the center of 20 cm of tissue-equivalent material. She takes one with full-field exposure and one with the x-ray beam restricted to the area of the test pattern. As the films develop, the image will be better in the one taken with the _____ because it results in _____ because of a smaller _____.

15. The x-ray beam is restricted to reduce _____ and improve _____.

16. Sharon is concerned about counteracting scatter radiation among her mammography patients. She discovers that the key to improving spatial resolution is through use of a _____ device because it reduces _____, _____, and _____ to improve image contrast.

17. Under no circumstances should the x-ray beam exceed the size of the

_____.

Answer each of the following on a separate sheet of paper.

18. The following problem lends itself to collaboration with a partner: "Carolyn is trying to take an AP film of a patient's abdomen, but the normal technique factors are not proving to be sufficient to acquire an adequate image. Argue the pros and cons of two choices Carolyn seems to face at this point. If you choose to do this with a partner, prepare your points together and then be prepared to present them to the rest of the class.

19. At the 50-kVp level, what percentage of the x-ray beam is scattered through Compton interaction? What percentage is scattered through photoelectric interaction?

20. Jeff performs a procedure demanding 60 kVp; Leslie is using 110 kVp in a separate procedure. Refer to Table 17-1 to answer the following questions:
    a. What is the difference in Compton scatter radiation resulting from these two kVp levels?
    b. Photoelectric interaction in Jeff's case is 70%; in Leslie's case it's 23%. How could contrast be affected on each of these radiographs?
    c. What is the trade-off when percent transmission of the remnant beam reaches 7% in Leslie's procedure?

21. What is meant by remnant radiation? Describe its sources.

Calculate the following, based on Table 17-1.

22. Davis uses 50 kVp in a procedure; Jackie uses 110 kVp. What is the difference in photoelectric interaction between the two? How will this affect the contrast of each radiograph?

23. Jackie repeats her procedure at 90 kVp. What percentage of the x-ray beam is scattered through Compton interaction?

24. With his next patient, Davis must increase kVp to 70. What will happen to image contrast, as compared with his last procedure (see question 28)?

25. How does the aperture diaphragm work? What are its major components?

26. Draw an illustration of the x-rays that interact with the patient.

27. Bill is restricting the x-ray beam using an aperture diaphragm. He wants to be sure he has an unexposed border around the edge of the new radiograph. Why?

28. Create a diagram series that will illustrate clearly just exactly what occurs in cone cutting.

29. A dental x-ray unit has been using 20-centimeter plastic pointer conew, but has not found these satisfactory. (a) What is probably the problem? (b) What is a possible solution?

30. Describe how off-focus radiation is controlled.

31. Create a flow chart or diagram that demonstrates how light localization is accomplished as part of a variable-aperture collimator. Rather than labeling your own, it may be helpful to exchange with a partner and label each other's flow chart's to show how key components in the collimator play a role in light localization.

32. What is the function of an extension cone? What kinds of problems can arise with the use of extension cones? What type of procedure are they used for?

33. How do PBL devices work?

34. Tim is using a light-localizing variable-aperture collimator, but the light field and x-ray beam are not coinciding. What should he do?

CHALLENGE QUESTIONS
. . . .

1. Eliot is aware that lowering kVp levels will reduce scatter radiation to a patient; therefore, he has resolved to take all radiographs at the lowest reasonable kVp. Dennis does not agree. Molly is called in on the debate. After listening to both sides, she says, "I agree with Dennis, but not for the same reason." Can you come up with three lines of rationale that would make everyone's argument true?

2. With a partner, prepare a presentation that analyzes the uses and limitations of extension cones and cylinders. Be sure to address the following issues: (a) their limitations, (b) their uses today in comparison to past uses, and (c) specialist applications. If possible, with your instructor's assistance, you may be able to borrow samples to supplement your presentation. If this is not possible, you can create simple cardboard models. Conclude by preparing and administering a mini-quiz to the rest of the class.

3. The following exercise will be done in several steps.

   Step 1:   Create a simplified diagram of a light-localizing variable-aperture collimator. Do not feel that you have to reproduce the image in Figure 17–17. Instead, the more original (though accurate) your illustration, the more challenging this exercise will be for your colleagues.

   Step 2:   Next, as the drawing nears completion, you may decide to (1) leave out one component, (2) omit or mix up several labels, or (3) use a combination of these "traps."

   Step 3:   Exchange illustrations with another student and "fix" each other's illustration.

   Step 4:   Repeat Steps 1–3 without consulting your previous diagrams or your text. By the time you do this exercise a second time without consulting your text, you will be very familiar with the working components of a light-localizing variable aperture collimator.

   Step 5:   Finally, use this second, complete illustration as a guide while you write a brief description of how the variable-aperture collimator works.

The Grid

Circle the correct answer to each of the following.

1. The Compton effect:
   a. results in lack of useful information recorded on the film.
   b. increases film fog.
   c. reduces image contrast.
   d. all of the above.

2. Grid ratio can be understood as:
   a. the product of the line pair thickness and height of the grid.
   b. the thickness of the grid material (T) plus the thickness of the interspace (D).
   c. the height of the grid divided by the interspace thickness.
   d. the product of the thickness of the grid material (T), the thickness of the interspace material (D), and the height of the grid (h).

3. The higher the frequency of a grid:
   a. the thinner the strips between its interspace material must be.
   b. the higher the grid ratio.
   c. the higher the deviation that is allowed.
   d. none of the above.

4. High-ratio grids:
   a. are made by reducing the height of the grid material.
   b. are made by reducing the width of the interspace.
   c. have the advantage of lower cost and reduced patient exposure than low-ratio grids.
   d. do not require higher exposure factors.

5. The number of grid strips or grid lines per inch or centimeter is called:
   a. line pair.
   b. line pair test pattern.
   c. interspatial ratio.
   d. grid frequency.

6. The amount of increased technique required to produce the same density when using a grid:
   a. is called the Bucky factor.
   b. also reflects how much of an increase in patient dose accompanies the use of a particular grid.
   c. is called the grid factor.
   d. all of the above.

7. A contrast improvement factor of 1:
   a. would mean a grid had been used.
   b. would double with the use of a grid.
   c. would mean no improvement whatsoever.
   d. would mean that the area is irradiated.

8. The grid's ability to improve radiographic contrast:
   a. acts as one of the factors in the contrast improvement factor.
   b. is specified by the ratio of the contrast of an image made with the grid to the contrast of an image made without the grid.
   c. is expressed as grid ratio.
   d. is called the Bucky factor.

9. The contrast improvement factor:
   a. is usually measured at 100 kVp.
   b. is the product of the x-ray emission spectrum times patient thickness.
   c. is the result of dividing the x-ray emission spectrum by the area irradiated.
   d. is generally lower for high-ratio grids.

10. The contrast seen in a radiograph made with a grid:
    a. is its grid ratio.
    b. is referred to as the grid factor, or grid ratio.
    c. when placed in a ratio against the contrast seen in a radiograph without a grid, constitutes what is known as the contrast improvement factor.
    d. is approximately half what it would be if the radiograph were made without a grid.

11. With increasing grid ratio:
    a. the amount of remnant radiation becomes less than the amount penetrating the grid.
    b. the Bucky factor decreases.
    c. penetration of scatter through the grid becomes less likely; therefore, the Bucky factor increases.
    d. the penetration of primary radiation through the grid increases proportionately.

12. At low kVp levels:
    a. aluminum-interspace material decreases the absorption of primary x-rays in the interspace.
    b. fiber-interspace grids are nonhygroscopic.
    c. patient doses, with use of aluminum-interspace grids, may be decreased by more than 20%.
    d. higher mAs factors are required with aluminum-interspace grids.

13. Which of the following statements about grid strips is/are accurate?
    a. Aluminum is preferred because it provides rigidity for the grid and helps keep out moisture; it is preferred over lead because of lead's high atomic number.
    b. Of tungsten, platinum, and gold, only tungsten is as useful as aluminum.
    c. Tungsten, platinum, and gold are preferred, but uranium and lead are not as effective as aluminum.
    d. The high atomic number and high mass density of lead make it preferable.

14. Aluminum-interspace grids:
    a. have a higher atomic number than those with plastic fiber interspaces, providing some selective filtration of x-rays absorbed in the grid material.
    b. produce more visible grid lines on the radiograph.
    c. need higher mAs factors.
    d. absorb as much moisture as those with plastic fiber will.

Indicate whether the following are true or false.

15. T F An off-level grid error occurs when the grid is shifted laterally and is thus "off level."

16. T F Lateral decentering results in grid cutoff and lower optical density.

17. T F Moving grids help minimize the distance between patient and film, improving image clarity.

18. T F Linear grid cutoff is most pronounced when the grid is used with a short SID or a large image receptor.

19. T F The attenuation of primary x-rays becomes greater near the edges of the grid.

20. T F With a linear grid, optical density decreases toward the central axis of the film.

21. T F Heavy grids gain in contrast improvement factors but necessarily have a loss in selectivity.

22. T F High-ratio grids have high improvement factors.

Calculate the following problems on a separate sheet of paper.

23. Peter is using a grid constructed with 55 μm grid strips and a 375 μm interspace. What percentage of incident x-rays will be absorbed by this grid?

24. Ralph takes two images. The first one, taken without a grid, measures a contrast of 1.6. With a grid, the same image is taken and results in a radiographic contrast of 3.5. What is the contrast improvement factor of Ralph's grid?

25. What is the grid frequency of a grid with a 240-μm interspace thickness and a 60-μm grid strip thickness in centimeters? in inches?

26. Mike is about to perform a procedure requiring high kVp. The grid most readily available at the moment has lead strips that are 30 μm thick. These are separated by sections of interspace material that are each 300 μm thick. The height of the grid is 1.5 millimeters. (a) What is the grid ratio? (b) Is this grid appropriate for Mike to use at this point?

27. An 18:1 parallel grid is positioned for a chest radiograph at 200-centimeter SID. What is the distance to grid cutoff?

28. A 14:1 parallel grid is positioned for a chest radiograph at a 180-centimeter SID. What is the distance to grid cutoff?

29. Define grid. Who invented grids and when? Define the ideal grid.

30. Draw an illustration showing grid ratio.

31. Write the formulas for:
    • grid ratio
    • grid frequency
    • contrast improvement factor
    • Bucky factor
    • selectivity

32. Draw a cross-section of a linear grid and a focused grid, including tube and x-ray beam, using normal SID, then using a too short SID.

33. Discuss three interrelated factors that must be examined when selecting a grid with the proper ratio. Elaborate on how these factors affect such a decision. Finally, offer a general guideline for establishing an acceptable grid ratio.

34. Discuss when grid ratios up to 8:1 are used. When are grid ratios over 8:1 used?

35. What are the three factors that must be considered when selecting a grid?

36. Hillary is talking about the air-gap technique to a group of newer students she is tutoring. Freddie overhears her calling it "air filtration." This drives him crazy, and even though she is in the middle of tutoring, he finally breaks in and says, "I'm sorry, I just have to put a stop to this." What is Freddie's problem? Is he correct in wanting her to stop calling it air filtration? Why might Hillary feel justified in calling it that? Which side would you take?

37. What three factors affect the intensity of scatter?

38. Explain the advantage a crossed grid has over a linear grid. Exactly how does it accomplish this? What are its disadvantages?

39. Melanie is using a high-frequency grid and finds that the patient dose is increased. How can she counteract or minimize this?

40. Create three scenarios using one of the grids discussed in Table 18-3. Describe the advantage that leads you to select this grid, and then describe a shortcoming or disadvantages.

41. A radiography student has a choice between two separate grids. One has a ratio of 8:1; the other has a ratio of 14:1. The procedure he is about to perform requires a high kVp. (a) Which grid may be more useful? (b) Which would most likely be used with general-purpose equipment?

42. Memorize Table 18-7.

CHALLENGE QUESTIONS
. . . .

1. Ron has been using a grid with 60-μm strips and a 300-μm interspace. He estimates that 20% of the grid absorbs x-ray photons. Steve agrees, adding that, conversely, 20% of incident x-rays will be absorbed by the grid. Carolyn believes that the percentage is actually not that high. "You have forgotten something," she says. Sally agrees with this statement but says, "Actually, Carolyn, the percentage will be even higher." Who is right? Why? Show your calculations with your answer.

2. Robin and Eliot are using grids that have identical grid ratios. They know that selectivity is related to grid ratio and that selectivity is primarily a function of the construction characteristics of the grid—as is the grid ratio—rather than the characteristics of the x-ray beam. Thus, they predict that their grids will produce the same selectivity. Do you agree? Why or why not?

3. Solve the following three-step problem.

   Step 1:   You are a sales representative from a company that manufactures grids with aluminum interspaces. Recently, your boss asked you to prepare to travel to a radiologists' convention where your company will have a booth for two days. Aware of the ongoing debates about whether aluminum or plastic fiber interspaces are better, anticipate all of your potential customers' questions and criticisms. Research articles in professional journals—as well as any promotional material you may find—to discover as many arguments or points as possible for both sides.

   Step 2:   List any negatives or questions that may be raised about your product. Then, prepare arguments to counteract each.

   Step 3:   After you have finished, answer this question: Would you be comfortable representing this product, or would you prefer (now that you see all the arguments) to join the other side of the aluminum-vs.-plastic fiber debate?

   If you are doing this exercise with a partner, each should research and complete this exercise for opposing viewpoints; be prepared to possibly present your results in a debate format, with each of you representing different companies, as a catalyst for open class discussion afterward.

4. With a partner, prepare a demonstration of the differences between the following: a linear grid, a crossed grid, a focused grid, a single-stroke grid, reciprocating grid, and an oscillating grid. Prepare audiovisuals such as (1) diagrams of construction and (2) charts showing advantages and disadvantages of each. Is it possible for you or your instructor to borrow any real sample grids for instructional purposes? Finally, close your demonstration with a quick quiz that you and your partner prepare ahead of time.

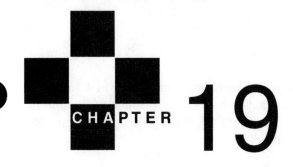

CHAPTER 19

Radiographic Quality

Indicate whether the following are true or false.

Film X has a much steeper characteristic curve than film Z. What do we know about each?

1. T F When using film X, more radiographs may be taken near the high, or shoulder, end, since a wider range of exposure will appear on the x-axis.

2. T F It will be more difficult to obtain adequate contrast on body parts from "toe" to "shoulder" when using film X.

3. T F The steeper the curve, the higher the contrast, so film X has higher contrast.

4. T F The curve for head radiography cannot be determined for film X or film Z, but film X has a narrower range of usefulness.

5. T F Film X will be more affected by the size, shape, and x-ray–attenuating characteristics of the anatomic part.

Jesse takes two radiographs and finds that fog level is worse on the second radiograph than on the first. How might this best be explained?

6. T F Radiograph 2 may have had a development time as little as 5 seconds longer.

7. T F Radiograph 1 may have been exposed to a lower development temperature.

8. T F If temperature was the only factor that changed, no change would be evident at a temperature change less than 8 degrees.

9. T F If time was the only factor that changes, no change would be evident at a time change less than 90 seconds.

10. T F Fog is generally a product of either an incorrect composition of processing chemical solutions or the degree of chemistry agitation during development. These have a much greater influence than time and temperature of development.

Paul uses an x-ray film that requires less exposure than does Jack's. Which of the following must also be true?

11. T F We can know for certain only that Paul's film would appear on a log relative exposure scale.

12. T F Paul's film requires more mAs than Jack's to produce a given optical density.

13. T F The characteristic curve of Paul's film would be positioned to the right of Jack's film along a log relative exposure scale.

14. T F Jack's film, because it requires more exposure, might be of lesser quality because of increased radiographic noise.

15. T F Paul's film is faster than Jack's.

Michelle is using high-contrast film; Gina is using low-contrast film. Which of the following are true?

16. T F Gina's film has a narrow latitude.

17. T F Gina's film has a long gray scale.

18. T   F   Michelle's film has a narrow latitude.

19. T   F   Gina's film will have a steeper slope on its characteristic curve than Michelle's will.

20. T   F   Michelle's film will always produce a higher radiographic contrast than Gina's will.

Calculate the following problems on a separate sheet of paper.

21. A radiographic film has an optical density of 3. What does this say about the actual number of light photons that are capable of penetrating the x-ray film?

22. The characteristic curve of a given film screen shows that 23 mR are needed to produce an optical density of 1 on that image receptor. What is the image-receptor speed?

23. How much exposure is required to produce an optical density of 1 on a 500-speed image receptor?

24. Gina successfully takes a radiograph requiring 140 kVp at 7 mAs, using a 100-speed image receptor. What radiographic technique should be used with a 200-speed image receptor?

25. Ken successfully takes a radiograph requiring 120 kVp at 9 mAs with a 150-speed image receptor. What radiographic technique should he use with a 250-speed image receptor?

26. If a heart measures 10.7 centimeters from side to side and its image on a chest radiograph measures 14.1 centimeters, what is the magnification factor?

27. Jack is using an x-ray tube target that has a 1.6-mm effective focal spot to image an object in a chest cavity estimated to be 6 cm from the anterior chest wall. If the radiograph is taken at 180 cm SID, with a table-top film separation of 5 cm, what will be the size of the focal-spot blur?

28. A film that has a film contrast of 4.1 is used to radiograph a long bone that has a subject contrast of 4.3. What is the radiographic contrast?

Answer each of the following on a separate sheet of paper.

29. Discuss the importance of high quality radiographs.

30. Define:
    - radiographic quality
    - resolution
    - noise
    - speed

31. Explain what a quality control program refers to.

32. What are the three factors that affect radiographic quality?

33. How is the characteristic curve for radiographic film derived?

34. Draw an illustration of the characteristic curve and label its parts.

35. What is the base density value?

36. What value should fog density not exceed?

37. What is the characteristic curve used for?

38. Name and describe two types of radiographic factors.

39. What is the diagnostically useful optical density?

40. Describe factors affecting radiographic contrast. Which factor is easier to manipulate to get the desired effect?

41. What does the slope of the characteristic curve indicate?

42. What is average gradient? How is it used?

43. What are the development and processing factors that affect the finished radiograph?

44. How do the factors of development time and temperature affect the characteristic curve?

45. What is the relationship between film speed and reciprocal roentgens?

46. Define latitude; how does change in latitude affect the characteristic curve?

47. Why do mammograms need such a short SID?

48. Margie has produced a radiographic image of a patient's hand, which was positioned laterally to the central axis. Mark has produced an image of a patient's chest, which was also positioned laterally to the central axis. Both used the appropriate kVp and SID. However, one image shows dramatically greater distortion than the other. (a) All things being equal, predict whose image is most likely to show the greater distortion. (b) Explain your reasons.

49. Alan is asked to take an AP radiograph of a patient who has sustained a bullet wound—the projectile is believed to still be in the patient. Alan is careful, but still the image does not show the projectile very well. The bullet appears circular, not conical with a rounded tip. (a) What kind of distortion has occurred? Explain what has happened. (b) Can Alan complete this exam without moving the patient? How?

50. What causes focal spot blur?

51. Describe the three main causes of focal-spot blur. (a) Explain each. (b) How can heel effect influence focal-spot blur? (c) What is the most recommended strategy for minimizing focal-spot blur?

52. List examinations that take advantage of the heel effect. Include, for each, positions toward the cathode (-) and anode (+).

53. Compare and contrast the effects of varying kVp from one radiographic image to the next. Is one range more desirable than the other?

54. Explain how a radiographic technique that produces low subject contrast (higher kVp) allows for wide latitude in exposure factors.

55. How do you reduce motion unsharpness?

CHALLENGE QUESTIONS
. . . .

1. List the general principles that should be considered when selecting the proper film-screen combination for a radiographic examination.

2. Why is it important to keep exposure times as short as possible?

3. What are the priciple advantages of the use of high kVp techniques?

4. Create a chart that outlines general principles to consider before choosing appropriate film-screen combinations.

5. What effect does kVp have on the *quantity*—rather than quality—of the x-ray beam? What effect does mAs have on this same factor? Finally, how does kVp affect optical density and fog? How does mAs affect optical density?

6. How do changes in SID and filtration affect radiographic quality?

7. Recreate the principle headings in Table 19-3. Then challenge yourself, each day, to fill out several columns accurately.

8. A particular radiograph transmits 0.32% of incident light as determined with a densitometer. Using Table 19-1, determine the optical density.

9. The light incident on a particular radiograph has a relative value of 1500. The light transmitted through the radiopaque bony stuctures on the film has an intensity of 375. Using Table 19-1, what is the optical denisty?

10. With another student, prepare a discussion that relates to Figure 19-4. Explain the relationship among exposure, log relative exposure, and mAs.

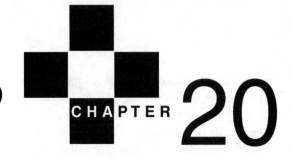

CHAPTER 20

Radiographic Exposure

■ ■ ■ ■ ■ ■ ■ ■ ■ ■ ■ ■ ■ ■ ■ ■

Circle the correct answer to each of the following.

1. Adjusting the amount of kVp is a way of controlling:
   a. the scale of contrast on the finished radiograph.
   b. radiation quantity.
   c. magnification.
   d. single-phase, three-phase, and high-frequency radiation.

2. Changes in mA change x-ray quantity:
   a. qualitatively.
   b. quantitatively.
   c. proportionately.
   d. in inverse proportion.

3. When exposure time is reduced:
   a. patient radiation exposure is reduced.
   b. mA must be decreased proportionately.
   c. the single-phase unit can produce an exposure time of as little as 8 milliseconds.
   d. mA is also reduced.

4. Which of the following milliamperage settings are usually available in those units designed for private offices?
   a. 25 mA and 50 mA
   b. 50 mA and 100 mA
   c. 800 mA, 1000 mA, and 1200 mA
   d. 1200 mA and 1400 mA

5. Which best describes the relationship between mA and exposure time?
   a. Time and mA are directly proportional.
   b. As mA is increased, it requires a corresponding decrease in time.

   c. Time is the key factor in the control of optical density on the radiograph.
   d. The product of time and milliampere seconds is the mA.

6. Milliampere seconds:
   a. are the product of kVp and time.
   b. measure the x-ray tube current.
   c. represent the product of x-ray tube current and exposure time.
   d. is not a selection option on a falling-load generator; instead mA and exposure time are selected individually.

7. Source-to-image receptor distance (SID):
   a. has an inversely proportional effect on radiation quality.
   b. influences mAs in accordance with the direct square law.
   c. has an inversely proportional effect on kVp.
   d. has no effect on skin entrance exposure, thanks to the distance maintenance law.

8. Small focal spots:
   a. provide for minimal possible exposure time.
   b. are microfocus tubes reserved for fine-detail radiography.
   c. minimize motion unsharpness.
   d. prevent filament burnout.

9. The use of longer SID is based on achieving:
   a. lowered patient dose.
   b. less kVp.
   c. more magnification.
   d. less focal-spot blur.

10. Which of the following are true regarding filtration?
    a. Radiographic technique charts are formulated at the lowest filtration position.
    b. Equipment is usually placed into service with the highest allowable added filtration.
    c. Contrary to popular opinion, mirrors do not provide any additional aluminum equivalent.
    d. The total filtration required is 2.5 millimeter aluminum plus an additional 1 millimeter provided by the variable-aperture light-localizing collimator.

Calculate the following problems on a separate sheet of paper.

11. Carole has been monitoring patient exposure carefully. For her next radiograph, she selects the 450-mA station. What will be the electron flow from cathode to anode?

12. At 200 mA, the entrance skin exposure (ESE) is 752 mR. Freddie is trying to achieve an ESE of no more than 2300 mR, while selecting the highest mA station possible. His choices of mA station selections are 600, 700, and 800. Which station selection is Freddie's best option?

13. Change the following fractional exposure times to seconds and milliseconds:
    • 4/5
    • 1/2
    • 1/5
    • 1/20
    • 1/120

14. Dale will use a radiographic technique that calls for 500 mA at 75 milliseconds. What is the mAs?

15. Michelle will use a radiographic technique that calls for 600 mA at 300 milliseconds; Dylan will use a technique needing 200 mA at 500 milliseconds. Whose procedure will require the higher mAs?

16. Dylan is taking a radiograph of a small child. The radiograph requires 200 mA and 400 milliseconds. However, the child is afraid. Dylan wants to shorten the exposure time to 200 milliseconds. What new mA will Dylan need?

17. Ellie selects a technique of 300 mAs. The operating console is automatically adjusted to the the 800 mA station. Bill selects a technique of 400 mAs on a console that is automatically adjusted to 600 mA. Whose technique will use the shorter exposure time?

18. Jack performs an exam calling for 70 kVp at 35 mAs. It results in an entrance skin exposure (ESE) of 120 mR. Jack's next patient is examined at 70 kVp/30 mAs. What will be the ESE this time?

19. John sets up an exam that uses 200 mAs at 300-centimeters SID. His instructor suggests he change the distance to 150-centimeters SID. John thinks about this. What should the new mAs be for this projection?

20. An exam calls for 140 mAs at a 200-cm SID. If the SID is changed to 120 cm, what is the new mAs?

21. An exam calls for 120 mAs at a 180-cm SID. If the SID is changed to 90 cm, what is the new mAs?

22. An exam calls for 100 mAs at a 160-cm SID. If the SID is changed to 100 cm, what is the new mAs?

MATCHING

In each of the following scenarios, identify which type of generator is being used:

23. _____ Pam's unit produces and emits x-rays only half of the time.

24. _____ Dan's generator could be either 6-pulse or 12-pulse; he's not sure which one it is . . .

25. _____ Terri's generator produces a voltage waveform that is nearly constant with less than 1% ripple.

26. _____ Lois uses a mammography system; Rick uses a mobile unit.

27. _____ Patty's machine requires only half the exposure time of Pam's and has no dead time.

28. _____ Henry's and Molly's generators come in two forms that differ only in the manner in which the high-voltage step-up transformer is engineered in each.

a. half-wave rectification

b. full-wave rectification

c. three-phase power

d. high-frequency generation

■ ■ ■ ■ ■ ■ ■ ■ ■ ■ ■ ■ ■ ■ ■ ■

Answer each of the following on a separate sheet of paper.

29. What are the primary factors used to control beam quality and quantity?

30. What is the relationship between kVp and beam penetrability?

31. Write the equation for number of electrons/second.

32. Discuss the standardization of SID.

33. When is the small focal spot most commonly used?

34. What focal spot sizes do mammography units have?

35. Study and recreate Table 20-30. Exchange partially finished tables with another student and complete.

36. Memorize Table 20-4.

CHALLENGE QUESTIONS
■ ■ ■ ■ ■ ■ ■ ■ ■ ■ ■ ■ ■ ■ ■ ■

1. To reinforce the fact that in a properly calibrated generator, it is possible to produce the same mAs (and therefore, the same optical density) with various combinations of mA and time, reproduce by hand Table 20-2, leaving out key elements in columns 1, 2, and 3 (mA, milliseconds, and seconds), so that these will have to be recalculated to complete the equation. Exchange incomplete tables. Calculate to discern the missing elements; naturally, all completed values will equal 10 mAs when multiplied.

2. Prepare a chart that outlines characteristics, uses, and general differences among the types of generators. The trick, of course, is to make it incomplete. Exchange charts with a peer and complete.

3. Assess the radiographic units at your clinical site. What is the standard SID? What filtration is used? What are the sizes of focal spots? What type of high voltage generation is used?

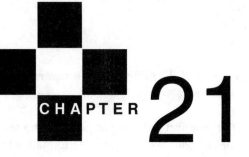

CHAPTER 21

Radiographic Technique

1. Label each of the four body types shown here.

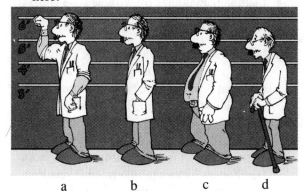

a   b   c   d

a. _____

b. _____

c. _____

d. _____

Circle the correct answer to each of the following.

2. Which of the following is incorrect regarding radiographing suspected pathology?
   a. Atrophy makes the tissue more radiolucent.
   b. Some pathology can increase mass density.
   c. If cancer is present and has metastasized, the tissue may be more radiopaque.
   d. Pneumothorax, emphysema, and pneumonia will make the lungs more radiolucent.

3. To minimize distortion as much as possible, what factors will most affect this outcome?
   a. SID, OID, motion, and especially focal-spot size
   b. development time and temperature, image receptor speed, and especially kVp
   c. mainly mAs; secondarily, collimation, distance, and grid ratio
   d. patient positioning and alignment of tube, anatomic part, and image receptor

4. What factors should be considered in achieving proper optical density?
   a. mass density, SID, grid ratio, and especially OID
   b. distance, thickness of part, kVp, and especially mAs
   c. motion, alignment of tube, anatomic part, and image receptor
   d. focal-spot size more than any other factor

5. In preparing to take a chest x-ray to image lung tissue, which of the following is incorrect?
   a. The chest has low mass density because of the lungs.
   b. The chest has high mass density becuase of all the bony struture.
   c. Use high kVp and low mAs for this image.
   d. All of the above.

6. Harry is trying to achieve a shorter scale of contrast on his radiographs. Which piece of advice below should he ignore?
   a. Use a grid and collimation.
   b. Grids and collimation are great for removing scatter radiation, but neither can be relied upon to produce a radiograph of shorter scale contrast.
   c. You need to use an intensifying screen.
   d. A grid with a high ratio will increase the contrast, and that produces a shorter contrast scale.

7. Which of the following is correct? Contrast is:
   a. necessary for the outline of a structure to be visible.
   b. the result of differences in x-ray beam attenuation before it passes through various tissues.
   c. not determined by the relative penetrability among tissues.
   d. controlled primarily by mAs.

8. Optical density on a radiograph can be controlled by two major factors. They are:
   a. mAs and SID
   b. mAs and kVp
   c. SID and OID
   d. intensifying screens and kVp

9. Stacy is asked to "increase contrast" in an image she has just taken with disappointing results. Which of the following is correct?
   a. Make the range of optical densities more black and white, with a greater difference in adjacent structures.
   b. Increase the range of degrees of gray visible in this image.
   c. Produce a radiograph with a longer contrast scale.
   d. Increase kVp.

Calculate the following problems on a separate sheet of paper.

10. When Daryl makes an exposure at 58 kVp/14 mAs, the resulting contrast scale is too short. Use the fifteen-percent rule to suggest what the repeat technique should be.

11. You have changed your mind about what Daryl (in the previous question) should do. Apply the five-percent rule instead, for less abrupt technique compensation.

12. Assume that a phantom body part measures 20 centimeters thick. If you were setting up a variable-kVp technique chart, using a single-phase high-voltage generator, what kVp would you use to begin the chart's construction? What if you were using a three-phase high-voltage generator? a high-frequency high-voltage generator?

Answer each of the following on a separate sheet of paper.

13. "High-contrast radiographs produce shorter scales of contrast." Is that true? Explain why or why not.

14. List the pathologies from Table 21-3 (p. 260) that are radiolucent or radiopaque.

15. What is a radiographic technique chart or guide? Include the following in your answer: (a) What is its purpose? (b) How are such charts constructed? (c) How are they used?

16. Dennis is asked to establish a radiographic technique chart for his facility's exam rooms. He chooses a chart from a reliable textbook, duplicates it, and displays it in each exam room. Wendy, his supervisor, says, "Nice try, Dennis." What is her point?

17. Bernie is developing a variable-kVp chart for his department's exam rooms. Phyllis stops him, saying, "Why waste your time, Bernie? Wouldn't you be better off creating a fixed-kVp technique chart? How would you respond if you were Bernie?

18. Copy Table 21-7 and fill in the missing image quality factors later.

19. Create a table that demonstrates factors that must be considered when preparing the radiographic exposure chart for an automatic x-ray system. Include the rationale for each factor selection.

20. Jack has never used a phototimer before. Explain how this device works.

21. Jack, from the previous question, asks you how microprocessors differ from phototimers. (a) What will you say? (b) How can a microprocessor be used to reduce motion blur?

CHALLENGE QUESTIONS

▪ ▪ ▪ ▪ ▪ ▪ ▪ ▪ ▪ ▪ ▪ ▪ ▪ ▪ ▪ ▪ ▪ ▪

1. You have been asked to produce a checklist to help your colleagues evaluate the image quality of their radiographs. For each image quality factor you are able to identify, write at least two questions that will help students assess the quality of any image.

2. Through your instructor, select several radiographs that demonstrate varying degrees of optical density. Describe these to the rest of the class, explaining (a) what causes the darkest and lightest areas, (b) the numerical equivalencies, in optical density, of black areas as opposed to clear areas, and (c) the exact meaning of optical density. If you are able to obtain radiographs that have either over- or underexposures, point these out as well. (d) Explain how these can occur.

3. With your instructor, use Figure 21-11 to help you prepare and reproduce (or *try* to reproduce) your own scale of contrast step-wedge experiment.

4. Research and establish a medium-size measurement for any anatomic part in an average-sized adult. Present this measurement as a medium-sized phantom for a fellow student to use as the basis for planning preparation of a fixed-kVp radiographic exposure chart. Exchange these phantom measurements. Describe how you would create a single line of a fixed-kVp radiographic chart under the assumption that the measurement you have received represents a medium-sized anatomic part. How would this procedure vary in preparing a high-kVp chart?

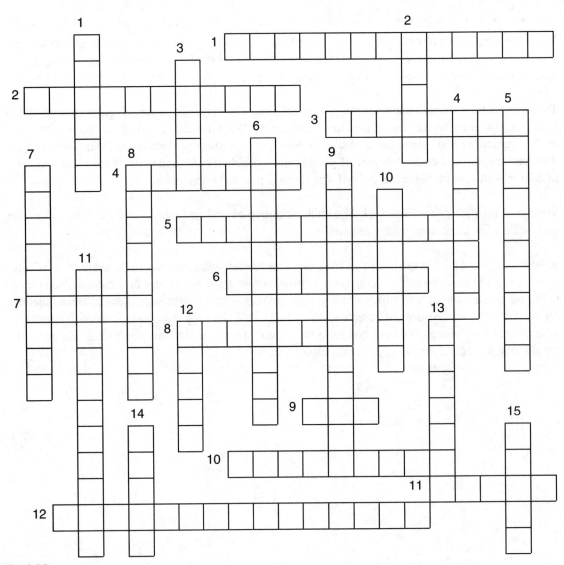

ACROSS

1. To change kVp and mAs, a good guideline is to remember that mAs is changed according to the _____ _____ in order to provide the optical density required.
2. The degree of variation on a radiograph is a result of differences in _____ of the x-ray beam as it passed through various tissues of the body.
3. Changing from a low-ratio grid to a high-ratio grid will _____ the contrast.
4. Your department installs new intensifying screens. "This is great," you tell a colleague. "This means that now I'll be able to obtain _____ scales of contrast."
5. A patient who has a big frame and requires more technique is _____.

6. The difference on a radiograph between lung tissue and the ribs is an example of high subject _____.
7. Henry's radiograph shows an image of a hand that is smaller than the patient's actual hand. This may have happened because Henry did not properly _____ the part, resulting in foreshortening.
8. A patient asks, "What is the black area? Air?" You tell her it is from silver _____ crystals.
9. The simplest way to increase the optical density on a chest radiograph is to increase the _____.

10. If a radiograph has low contrast as a result of using a high-kVp exposure technique, you might say that the image shows a ____ ____ of contrast.

11. You have been given a box of old radiographs. Your instructor has asked you to select a radiograph that will clearly demonstrate both short and long scales of contrast. You will therefore be evaluating the ____ of optical densities in each image.

12. An advantage of fixed-kVp charts is that they produce scales of contrast that are consistent within ____ ____.

DOWN

1. If the radiographic image is not quite as sharp as hoped using an intensifying screen and a small focal spot, a possible cause could be patient ____.

2. To accurately determine the specific technical factors needed for radiographic procedures, use a radiographic technique ____.

3. What is the mathematical representation of optical density? It is the logarithm to the base 10 of the ____ of light incident on a film to the light transmitted through the film.

4. The best way to determine satisfactory contrast is to check for variation optical density between ____ anatomic structures.

5. Poor alignment of the image receptor or the x-ray tube, causing the part to appear larger, is called ____ of the image.

6. The blackening on a radiograph is a result of ____ of silver-bromide crystals in the film emulsion.

7. If the exposure is terminated when the proper optical density on the image receptor has been reached, an ____-exposure system is being used.

8. If a student holds up a radiograph, points to the structural lines or borders of tissues in the image, and is concerned with the amount of clarity or blur of the image, the student is talking about the image's ____.

9. Mediastinal structures tend to have ____ mass density, when compared to lung tissue or bone.

10. In order to expose a radiograph properly, a radiographer must consider not only part thickness and pathology but also the mass ____ of the part.

11. The ____ rule is associated with a 5% increase in kVp and a 30% reduction in mAs.

12. ____ on a radiograph reflects an optical density of 3 or greater.

13. Molly and Henry have produced radiographs with varying contrasts. Molly's image is high contrast; Henry's is low contrast. Molly's radiograph has a ____ scale from black to white.

14. When using a computer-assisted automatic-exposure control system, the anatomic part must be placed over the ____-timing device to ensure proper exposure.

15. Film fog may be caused by radiation or ____.

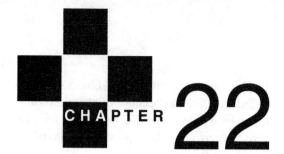

CHAPTER 22

Alternative Film Procedures

Circle the correct answer in each of the following.

1. A tomographic examination is designed to:
   a. bring into focus anatomy of interest while blurring structures above or below.
   b. expose the entire length of film.
   c. give a panoramic view.
   d. shorten exposure time.

2. For magnification radiography,
   a. a large focal spot is required to avoid destroying the diagnostic value of the radiograph.
   b. the large OID makes grid use unnecessary.
   c. the use of a grid is recommended to eliminate the significant air gap.
   d. a decreased patient dose is a distinct advantage.

3. Choose the answer below that will make this statement correct: "In tomography, the larger the tomographic angle—"
   a. the larger the area that will be presented in focus.
   b. the farther away structures outside the object plane will appear.
   c. the thinner the section of tissue that is clearly shown.
   d. the smaller the patient dose will be.

4. Which is incorrect? Grids used in tomography:
   a. must be linear.
   b. must have their grid lines oriented in the same direction as the tube movement.
   c. must change with the movement of the tube head in multidirectional tomography.
   d. must remain fixed, eliminating all rotation during multidirectional tomography.

5. Which of the following is incorrect? The tomographic angle:
   a. refers to the angle of movement of the x-ray tube and image receptor.
   b. determines section thickness during tomography.
   c. determines what tissue will not be blurred during tomography.
   d. refers to the fulcrum or pivot point in the object plane.

6. Which of the following is incorrect? In tomography:
   a. a vertical rod fixes the x-ray tube head to the table Bucky device.
   b. the x-ray tube and image receptor are not linked, thus enabling them to both move at the same time.
   c. the anatomy of interest is not actually focused but has its contrast enhanced by the blurring of structures above and below.
   d. the x-ray tube and image receptor move in opposite directions.

7. Tomography affects patient dose by:
   a. reducing exposure time with high-speed film.
   b. keeping the x-ray tube on during the entire tube travel, thus increasing patient exposure.
   c. decreasing kVp, thus decreasing dose.
   d. using consistent rhythmic tube movement for uniform, efficient exposure.

8. Tomography improves radiographic contrast by:
   a. eliminating fogging and blurring of the primary and surrounding tissues.
   b. blurring overlying and underlying tissues.
   c. shortening exposure time.
   d. lengthening exposure time.

9. Claire is interested in experimenting with multidirectional tomography, so her instructor tells her to work only with the movement(s) that result(s) in the sharpest tomographic image. Therefore, Claire will perform procedures involving the:
   a. circular movement.
   b. linear movement.
   c. hypocycloidal movement.
   d. elliptical movement.

10. Assume that you have been asked to create a stereoradiograph for purposes of historic interest for a convention on contemporary CT and MR technology. In what order would the following factors become important during the process of making a stereoradiograph?
    a. Mark the new film to identify the direction of the tube shift.
    b. Shift the tube to the opposite side and expose the second radiograph.
    c. Aim for a tube shift to SID ratio of 1:10.
    d. Shift the tube half the required distance and expose the film.
    e. Process each film under identical conditions.

Calculate the following problems on a separate sheet of paper.

11. If you are making a stereoradiograph at 200 centimeters SID, what should be the amount of tube shift on either side of the midline?

12. You take a magnified radiograph at 120 centimeters SID with the object positioned 30 centimeters from the image receptor. The image measures 20 millimeters. What is its actual size?

Answer each of the following on a separate sheet of paper.

13. What features does a radiographic room have if nephrotomography can be performed with the equipment?

14. If radiographs are not able to show a suspected calcification because of superimposition, which alternative film procedure might be used to avoid superimposition on a radiographic image?

15. You and a colleague find a box of old stereoradiographs. You'd like to look at them, but no one knows where to find a stereoscope. However, your colleague suggests you try an "alternative" viewing technique. Describe both methods.

16. Write a brief presentation that would illustrate the advantage of using a book cassette for tomography.

17. Henry's patient needs an examination of the mandible. During the examination, the image receptor rotates around the patient with the slit collimator exposing the film. What procedure is Henry probably using?

18. Patrick wants to use linear tomography on a patient's lower leg, but he is unsure how to align it to achieve the best image possible. What advice does the instructor give him?

19. Patrick completes his tomogram but is disappointed that it appears streaked. Why did this happen? He retakes the image and finds that he cannot get the in-focus section to appear as distinctly as he wants it to. In fact, the degree of blurring appears uneven over the radiograph. What's going on? What suggestions might you make to Patrick?

20. Tracy has been experimenting with linear tomography. As she keeps reducing the tomographic angle, Clint predicts that the section thickness will become thinner and thinner. At zero angle, he says, there will be no clear image. Clark says that the image will become completely blurred. Claire predicts that it will cease to be tomography, but there will be a usable image. Who is right? Why?

21. What procedures have largely replaced tomography? Why? Why can we say that these procedures provide examples of virtual reality?

22. How does the tomographic angle affect the anatomic section that will be in focus?

23. Why is stereoradiography not used much today?

CHALLENGE QUESTIONS

1. With a partner, prepare a brief presentation that demonstrates the differences in the five basic types of tomographic movements. What are the advantages or uses of each?

2. If you can, bring examples of stereograms to class. These are available in books or even in the form of post cards and greeting cards. Pool as many of these as you can and practice viewing them.

3. Using Figures 22-4 and 22-5, explain tomographic theory.

4. Research several or all of the special procedures discussed in this chapter and create a time line that puts their historical development and present uses into time perspective.

5. Experiment using a hand or foot phantom, and produce images such as those shown in Figure 22-9.

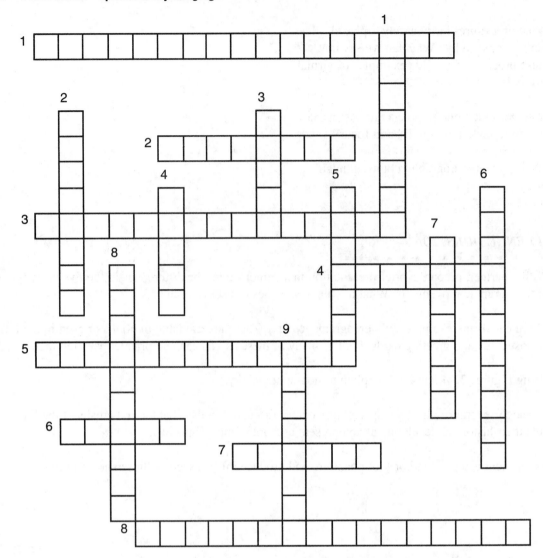

ACROSS

1. _____ is particularly helpful in locating foreign bodies.
2. Tomography achieves radiographic contrast by _____ structures above and below the object plane.
3. Tomography may be ordered when a diagnosis cannot be made with conventional radiography because of _____.
4. The larger a tomographic angle is, the _____ the imaged section will be.
5. One of the two multidirectional movements that produce the sharpest tomographic images is the _____ movement.
6. In magnification radiography, it is preferable to use a _____ focal spot.
7. In _____ tomography, the grid lines should be parallel with the length of the table.

8. Despite the fact that CT and MRI have replaced most plain-film tomographic exams, _____ is still frequently performed, even in modern departments.

DOWN

1. The most important requirement for viewing stereoradiographs is to be sure the radiographs are viewed in the same _____ in which the radiographs were taken.
2. Magnification radiography is used principally by _____ radiologists.
3. _____ are not needed in magnified radiography.
4. In multidirectional tomography, the image receptor should be remain _____.

5. When CT and MRI images can be viewed from any direction, the phenomenon can be called _____.
6. Many radiologists are proficient at crossing their eyes to perform _____.
7. During exposure in linear tomography, the changes in x-ray tube–to–patient distance and in the angulation of the x-ray beam can result in a lack of _____ optical density.
8. In _____, the section of tissue between two select parallel planes is all that will be in focus.
9. In making stereoradiographs, make sure the tube shift is across any _____ linear structures.

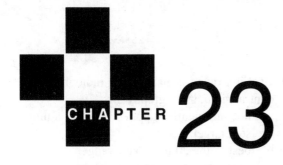

CHAPTER 23

Mammography

1. In the figure below, identify each lettered component by assigning it to the appropriate term on the right.

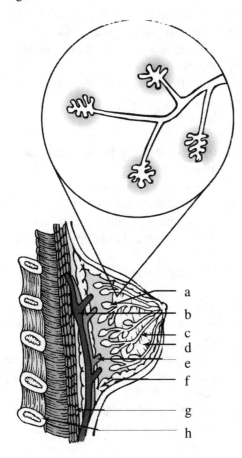

_____ artery

_____ connective tissue

_____ duct

_____ lobules

_____ pectoralis major muscle

_____ retromammary adipose tissue

_____ rib

_____ vein

a
b
c
d
e
f
g
h

- - - - - - - - - - - - - - - - - - - -

Circle the correct answer to each of the following.

2. Normal breasts consist of:
   a. fibrous tissue.
   b. glandular tissue.
   c. adipose tissue.
   d. b and c.
   e. all of the above.

3. Erika is evaluating a mammogram of a patient who has reported a "lump." If a malignancy is present, it will be seen in the mammogram as:
   a. a distortion of the normal duct and connective tissue patterns.
   b. calcifications greater than 500 μm in size.
   c. fibrous tissue.
   d. a and b.
   e. none of the above.

4. Conventional radiographic technique is useless in examining the breast because:
   a. mass densities of breast components are so similar.
   b. the atomic numbers of breast components are so similar.
   c. Compton scattering predominates.
   d. a and b.
   e. all of the above.

5. X-ray absorption caused by differences in mass density is:
   a. directly proportional for Compton interactions.
   b. proportional to the cube of the atomic number.
   c. simply proportional.
   d. a and b.
   e. b and c.

6. In mammography, compression of the breast:
   a. prevents motion blur.
   b. prevents superimposition and brings all tissue closer to the image receptor.
   c. makes the optical density of the image more uniform while reducing patient dose and scatter radiation.
   d. b and c.
   e. all of the above.

7. Mammographic x-ray tubes are manufactured with a _____ target.
   a. tungsten
   b. molybdenum
   c. aluminum
   d. a and b.
   e. all of the above.

8. L-characteristic x-rays are of no value in mammographic imaging because:
   a. their photons are not absorbed.
   b. their energy is too low to penetrate the breast.
   c. they enhance differential absorption in breast tissue.
   d. a and b.
   e. all of the above.

9. Useful x-rays for maximizing radiographic contrast in mammography are:
   a. not sufficiently supplied by using a tungsten target.
   b. best in the 20 to 30 keV range.
   c. possible in the 12 keV range.
   d. a and b.
   e. all of the above.

10. The difference in emission spectra between molybdenum and tungsten is due to:
    a. the difference in their atomic numbers.
    b. thinner target tissue.
    c. the difference in keV used with each.
    d. a and b.
    e. all of the above.

11. For mammography, it is important that the x-ray tube window:
    a. is not made of beryllium.
    b. does not attenuate the x-ray beam.
    c. has a total beam filtration of less than 5.0-millimeter aluminum equivalent.
    d. b and c.
    e. all of the above.

12. The use of a 4:1 ratio grid in mammography:
    a. requires a grid frequency of at least 30 lines per centimeter.
    b. roughly doubles the patient dose, compared to nongrid screen-film mammography.
    c. can compromise spatial resolution but does increase patient dose.
    d. a and b.
    e. all of the above.

13. Phototimers for mammography:
    a. measure x-ray intensity at the image recepter but not x-ray quality.
    b. are referred to as automatic-exposure control devices.
    c. are positioned between the Bucky device and the image receptor.
    d. a and b.
    e. all of the above.

14. The detectors in a mammographic photo-timer:
    a. are filtered precisely the same to prevent distortion.
    b. allow the AEC to determine beam quality.
    c. allow an assessment of breast composition.
    d. a and b.
    e. b and c.

15. Not commonly used for mammography, double-emulsion low-crossover film matched with two screens:
    a. cuts patient dose in half, when compared with single-emulsion systems.
    b. compromises image quality.
    c. can result in blur from crossover.
    d. b and c.
    e. all of the above.

16. In mammography, the _____ must always be next to the screen, while the _____ must be closest to the x-ray tube.
    a. film base; emulsion surface of the film
    b. grid; film base
    c. emulsion surface of the film; film itself
    d. none of the above
    e. any of the above

17. Magnification mammography:
    a. should not use a focal-spot size greater than 0.3 millimeters.
    b. magnifies the image while maintaining no change in patient dose.
    c. produces images twice the normal object size.
    d. a and b.
    e. all of the above.

18. A charged couple device (CCD):
    a. is an image receptor.
    b. converts light from the intensifying screen into a digital image.
    c. converts visible light electrons into protons whose signal is read in pixel-fashion to form an image.
    d. a and b.
    e. all of the above.

Complete the chart below.

19.

Target X-ray Tube Material	Preferred Filter	Rationale
Tungsten		
Molybdenum	Molybdenum or rhodium	
Rhodium		Provides a slightly higher quality x-ray beam of greater penetrability. Preferred for thicker, more dense breasts.

Answer each of the following on a separate sheet of paper.

20. What is the difference between diagnostic mammography and screening mammography?

21. In adding information to a patient's record, a student notices that the woman's very first mammogram is still in her files, despite the fact that it is nearly twenty years old now. Should this old information be discarded?

22. Explain why x-ray mammography requires a low-kVp technique.

23. Identify the three types of image receptors that have been used for mammography. Which is preferred and why?

CHALLENGE QUESTIONS
■ ■ ■ ■ ■ ■ ■ ■ ■ ■ ■ ■ ■ ■ ■ ■ ■ ■ ■

1. Use the illustration below to point out distinct advantages of the use of compression in mammography by drawing arrows and adding notes.

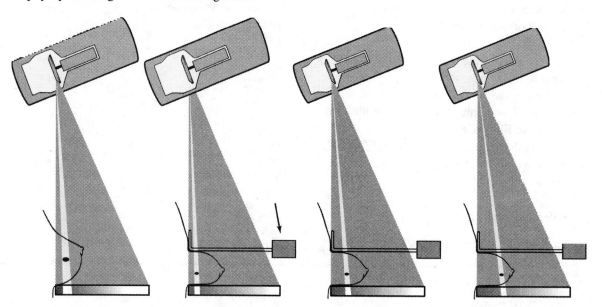

2. Two friends meet unexpectedly in a waiting room while waiting to get their mammograms. Since they haven't seen each other in a while, they agree to wait for each other at the clinic and go out for coffee afterwards. Helen comes out first and notices that Elaine's exam is taking a lot longer than hers. Later, over coffee, Helen asks, "Did something go wrong?"

"No," Elaine says, "everything went just fine."

"Well, did they have to redo it or something?"

"No. They took several different views of each breast, very efficiently, and I came right out. Why? Did you wait a long time?"

"Well, not too long, but—wait a minute. Did you say they took several views?"

"Of each side, yes."

Helen frowns. "They only took one x-ray on each side when I was in there." Helen looks at Elaine. "Maybe I got cheated."

Is Helen right? What possible explanation could there be for Elaine's more extensive examination? Based on the clues given here, what assumptions could you make about the rationale for the differences in their exams?

3. Why is the heel effect disregarded in mammography?

4. Copy and fill in Table 23-3, "Features of a Mammography Unit."

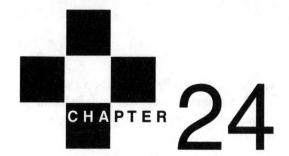

Mammography Quality Control

Indicate how often each function below should be evaluated: D = daily; W = weekly; M = monthly; Q = quarterly; and S = semi-annually.

1. _____ analysis of fixer retention in film

2. _____ compression

3. _____ darkroom cleanliness

4. _____ darkroom fog

5. _____ phantom images

6. _____ processor quality control

7. _____ repeat analysis

8. _____ screen cleanliness

9. _____ screen-film contact

10. _____ viewboxes and viewing conditions

11. _____ visual checklist

Circle the correct answer to each of the following.

12. Continuous quality improvement is:
    a. the medical physicist's evaluation of the radiographic and mammographic equipment and processing.
    b. the radiologist's responsibility to oversee and link different aspects of quality control.
    c. is the hospital or clinic's administrative plan for quality control and quality assurance.
    d. a and c.
    e. a and b.

13. The medical physicist's responsibilities include, among others:
    a. supervising patient education and monitoring continuous quality improvement (CQI).
    b. advising mammographers on quality control and consulting with the service engineer.
    c. inspecting the mammographic unit assembly and evaluating image quality.
    d. b and c.
    e. all of the above.

14. The mammographer:
    a. handles the most hands-on, day-to-day execution of QC.
    b. monitors all control charts and logs for possible problematic trends.
    c. supervises patient tracking.
    d. a and b.
    e. all of the above.

15. The first step in a processor QC program is to:
    a. wipe the darkroom clean, beginning with the floor.
    b. establish operating control levels for the processing system.
    c. wipe down the processor and passbox.
    d. expose a sheet of control film with a sensitometer.

16. When processing a sensitometric strip:
    a. the least exposed end is fed into the processor first.
    b. the same side of the feed tray is used with the emulsion side down.
    c. the delay between exposure and processing should be similar each day.
    d. a and c.
    e. all of the above.

17. The mid-density step:
    a. has an average optical density closest to 1.5 but not less than 1.
    b. is the same thing as the speed index.
    c. has an average density closest to 2.2.
    d. a and b.
    e. b and c.

18. The density difference is:
    a. the difference between the step with average density closest to 2.2 and the step with average density closest to but not less than 0.45.
    b. the same thing as the speed index.
    c. the same thing as the contrast index.
    d. a and b.
    e. a and c.

19. The average density from an unexposed area of strips is the:
    a. base plus fox (B + F).
    b. speed index.
    c. mid-density (MD).
    d. density difference (DD).
    e. contrast index.

20. The constancy of image contrast:
    a. is evaluated by the MD.
    b. is evaluated by the DD.
    c. may vary within + 0.15 of the control value.
    d. a and c.
    e. b and c.

21. The B + F:
    a. evaluates the level of fog present in the processing chain.
    b. may vary within +0.05 of the control value.
    c. of the new film should not exceed the B + F of the old film by more than 0.02.
    d. a and c.
    e. all of the above.

22. Because mammography viewboxes have considerably higher luminance levels than conventional viewboxes:
    a. no mammogram should be completely masked.
    b. it is important to ensure that bright lighting is available.

    c. no extraneous light from the viewbox should enter the eye during viewing of mammography test images.
    d. a and c.
    e. a and b.

23. When taking a phantom image, ensure that:
    a. the technique is that used for a 50% fatty, 50% dense compressed breast.
    b. a densitometer is used to measure the optical density for the density disk, but not for the background.
    c. the exposure time or mAs stays within a range greater than 1.2 with an allowed range of ±0.2.
    d. 28 kVp is used at all times, with a density difference of 0.4 with an allowed range of ±0.05.
    e. none of the above.

24. A score of 0.5 could be assigned to:
    a. a fiber if its entire length is visible.
    b. a fiber if less than half of it is visible.
    c. a speck group if at least two of six specks are visible.
    d. a mass with a density difference seen at the correct location with a circular border.
    e. none of the above.

25. In scoring a phantom image, the minimum number of objects required to pass ACR accreditation is:
    a. four fibers, three speck groups, and three masses.
    b. three fibers, four speck groups, and three masses.
    c. four fibers, four speck groups, and four masses.
    d. three fibers, three speck groups, and four masses.
    e. none of the above.

26. Elements included in a monthly visual check might include:
    a. repeat analysis.
    b. phantom images.
    c. mechanical rigidity and stability.
    d. MD, DD, and B + F.
    e. none of the above.

27. An archival quality check:
    a. determines the rate of repeat or rejected images against the total number of usable images on archive.
    b. determines the amount of residual fixer in the processed film.
    c. is the quarterly collection and analysis of phantom images stored in archives.
    d. is more commonly referred to as the quality control visual check.
    e. none of the above.

28. The purpose of a screen-film contact test is to:
    a. determine the performance rate of both screen and film.
    b. determine the amount of contact between the screen and film in each cassette.
    c. determine the safelight filter brightness.
    d. none of the above.

29. In a successful compression check:
    a. pressure should never exceed 40 pounds in the automatic mode.
    b. both modes should be able to compress between 25 and 40 pounds.
    c. both modes should be able to hold optimal compression for at least 15 minutes.
    d. a and b.
    e. all of the above.

30. Number each of the following steps in a processor quality control (QC) program.

    _____ Begin determining and plotting the MD, DD, and B+F daily.

    _____ Clean the processor tanks and racks, then supply proper replenisher, fixer, developer, and developer starter fluids.

    _____ Establish operating control levels.

    _____ Expose a sheet of control film with a sensitometer, and measure the delay between exposure and processing; this should be similar each day.

    _____ Record the base plus fog (B + F).

    _____ Measure and mark the mid-density (MD) step, or speed index, and the density difference (DD), or contrast index.

    _____ Warm up the processor to the correct temperature.

31. Number each of the following steps in a screen-film contact test.

    _____ Place cassette on top of the cassette holder assembly with the test tool directly on top of the cassette.

    _____ Select between 25 and 28 kVp for an optical density between 0.7 and 0.8 near the chest wall or place a piece of acrylic between the x-ray tube and cassette.

    _____ Load and allow cassette to be upright for 15 minutes to allow trapped air to escape.

    _____ Clean and air dry cassettes and screens.

    _____ Expose for at least 500 milliseconds and view from a distance of at least 3 feet after processing.

    _____ Raise the compression paddle as high as possible.

32. The _____ is determined to evaluate the constancy of image-receptor speed, and the _____ is determined to evaluate the constancy of image contrast.

33. DD and MD values may reasonably vary within _____ of the control values; if either is out of this control limit, the cause should be corrected. If either value falls outside a _____ range of the control value, repeat the test.

34. The B + F evaluates the level of
_____ present in the pro-
cessing chain. This value is allowed to vary
within _____ of the con-
trol value.

35. When scoring phantom images, once an
accredited phantom has been used and established, the score of phanom objects counted
on subsequent phantom images for each type
of object should not decrease by more than
_____. The minimum number of
objects required to pass ACR accreditation is
_____ fibers, _____ speck
groups, and _____ classes.

***Answer each of the following on a separate
sheet of paper.***

36. Describe how one should prepare the darkroom each day. What steps can be taken to
assure cleanliness?

37. Chris, the QC mammograper, has opened a
new box of test film for a crossover with the
old film. After exposing the sensiometric
strip and leaving, she returns after a couple
of hours to finish the job. (a) What manufacturer recommendations are particularly
important at this point? (b) Point out any
potential problems in Chris's procedure.

38. Next, Chris is asked to perform an archival
quality check. (a) What is the purpose of this
task? How often is it usually done? How are
the results used? (b) Describe the process.

39. On her first try at doing an archival quality
check, Chris notices that the spot on her test
film darkens, making it difficult to know how
to score it accurately. What might she have
neglected to do?

40. Create a concise checklist that could be
posted in your mammography facility's darkroom to guide radiographers in analyzing
darkroom fog.

CHALLENGE QUESTIONS

. . . .

1. Discuss the specific roles and duties of the members of the mammography QA/QC team. Define
ACR and MSQA.

2. Janet, a QC mammographer, finds that the B+F of the new film exceeds that of the old film by more than
0.02. She records this and adjusts the control values accordingly. Is there anything else she should do?

3. Create a chart for interpreting objects on a mammography phantom image. The chart should allow
anyone who uses it to quickly determine the varying possible scores for (a) a fiber, (b) a speck
group, and (c) a mass.

4. Gina has been asked to conduct a repeat analysis. Because she is new to this facility, she says, "You
realize, of course, that because this is a new facility, you may not have had enough patients yet for
me to perform this analysis."
   a. What purposes can a repeat analysis serve? Which is most important?
   b. What did Gina mean when she said "—you may not have had enough patient yet—"? How
      many patients are needed? Why?
   c. Describe the process Gina will use.

5. Gina determines that 640 films were exposed, and 24 of these were repeated. What is the repeat
rate? Is this an acceptable rate? What is an acceptable rate?

6. Gina comes back the next quarter to do another repeat analysis. This time she finds that 851 films
were exposed and 14 were repeats. Determine the repeat rate this time around. Is this an acceptable
rate?

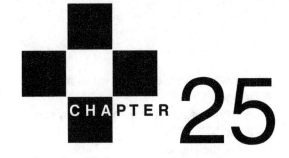

CHAPTER 25

Fluoroscopy

1. Match the letters in the illustration below to their corresponding labels on the right.

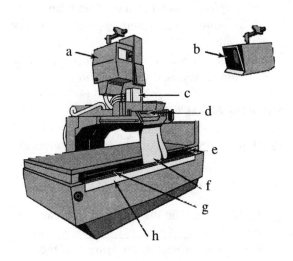

_____ Bucky diaphragm for overhead film

_____ Bucky slot cover

_____ cine or spot film camera

_____ fluoroscopic x-ray tube under table

_____ image intensifier tube

_____ protective curtain

_____ spot film cassette

_____ video monitor

Circle the correct answer to each of the following.

2. Phototopic vision:
   a. is that enabled by cones, which are used primarily for daylight vision.
   b. is that enabled by rods, which are used primarily for daylight vision.
   c. is that enabled by cones, which are used primarily for night vision.
   d. is that enabled by rods, which are used primarily for night vision.

3. Cones:
   a. are primarily responsible for phototopic and scotopic vision.
   b. are less effective than rods at contrast perception.
   c. are more effective than rods in visual acuity.
   d. are less effective than rods when it comes to contrast perception.

4. Photoemission occurs:
   a. when photocathode compounds emit electrons in response to being stimulated by light.
   b. when electrons are emitted from the photocathode after heat stimulation.
   c. in proportion to the intensity of the incident x-rays.
   d. a and c.
   e. b and c.

5. The process of focusing electrons emitted over the face of the image-intensifier tube:
   a. demonstrates electron optics.
   b. is controlled by the electrostatic focusing lenses.
   c. results in the electrons arriving at the output phosphor with high kinetic energy, and with the image of the input phosphor in minified form.
   d. a and b.
   e. all of the above.

6. The increased illumination of the image once it reaches the output phosphor is due to:
   a. the multiplication of the light photons at the output phosphor compared with the x-rays at the input phosphor.
   b. the image minification from input phosphor to output phosphor.
   c. thermionic emission.
   d. a and b.
   e. all of the above.

7. The brightness gain is:
   a. the product of the minification gain and the flux gain.
   b. the ratio of illumination intensity between the input phosphor and photocathode.
   c. the ratio of the square of the diameter of the input phosphor to the square of the diameter of the output phosphor.
   d. a and b.
   e. all of the above.

8. The conversion factor in fluoroscopic intensification is:
   a. the ratio of the square of the diameter of the input phosphor to the square of the diameter of the output phosphor.
   b. the proper way to express intensification.
   c. the ability of the image-intensifier tube to increase the illumination level of the image.
   d. a and b.
   e. all of the above.

9. The conversion factor in fluoroscopic intensification is:
   a. approximately 10-5 times the brightness gain.
   b. is equal to the output phosphor illumination divided by the input exposure rate.
   c. the product of the minification gain and the flux gain.
   d. a and b.
   e. none of the above.

10. The vidicon:
    a. is the television camera tube least often used in television fluoroscopy.
    b. converts the light image into an electronic signal that is then sent to the monitor where it is reconstructed as an image.
    c. is a type of plumbicon, or electron gun.
    d. a and b.
    e. all of the above.

11. The photo-spot camera:
    a. does not require significant interruption of the fluoroscopic exam.
    b. exposes several frames when activtated.
    c. requires more patient exposure than spot film.
    d. requires additional heat load on the x-ray tube associated with spot films.

Fill in the blanks below.

12. Illumination levels are measured in units of _____ and _____.

13. Light incident on the eye must first pass through the _____, a transparent protective covering, and then through the _____, which focuses the light onto the _____. The _____ behaves like a diaphragm, contracting or dilating as it adjusts to light and dark.

14. Cones, which are capable of responding to _____ light levels, are concentrated in the _____, whereas rods, which are sensitive to _____, appear in the _____.

15. Output phosphor size is fairly standard at _____ centimeters; input phosphor size varies from _____ to _____ centimeters.

16. The brightness gain is the ratio of the illumination intensity at the _____, measured in _____.

17. Image intensifiers have conversion factors ranging from _____ to _____. This corresponds to brightness gains at _____ to _____.

18. Use of the smaller dimension of a multifield image-intensifier tube always results in a magnified image with a magnification factor in _____ proportion to the _____.

19. In general _____ kVp and _____ mA are preferred for fluoroscopy.

20. Good spatial resolution is associated with _____ lp/mm.

21. In the fluoroscopic image monitor, _____ resolution is determined by the number of lines. _____ resolution is determined by bandwidth or bandpass, which describes the number of times per second that the _____ can be _____. The _____ the bandpass, the better the resolution.

Calculate the following problems on a separate sheet of paper.

22. What is the brightness gain for a 17-centimeter image-intensifier tube having a flux gain of 140 and a 2.5-centimeter output phosphor?

23. How magnified is the image of a 23/15/10 image intensifier in the 10-centimeter mode compared with the 23-centimeter mode?

24. A 25/17/12 image-intensifier tube is used in the 12-centimeter mode. How much higher is the patient dose in this mode compared with the 25-centimeter mode?

Answer each of the following on a separate sheet of paper.

25. Describe the structure and actions of the input phosphor layer.

26. Why is a potential difference of about 25,000 volts maintained across the tube between photocathode and anode?

27. In multifield image intensification, what happens to that portion of the image resulting from the periphery of the input phosphor?

28. Why is spatial resolution better in multifield image intensification?

29. You have been asked to present to your facility's staff a brief discussion on the advantages and disadvantages of installing and using a television monitoring system. What will you be sure to include in your presentation?

30. What is one of the most important things to remember in handling a lens coupling system?

31. Explain how bandpass is expressed. What does this measure tell us about horizontal resolution?

32. Explain the cassette spot-film exposure process, describing, as well, the distinction between one-on-one and two-on-one modes.

33. Copy Table 25-1, leaving kVp blank. Fill this in later.

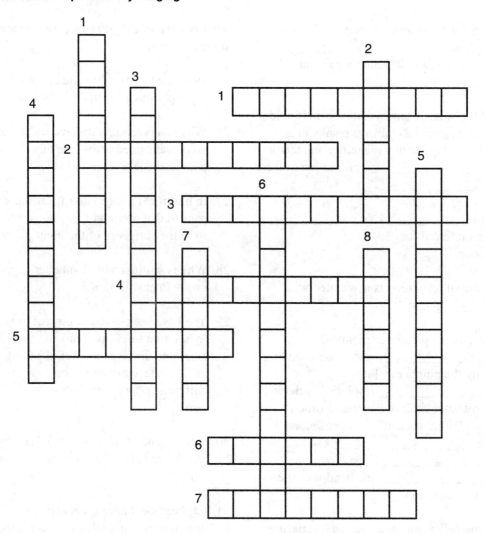

ACROSS

1. Type of television camera tube used in television fluoroscopy.
2. Daylight vision, involving the cones.
3. Produced studies on illumination that resulted in the development of the image intensifier in the 1950s.
4. Type of electron emission occurring after heat stimulation.
5. Night vision, involving the rods.
6. Invented the fluoroscope in 1896.
7. Ability to detect differences in brightness.

DOWN

1. Property that describes the number of times per second that an electron beam can be modulated or changed; used to determine horizontal resolution.
2. Ability to perceive fine detail.
3. Photoemissive surface composed of cesium and antimony compounds that emit electrons when stimulated by light.
4. Ability of the image-intensifier tube to increase the illumination level of an image.
5. Reduction in brightness at the periphery.
6. Ratio of the square of the diameter of the input phosphor to the square of the diameter of the output phosphor.
7. Input phosphor with which x-rays interact after exiting the patient and the glass envelope.
8. Line of varying intensity of light.

CHALLENGE QUESTIONS

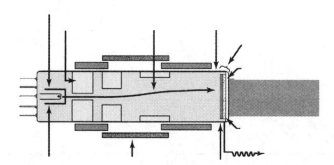

1. Use this diagram as the basis for a discussion of how the internal elements of a vidicon television camera tube operates. Label principal parts as you refer to them in your discussion.

2. Describe how multifield image intensifiers reduce the field of view and thereby magnify the image.

3. Explain how a magnified image from multifield image intensification affects patient dose, noise, and contrast resolution.

4. Create a chart to help demonstrate the advantages and disadvantages of the two methods commonly used to couple the television camera tube to the image-intensifier tube.

5. Prepare a concise demonstration of how the image on the television monitor is formed. Include the following aspects in your discussion: (1) How are the electron beams—the constant one of the television camera tube and the modulated one of the television picture tube—kept synchronous? (2) How does the movement of these electron beams produce a raster pattern on the screen?

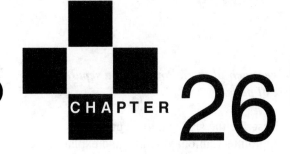

- - - - - - - - - - - - - - - -

1. Match each item below to its appropriate use.

_____ Cobra (or C2) catheter

_____ guidewire

_____ headhunter (H1) tip

_____ J-tip

_____ pigtail catheter

_____ Simmons catheter

a. used for the femoral approach to the brachio-cephalic vessels

b. highly curved for approach to sharply angled vessels such as the celiac axis

c. used for introduction into renal and mesenteric arteries

d. has side holes for ejecting contrast media into a compact bolus

e. allows the safe introduction of a catheter into a vessel

f. deflects off edges of plaques and helps prevent dissection of an artery

- - - - - - - - - - - - - - - -

Circle the correct answer to each of the following.

2. Angiointerventional procedures require:
   a. high-voltage generators with three-phase, 12-pulse power.
   b. high-frequency generators.
   c. generators capable of at least 100 kW with low ripple.
   d. a and c.
   e. b and c.

3. Angiointerventional imaging:
   a. duplicates the control switches for couch positioning on a floor switch.
   b. requires tilt-tables.
   c. has eliminated the need for a bulky computer-controlled stepping feature.
   d. does not allow imaging from the abdomen to the feet after a single injection.

4. Cinefluorography:
   a. makes possible a lower patient dose than that required for recording images electronically.
   b. provides a higher image quality than those images recorded electronically.
   c. is least helpful in recording those procedures associated with cardiac catheterization.
   d. does not require synchronization, which would result in unnecessary patient exposure.

5. Serial changers are often used in pairs with two orthogonal x-ray sources in a configuration called:
   a. roll-and-cut film.
   b. rapid film changers.
   c. biplane imaging.
   d. bilateral serial changers.

6. The most popular type of serialographic changers used today are:
   a. roll-film changers.
   b. bulky cassette changers.
   c. cut-film changers.
   d. rapid film changers.

Fill in the blanks below.

7. Nonionic contrast media, because of its low concentration of ions, causes fewer physiologic problems; this low ion concentration is called _____.

8. Risks associated with angiography include _____, _____ and _____.

9. The angiointerventional x-ray tube has a _____ target angle, a _____ anode disk, and cathodes designed for _____ and serial radiography.

10. The size and construction of the anode disk determines the _____, which in turn influences the power rating.

11. Rapid flow requires _____ frames per second, whereas delayed films may be included at _____ seconds after injection.

Calculate the following problems on a separate sheet of paper.

12. An angiogram is performed with a 0.3-millimeter focal spot at 100 centimeters SID. The artery to be imaged is 30 centimeters from the image receptor. What is the magnification factor, focal-spot blur, and approximate spatial resolution?

Answer each of the following on a separate sheet of paper.

13. Describe the size requirements for an angiointerventional facility, and explain the rationale behind these requirements.

14. List individuals who may be present during a procedure in the angiographic suite and their functions.

15. Describe the x-ray tube apparatus needed for angiointerventional procedures.

16. Create a table that provide the appropriate size and rational for each of the following features: anode disk size, anode heat capacity, focal spot, and power rating.

17. Discuss advantages and disadvantages of both 16- and 35-millimeter film movie cameras used for cinefluorography.

18. What do we mean when we say that cinefluorographic systems are synchronized? What is the effect of this synchronization?

19. Explain Seldinger technique for arterial access.

CHALLENGE QUESTIONS

. . . .

1. Christa, RT (R) (CV), is about to set up a cinefluorography procedure for a catheterization study. She selects a frame rate of 7.5 frames per second. Before exposure, she ensures that the screens in the exposure chamber are separated in order to move a film from the supply magazine into position. Do you agree with all of her choices? Why or why not?

2. Next, Christa sets up for a renal study. Will the screens in the exposure chamber remain separated during the exposure as well? If so, what purpose does this serve? If not, why not?

   a. What is the frame rate for rapid flow?

   b. Will the screens in the exposure chamber remain separated during the exposure as well? If so, what purpose does this serve? If not, why not?

   c. After catheter placement during the procedure, a test injection is done under fluoroscopy before filming. What is the radiographer looking for? What purpose does this test serve?

   d. Describe what will be done during this same test.

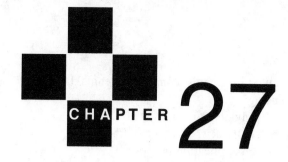

CHAPTER 27 Computer Science

Circle the correct answer to each of the following.

1. Which of the following was the first large-scale computer application in radiology?
   a. magnetic resonance imaging (MRI)
   b. computed tomographic (CT) scanning
   c. diagnostic ultrasound
   d. digital fluoroscopy

2. Geoffrey has provided his computer with a significant amount of patient data and operating instructions. The computer performs these operations on the patient data without any further intervention. This computer can be said to be:
   a. batch processing.
   b. microprocessing.
   c. performing large-scale integration.
   d. performing very large-scale integration.

3. Stored-program computers:
   a. must have their instructions (programs) and data stored in a separate system.
   b. are laid out so that the sequence of steps to be followed during any calculation is preestablished.
   c. handle only arithmetic functions.
   d. are made specifically to execute logic functions.

4. Second-generation computers:
   a. were vacuum-tube machines.
   b. incorporated large-scale integration (LSI).
   c. came in three sizes.
   d. were based on individually packaged transistors.

5. Very large-scale integration:
   a. is an extension of the third generation computers.
   b. is accomplished with vacuum-tube machines.
   c. places hundreds of thousands of circuit elements on a chip.
   d. is the same thing as a microcomputer.

6. The microcomputer:
   a. is one of the smallest computers, larger only than the minicomputer.
   b. uses several microprocessors and has a larger capacity and flexibility than the minicomputer.
   c. appears as a personal computer, a word processor, and a control for many industrial processes.
   d. a and c.
   e. b and c.

7. In a PC, the microprocessor:
   a. is built around the primary control center for a computer.
   b. is a single, very large-scale integrated circuit on a silicon chip less than a centimeter on a side that contains hundreds of thousands of individual circuit elements.
   c. is the central processing unit, or primary control center.
   d. a and b.
   e. b and c.

8. The CPU:
   a. is the primary control center, supervising all of the other components of the computer.
   b. performs the mathematical manipulations and even stores information.
   c. is an electrical conductor called a bus.
   d. a and b
   e. none of the above.

9. The control unit:
   a. identifies the route of entry and directs the data to the arithmetic unit or to memory.
   b. transfers computational results to the output device selected.
   c. is the computer's basic overseer in charge of interpreting the user's program instruction in the proper order.
   d. a and c.
   e. all of the above.

10. A printer that maps digital information for each character onto a 300 x 300 dots-per-inch grid and then burns it into the paper at 200° C at 100 milliseconds per character is a:
   a. dot matrix printer.
   b. laser printer.
   c. thermal printer.
   d. inkjet printer.
   e. bubblejet printer.

11. Data transmission between computers is routinely accomplished through the use of:
   a. a modem (modulator-demodulator).
   b. optical scanners.
   c. bauds.
   d. compilers.

12. Adam is using a computer program that recognizes symbolic instructions and translates them into the corresponding binary code. Emma is using a program that is translating an application program based on Pascal into a form that will be accepted directly by the CPU. She tells Adam that her program will "make program development easier and more interactive." Adam is probably using a(n) _____; Emma is problem using a(n) _____.
   a. assembler; interpreter
   b. compiler; interpreter
   c. interpreter; assembler
   d. assembler; compiler

13. Dennis' lab frequently uses a program that permits the computer to perform the specific task of reconstructing an image from an x-ray transmission pattern. It was written in one of many high-level computer languages and then translated into a corresponding machine-language program that is now exe-cuted by Dennis' computer. Dennis' lab is using:
   a. a bootstrap.
   b. FORTRAN.
   c. an application program.
   d. BASIC.
   e. systems software.

14. Number the following to show an accurate sequence of events in the development of the computer—from the abacus on.

   _____   Babbage designs an analytical engine to perform general calculations automatically.

   _____   Computers incorporate very large-scale integration.

   _____   Eckert and Mauchly develop the ENIAC (electrical numberical integrator and calculator).

   _____   Eckert and Mauckly develop UNIVAC, which is the first commercially successful general purpose stored-program electronic digital computer.

   _____   Harvard University experts develops the Mark I.

   _____   Hollerith designs a data recording system that stores information as holes on cards that are interpreted by machines with electrical sensors.

   _____   Integrated circuits are introduced, which consist of many electronic elements fused onto a chip.

   _____   Pascal and Leibniz build mechanical calculators with pegged wheels to automatically perform arithmetic functions.

   _____   Shockley at Bell Labs develops the transistor which makes possible the development of the stored-program computer.

15. Label each of the lettered boxes below to demonstrate the sequences of software manipulation needed to complete an operation.

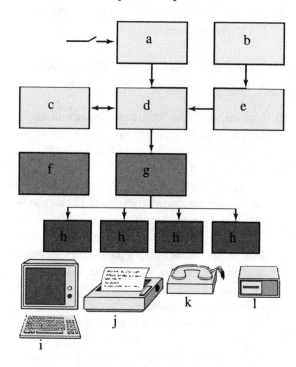

a. _____

b. _____

c. _____

d. _____

e. _____

f. _____

g. _____

h. _____

i. _____

j. _____

k. _____

l. _____

■ ■ ■ ■ ■ ■ ■ ■ ■ ■ ■ ■ ■ ■ ■

Fill in the blanks below.

16. _____ evaluate an intermediate result and perform subsequent computations, depending on that result.

17. _____ speed up the transfer of bulk data between main memory and external devices, bypassing the CPU.

18. The RAM primary memory is sometimes called _____. There are two principle types:

_____, which retains its memory, even if power to the computer is lost, and _____, structured in a parallel fashion, which increases computer speed. ROM usually contains the primary _____, called _____, which get the computer going when it is first turned on.

19. In VDTs, _____ is the display normally encountered. This is a series of _____ that conveys information. The characters needed for the display of text are generated by patterns of dots from a _____. If _____ is also available, one can display the results of numeric computations graphically. VDTs are either programmable _____ or _____ devices.

20. Hard disks are _____ in nature. The data are grouped in _____, each of which is addressed. Some hard disks can hold _____ or more of data. Today optical disks (also called _____) are in use for _____ applications.

21. In computer language, a bit is a single
_____. Depending on the
microprocessor, a string of _____, _____, or
_____ bits will be manipulated simultaneously. Bits are often grouped into bunches of
_____, called _____. To
_____ is to translate from
ordinary characters to computer-compatible
characters or binary digits. The most popular
personal computers use _____- and _____-
bit microprocessors with 1 to 40
_____.

*Calculate the following problems on a separate
sheet of paper.*

22. Express the number 214 in binary form,
using Table 27-2 as a guide.

23. Express the number 630 in binary form,
using Table 27-2 as a guide.

24. For each of the decimal numbers below, calculate the binary and hexadecimal counterparts.

Decimal	Binary	Hexadecimal
4	_____	_____
11	_____	_____
23	_____	_____

*Answer each of the following on a separate
sheet of paper.*

25. How can a computer be considered artificial
intelligence?

26. Describe the evolution from magnetic core
memory to semiconductor memory. How has
the word core changed over time?

27. What is a flip-flop and how does it function?

28. Describe the difference between ROM and
RAM primary memory.

29. What do we mean when we say, "all primary
memory is addressed"?

30. List and describe various secondary memory
devices for computer hardware.

31. Explain the basic differences between the
decimal, duodecimal, and binary number systems. How do computers use the binary system?

32. Margie has been using a batch operating system on a main-frame computer, submitting
her batch jobs to a remote terminal connected to her computer by a cable or modem.
What mode of processing is she using?

33. Next, Margie goes to work for a research-
and-development institution, where she,
simultaneously with nearly a hundred other
users, works on the computer in sessions. In
a typical session, Margie presents a pass-
word, enters a program under the control of a
text editor, saves the program under a special, assigned name, and compiles and runs
the program. While the program is being run,
she and the computer may request information from each other; the process continues,
sometimes changing in response to the
results of these interactions. What type of
system is she using now?

34. Describe the way data move through a
pipeline processor. How does this differ from
an array processor?

CHALLENGE QUESTIONS

1. Generate a time line that integrates a mapping of chronological developments in the evolution of the computer with specific contributions made at certain stages. Try to highlight some of the more significant developments such as the transistor, the chip, etc. In other words, feature those developments that particularly revolutionized the way computers worked.

2. Hank creates a computer program that provides a series of instructions in order to organize the course of data through the radiology department computers. He is writing these in a higher-level language expressly to carry out some use function. Steve stops by the lab and says, "Are you still developing that systems software?" What is wrong with Steve's question? Explain.

3. Duplicate Table 27-4 to create your own expanded list of programming languages. Then reorder column 3 to create a matching exercise. Photocopy this for exchange with a colleague so that each of you have more than one version to practice on.

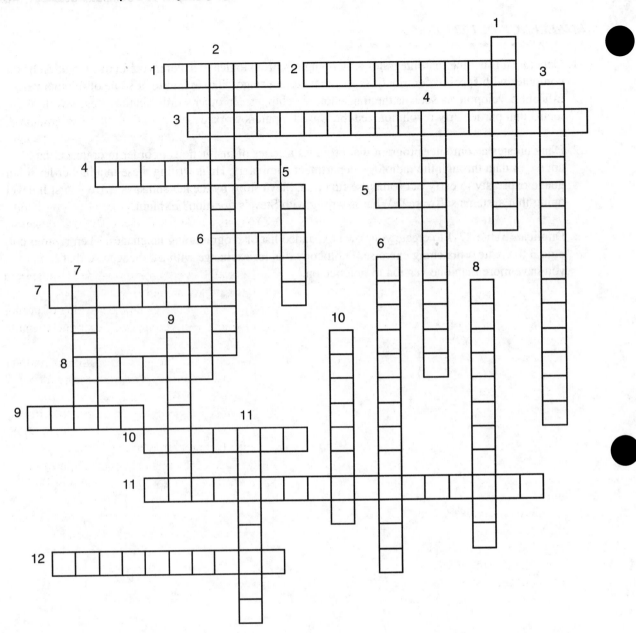

ACROSS

1. Type of memory that is retained even if power to the computer is lost.
2. Designed a system to record census data in 1890; started a company that eventually evolved into IBM.
3. System of many transistors and other electronic elements fused onto a chip.
4. One of two individuals who designed and built the first electronic digital computer.
5. I/O device consisting of a keyboard and cathode-ray tube display.
6. Tiny piece of semiconductor material, usually silicon.
7. Computer programs that tell the computer what to do and how to store data.
8. One of two mathematicians who built mechanical calculators using pegged wheels to automatically perform the four arithmetic fuunctions.
9. Type of data processing in which a computer performs operations on defined data without human input or intervention.
10. One of the individuals involved in developing UNIVAC, the first commercially successful general purpose stored-program electronic digital computer.
11. Primary control center unit built around a microprocessor.
12. Term indicating that a computer is powered by electrical devices rather than by a mechanical device.

DOWN

1. Leader of a team of scientists at the Bell Laboratories who, in 1948, developed the transistor.
2. Type of memory used for storing computational instructions or data that might change from time to time; sometimes called read-write memory.
3. Computer on a chip.
4. Device that identifies the route of entry and directs data from an input device to destinations; transfers computed results to the output device selected.
5. Operation in which information is transferred into primary memory.
6. Type of memory module consisting of groups of silicon chips etched with extremely small storage circuits.
7. Operation in which results of a computation is transferred from primary memory to storage or to the user.
8. Secondary memory device that stores digital data on a mirrored surface by modulating the reflective properties of that surface.
9. Designed an analytical engine to perform general calculations automatically in 1842.
10. Visible components of a computer.
11. Secondary memory device that stores data in a series of concentric magnetic tracks.

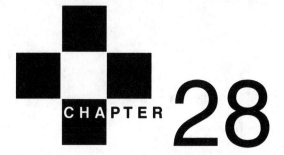

CHAPTER 28

Digital X-ray Imaging

Circle the correct answer to each of the following.

1. By what other name(s) can digital x-ray imaging be known?
   a. digital vascular imaging (DVI)
   b. digital subtraction angiography (DSA)
   c. digital fluoroscopy (DF)
   d. a and c
   e. all of the above

2. Digital fluoroscopy is:
   a. a digital x-ray imaging system that produces a series of dynamic images obtained with an area x-ray beam and an image intensifier.
   b. the static images produced with either a fan x-ray beam intercepted by a linear array of radiation detectors or an area x-ray beam intercepted by a light-stimulated phosphor plate.
   c. the use of existing CT gantry and computer to generate an image similar to a conventional radiograph.
   d. a and b.
   e. none of the above.

3. An image matrix is:
   a. a CT number or Hounsfield unit.
   b. a pixel.
   c. a layout of cells in rows and columns, each cell corresponding to a specific location in the image.
   d. a and b.
   e. none of the above.

4. The human eye can visualize _____ shades of gray; a computer can visualize a dynamic range in excess of _____.
   a. 2^1; 2^{10}
   b. 2^1; 2^5
   c. 2^5; 2^{10}
   d. 28; 2^{12}

5. Important, computer-controlled characteristics of a DF system include:
   a. image matrix size.
   b. system dynamic range.
   c. image acquisition rate.
   d. a and b.
   e. all of the above.

6. Continuously varying television camera output signals are converted to digital numbers by the:
   a. image matrix control.
   b. analog-to-digital converter.
   c. progressive mode.
   d. CCD.
   e. image intensifier.

7. Charles used to work in a lab with an 8-bit ADC. He has recently begun working at a new lab. This one uses a 10-bit ADS. Will Charles find this system more precise or less precise than the old one?
   a. He will find it more precise in that the conversion will range from 0 to 255.
   b. He will find it less precise in that the conversion will range from 0 to 255.
   c. He will find it more precise in that the conversion will range from 0 to 210.
   d. It is impossible to tell from the limited information provided.
   e. There will be no difference because ADS affects intensity, not precision.

8. In temporal subtraction:
   a. a single kVp is used.
   b. x-ray beam filter switching is preferred.
   c. motion artifacts are a problem.
   d. a and c.
   e. all of the above.

9. In energy subtraction:
   a. rapid kVp switching is required.
   b. contrast resolution at 1 millimeter at 1% is achieved.
   c. total subtraction of common structures is achieved.
   d. a and c.
   e. all of the above.

10. Energy subtraction:
    a. uses a single x-ray beam to provide a subtraction image resulting from differences in photoelectric interaction over time.
    b. is based on the abrupt change in photoelectric absorption at the K edge of the contrast media compared with that for soft tissue and bone.
    c. has the advantage of requiring only one emission spectrum by pulsing the x-ray beam at 70 kVp and then 90 kVp.
    d. eliminates the need for dissimilar filters on a fly wheel.
    e. all of the above.

11. The K absorption edge:
    a. refers to the binding energy of the two K-shell electrons of iodine during energy subtraction.
    b. is less than that for bone or muscle.
    c. is the large, abrupt increase in absorption when the incident x-ray energy becomes sufficient to overcome the K-shell electron binding energy of iodine.
    d. a and c.
    e. all of the above.

12. Compared to conventional radiographic images, SPR images:
    a. are virtually free of scatter radiation.
    b. are digital in form.
    c. have enhanced radiographic contrast due to reduced scatter radiation from fan beam collimation.
    d. a and c.
    e. all of the above.

13. The principal disadvantage of SPR is:
    a. poor spatial resolution.
    b. greater scattered x-ray photons.
    c. increased image noise.

d. a and c
e. all of the above.

14. In SPR:
    a. the more detectors there are per degree of fan x-ray beam, the better the spatial resolution.
    b. as the speed of translation is increased, fewer x-rays will be detected.
    c. as the speed of translation is increased, the more the image quality will decrease.
    d. a and c
    e. all of the above.

15. The image acquisition time in DR can be reduced by:
    a. using the area beam with an image receptor.
    b. using a fan beam.
    c. decreasing the translation time in SPR.
    d. a and c.
    e. all of the above.

Fill in the blanks below.

16. With conventional imaging, x-rays form an image directly on the _____. With digital techniques, x-rays form an electronic image on a _____, which is manipulated by a _____, temporarily stored in memory and displayed as a _____, each having a _____ of values.

17. Each cell of the image matrix is called a _____. In digital x-ray imaging, the value of the pixel determines _____. This value is used to provide _____ and to define _____. In CT scanning, the value of each pixel is a _____ that can be used to judge the _____ of the tissue represented.

18. For the same field of view (FOV), spatial resolution will be better with a _____ image matrix.

19. The range of values over which a system can respond is called its _____, which (in a digital system) corresponds to the _____ of each pixel. The _____ the dynamic range, the better the contrast resolution.

20. In hybrid subtraction, image acquisition follows the _____ mode procedure, but the mask and each subsequent image are formed by the _____ technique.

21. During translation in SPR, either the x-ray beam is _____ or the interrogation of the detector array is _____.

22. In DR, the requirement for a high heat capacity is due to _____ and _____.

23. The two basic designs used in the detector array of an x-ray tube-detector assembly include _____ and _____.

Calculate the following problems on a separate sheet of paper.

24. Claudia is working with a 1000-line system. How many pixels are contained in a 1000-line DF system?

25. Claudia switches to a 512-by-512 field of view (FOV). What is the pixel size of the system Claudia is using if it is operating in the 5-inch mode input phosphor?

Answer each of the following on a separate sheet of paper.

26. Discuss the advantages of digital fluoroscopy over conventional fluoroscopy.

27. Draw clear distinctions between digital fluoroscopy, scanned projection radiography, and computed radiography.

28. Why does a digital fluoroscopic monitoring station have three video screens?

29. Dan, the clinical vice president, has been asked to research video systems that may be purchased by his fluoroscopy department to set up a DF system. (a) What limits the usefulness of conventional video in digital techniques? (b) Describe the difference between interlace and progressive modes of reading video signals. Which one is preferred and why?

30. Cheryl, the fluoroscopy radiograper, has produced a digital fluoroscopic image in the 512-by-512 matrix mode. The speed with which it can be acquired, processed, and transferred to an output device is about 32 images per second. However, higher spatial resolution is required, so the 1024-by-1024 mode is requested. How will this affect data transfer time?

31. Micah, a CV technologist, is using a technique that helps him to take advantage of changing contrast media during the time of the exam; it requires no special demands on the high-voltage generator. Carla, another CV technologist, uses two different x-ray beams alternately to provide a subtraction image resulting from differences in photoelectric interaction. Which technique is each using? Offer advantages and disadvantages of each.

32. Micah uses image integration as part of his procedure. What mode must he be using? What is image integration? What advantage does it offer? What disadvantage does it introduce?

33. Micah discovers that his initial mask image was inadequate because of patient motion. What alternative does he have? What else could have caused an unacceptable mask image?

34. For the next patient, Micah will switch to TID mode. What is this? What is its principal application—can you predict what kind of patient he is to examine? Briefly describe the procedure he will use. What is its advantage over the previous mode? What is its main disadvantage?

35. Micah discovers that a subtracted image made in TID mode has a number of misregistration artifacts. How are these caused, and how can Micah fix this situation?

36. Describe how a latent image is made manifest in computed radiography (CR). What are the advantages and disadvantages of CR, as compared with conventional radiography?

37. Describe how a PACS system uses subtraction, edge enhancement, windowing, and highlighting. What other features can be used for careful visualization of precise regions of an image?

38. Explain how teleradiology and a PACS network operate. What impact does introducing a PACS system have on film storage?

CHALLENGE QUESTIONS

1. Eric has produced an excellent image with wide image latitude on a CRT console. However, the radiologist tells Eric that she prefers not to diagnose from a CRT console. She asks Eric to produce a film image from the one she sees on the CRT. How can Eric accomplish this? Identify and describe the process he will use.

2. This will be a student's first time assisting in a DF process. He has just discovered that the tube current is measured in hundreds of mA. "I think we've got the wrong part or something," he says. "Conventional fluoroscopy has tube currents of 5 mA or less. You'd better not use this one or you'll have a bit of a problem." Is this true? Has Dennis discovered a problem? If there is such a discrepancy, what will you do about such large currents?

3. During an inspection, an engineer informs Eric, a fluoroscopy supervisor, that although the DF system incorporates a three-phase generator, the interrogation and extinction times are a little less than 2 seconds each. Is this good news or bad? In the course of your answer, explain what interrogation and extinction times are.

4. Use the images below as aids as you contrast and list steps in both mask-mode DF and time-interval difference studies.

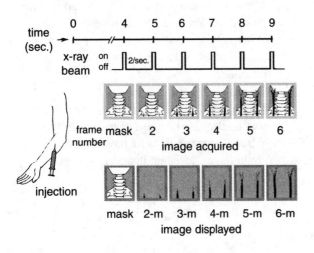

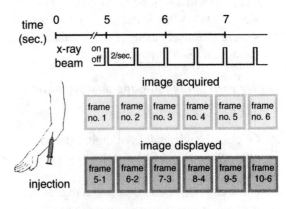

CHAPTER 29

Computed Tomography

1. Label the major components of a CT scanner system in the illustration below. Refer to this drawing as you summarize, on a separate sheet of paper, how a CT scanner system works.

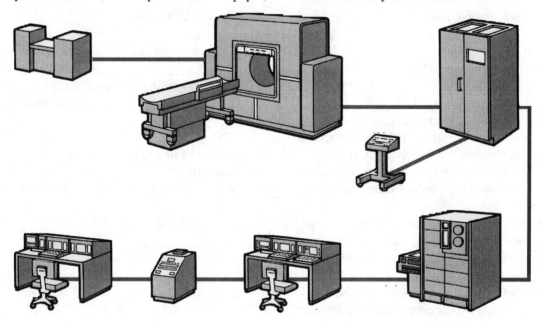

Circle the correct answer to each of the following.

2. A CT scan results in:
   a. an image that is parallel with the long axis of the body.
   b. sagittal and coronal images.
   c. a transverse (axial) image that is perpendicular to the long axis of the body.
   d. a transverse (axial) image that is parallel to the long axis of the body.

3. In computed tomography, when the source-detector assembly makes one sweep, or translation, across the patient, the internal structures of the body attenuate the x-ray beam according to their:
   a. mass densities and atomic numbers.
   b. radionuclide uptake.
   c. interface reflectivity.
   d. screen-film reception.

4. In its simplest form, a CT scanner consists of:
   a. an x-ray source emitting a finely collimated x-ray beam and an image-intensifier tube.
   b. a single detector, x-ray beam, and a film-screen combination.
   c. an x-ray source and a single detector, both moving synchronously in a translate-rotate mode.
   d. an x-ray source and a single detector, both stationary for correspondence with the screen-film receptor.

5. With the fan beam:
   a. a bow-tie filter is not needed to equalize the radiation intensity reaching the detector array.
   b. a disadvantage is increased scatter radiation.
   c. a pencil-sized x-ray beam is used.
   d. all of the above.

6. Third-generation scanners:
   a. involve the x-ray tube and detector array rotating concentrically around each other.
   b. can produce an image in as little as 3 seconds.
   c. use a curvilinear array containing many detectors and a fan beam that result in a constant source-to-detector path length.
   d. use a fan beam and a detector array, but only the fan beam views the patient at all times.

7. Post-patient collimation:
   a. determines the thickness of the tissue slice that is imaged.
   b. cannot take the place of a radiographic grid in conventional radiographic exams.
   c. determines the sensitivity profile.
   d. allows for better x-ray beam collimation to reduce the effect of scatter radiation.

8. In the fourth-generation CT scanners:
   a. there are many ring artifacts.
   b. both the x-ray source and the detector assembly rotate.
   c. radiation detection is accomplished through a fixed circular array of detectors.
   d. all of the above.

9. Fourth-generation CT scanners:
   a. use a fixed detector array.
   b. result in a constant beam path from the source to all detectors.
   c. do not allow each detector to be calibrated during each scan.
   d. all of the above.

10. The spatial resolution of a CT scanner is expressed as the:
    a. high-contrast edge (HCE).
    b. modulation transfer function (MTF).
    c. edge response function (ERF).
    d. none of the above.

11. For CT scanners, the number of line pairs per unit length is:
    a. the ratio of the image to the object.
    b. called the spatial frequency and is expressed in lp/cm.
    c. the opposite of the limiting resolution.
    d. none of the above.

12. In CT scanning, the x-ray linear attenuation coefficient is:
    a. the absorption of x-rays in tissue.
    b. a function of x-ray energy and the atomic number of the tissue.
    c. also determined by the mass density of the body part.
    d. all of the above.

Fill in the blanks below.

13. Third-generation CT scanners operate in the _____ mode with a fan x-ray beam-multiple detector array revolving _____ around the patient.

14. The _____ array is characteristic of first- and second-generation CT scanners; the _____ array is used in third- and fourth-generation units.

15. Ring artifacts can occur in _____ scanners because each detector views an _____ of anatomy during each scan.

16. The principal disadvantage of fourth-generation CT scanners is _____.

17. In the Toshiba design for a fourth-generation scanner, the x-ray source _____ and the stationary detector array _____.

18. _____ is a principal cause of CT scanner malfunction.

19. Rotate-only CT scanners operate with either a _____ or a _____ x-ray beam.

20. Modern CT scanners use multiple detectors in an array number up to _____ in two general classifications: _____ and _____.

21. _____ is the current crystal of choice for scintillation detectors.

22. In CT scanning, the prepatient collimator on the tube housing limits the _____ and thereby determines the _____ and _____. The postpatient collimator restricts the _____.

23. Tissue volume is determined by multiplying _____ by _____ of the CT slice. The diameter of the reconstructed image is the _____.

24. Each pixel is displayed on a video monitor as a level of _____ and on the photographic image as a level of _____.

25. Characteristics with numerical measurements of CT image quality include
_____,
_____,
_____, and
_____.

26. The important measures of scanner performance that can be evaluated with phantoms are _____,
_____, and
_____.

Indicate whether the following are true or false.

27. T F The time between the end of a scan and the appearance of an image is called the reconstruction time.

28. T F An array processor is slower than a microprocessor for image reconstruction.

29. T F A pixel is a two-dimensional representation of a corresponding tissue volume, known as a voxel.

30. T F The numerical information contained in a pixel is a CT number or Hounsfield unit.

31. T F With a CT scanner, the larger the pixel size and the lower the subject contrast, the higher the spatial resolution.

32. T F In simplistic terms, the MTF is the faithful reproduction of the image from the object.

33. T F The absolute object size that can be resolved by a scanner is equal to one third the reciprocal of the spatial frequency of the limiting resolution.

34. T F Increasing spatial frequency means better resolution of smaller objects.

Calculate the following problems on a separate sheet of paper.

35. Compute the pixel size for the following characteristics of a CT scanner used for brain scans.
   a. field of view 24 centimeters, 120-by-120 matrix
   b. field of view 32 centimeters, 512-by-512 matrix
   c. field of view 27 centimeters, 512-by-512 matrix

36. A CT scanner is said to be capable of 2 lp/cm resolution. What size object does this represent?

*Answer each of the following on a separate
sheet of paper.*

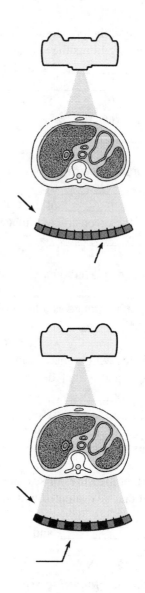

37. Use the figure on the right to explain why
    overall detection efficiency of a scintillation
    detector array is approximately equal to that
    of the gas detector array.

38. In computed tomography, how does the
    superimposition of the projections occur?

39. Describe differences in the operator's console
    and the physician's viewing console. How do
    physical differences reflect differences in
    function? Describe, for instance, how the
    operator can program for contiguous slices,
    intermittent slices, or spiral scanning.

40. Write the formula used to determine the
    value of a CT number and explain what each
    variable in the equation represents.

41. Use Table 29-1 to determine the approximate
    CT number and linear attenuation coefficient
    for each of the following.
    a. dense bone taken at 100 kVp
    b. gray matter taken at 150 kVp
    c. blood taken at 125 kVp

42. Describe factors that contribute to the loss in
    faithful reproduction with increasing spatial
    frequency in a CT scanner.

CHALLENGE QUESTIONS

1. Describe the capabilities a physician has with on-line computer software packages for CT images. If
   time allows, research into present and future technologies for CT scanning.

2. Claudia notices graininess on a CT image she has made. Her instructor attributes this graininess to
   noise. (a) What is "noise" in CT? What is it called in statistics? (b) In CT, what factors control
   noise? Which factor has the greatest effect in controlling (or contributing to) noise? (c) Reproduce
   the equation representing noise and interpret key symbols. (d) Describe how Claudia can check for
   system noise on a daily basis to prevent this from happening again.

3. CT scanners must be frequently calibrated so that water is consistently represented by CT number
   zero and other tissues by their appropriate CT values. (a) Describe the procedure involved in this
   calibration.

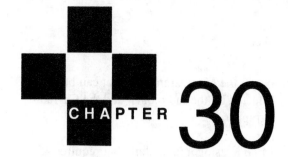

Circle the correct answer to each of the following.

1. The 180-degree algorithms:
   a. have the disadvantage of increased image noise.
   b. can produce breakup artifacts at high contrast interfaces when a cubic-spline interpolation algorithm is used.
   c. allow imaging at a pitch greater than one and improve sagittal and coronal reformatted views.
   d. all of the above.

2. The volume of tissue imaged is determined by:
   a. the examination time.
   b. couch travel.
   c. pitch and collimation.
   d. all of the above.

3. High z-axis resolution requires:
   a. 180-degree interpolation reconstruction.
   b. omitting thin-section collimation.
   c. selection of high pitch.
   d. a faster couch motion.

4. Limitation of spiral CT include:
   a. increased motion artifacts.
   b. decreased lesion detection.
   c. reduced z-axis resolution.
   d. all of the above.

5. The primary reason spiral CT reduces partial volume is that it:
   a. processes more data and more images.
   b. reconstructs at overlapping intervals.
   c. uses bigger x-ray tubes.
   d. increases with pitch.

Fill in the blanks below.

6. _____ estimates a value between two known values. _____ estimates a value beyond known values. During spiral CT, _____ of data is performed to reconstruct the image in any _____ plane.

7. Image reconstruction directly from a _____-degree segment will result in motion artifacts. _____ results in images free of such artifacts.

8. _____ is the relationship between the patient couch movement and x-ray beam collimation.

9. The section sensitivity profile for spiral CT widens as _____ is increased. It is also wider for _____-degree interpolation than for _____-degree interpolation.

10. Spiral CT is made possible by the use of _____ technology, which allows the gantry to rotate _____.

11. The principal advantage of spiral CT is the ability to image a large volume of anatomy in _____.

Calculate the following problems on a separate sheet of paper.

12. During a 360-degree x-ray tube rotation, the patient couch moves 9 millimeters. Section collimation is 6 millimeters. What is the pitch?

13. How much tissue will be imaged if collimation is set to 9 millimeters, scan time is 27 seconds, and the pitch is 1.5:1?

14. How much tissue will be image with 4-millimeter collimation, a pitch of 1.6:1, and a 16-second scan time at a gantry rotation time of 2 seconds?

Answer each of the following on a separate sheet of paper.

15. What are the two slip-ring designs used in spiral CT scanners? Describe their differences.

16. What are the functions of the three slip rings on a gantry?

17. Summarize how the design of the high-voltage slip ring differs among manufacturers.

18. Name the scan parameters that can be selected by the radiologist and the CT radiographer.

19. Mike is using a procedure that requires 45 seconds of imaging. However, the patient can hold her breath for only 20 seconds. What can he do?

20. Kate requires a longitudinally reformatted image. Discuss her display choices.

21. How does MIP reconstruct an image? What percent of the three-dimensional data points are used?

22. What is SSD? How does it work?

CHALLENGE QUESTIONS
■ ■ ■ ■ ■ ■ ■ ■ ■ ■ ■ ■ ■ ■ ■ ■ ■ ■

1. Mike wants to image some suspected lung calcifications. What Z-axis resolution should he specify? What other requirements must he meet in this procedure?

2. Allison uses spiral CT for examination of a calcified lung nodule; Bill uses conventional CT for the same exam.
   a.   How does the measurement of image quality, in general, compare between these two techniques? How does inplane resolution compare? Why?
   b.   Next, how will SSP and Z-axis spatial resolution compare? Why?
   c.   In Bill's image, the nodule was missed. How do you explain that? How can spiral CT avoid this?
   d.   Finally, explain how spiral CT uses multiplanar reformation.

Circle the correct answer to each of the following.

1. Quality control (QC):
   a. monitors radiology instrumentation and equipment.
   b. monitors patient-staff relationships.
   c. involves image interpretation and outcome analysis.
   d. all of the above.

2. The people on a diagnostic imaging QC team include:
   a. the QC radiographer.
   b. the radiologic engineer.
   c. the medical physicist.
   d. all of the above.

3. X-ray beam filtration:
   a. is the least important patient-protection characteristic.
   b. can be measured directly.
   c. is evaluated by measurement of the half-value layer (HVL) of the x-ray beam.
   d. none of the above.

4. The pinhole camera:
   a. is difficult to use and requires excessive exposure time.
   b. is the standard for measurement of effective focal-spot size.
   c. has significant limitations for focal-spot sizes less than 0.3 millimeter.
   d. all of the above.

5. Positive beam-limiting collimators:
   a. are used to measure focal-spot size.
   b. sense the size of the image receptor and adjust to that size.
   c. evaluate the accuracy of kVp.
   d. all of the above.

6. The distance indicator can be checked:
   a. visually.
   b. with an oscilloscope.
   c. with a tape measure.
   d. none of the above.

7. Exposure linearity is:
   a. the ability of a radiographic unit to produce a constant radiation output for multiple combinations of mA and exposure time.
   b. determined by using a precision radiation dosimeter to measure radiation intensity at various combinations of mA and exposure time.
   c. evaluated annually or after any significant change in the operating console or high-voltage generator.
   d. all of the above.

8. Jason evaluates screen film contact by radiographing a wire-mesh pattern. The image shows areas of blur. What might he do to correct this?
   a. Use a test phantom to spot the problem.
   b. Replace the felt or foam pressure pad under the screen; if this doesn't work, replace the cassette.
   c. Analyze and correct viewbox illumination.
   d. Measure and adjust light intensity using a photometer.

9. The assessment of linearity in CT:
   a. should show a linear relationship among the Hounsfield units.
   b. shows the electron density.
   c. should have a coefficient of correlation of 0.96% or more.
   d. all of the above.

10. When assessing quantitative CT, one should change:
    a. the CT scan parameters.
    b. the slice thickness.
    c. the reconstruction diameter.
    d. any of the above.

Fill in the blanks below.

11. Three steps involved in a QC program include _____, _____, and _____.

12. During collimation assessment, the misalignment must not exceed _____.

13. The spatial resolution of a radiographic imaging system is principally determined by the _____.

14. The test measurement of kVp should be within _____.

15. Exposure time should be within _____ of the indicated time for exposure times greater than 10 milliseconds. An accuracy of _____ is acceptable for exposure times of 10 milliseconds or less.

16. The entrance skin dose for an adult will average _____ per minute during fluoroscopy and will result in an average skin dose of up to _____ for most fluoroscopic examinations.

17. Most state statutes require that under normal operation the ESE rate shall not exceed _____ per minute. For angiointerventional procedure, the fluoroscope may be equipped with a high level control that will allow an ESE up to _____ per minute.

18. A measurement of the input exposure rate to the image-intensifier tube should be in the range of _____ per second.

19. In conventional tomographic quality control, agreement between the indicated section level and the measured level should be within _____ millimeters. When incrementing from one tomographic section to the next, the section level should be accurate within _____ millimeters, and constancy of _____ millimeter from one QC evaluation to the next should be achieved.

20. In CT quality control, a 20-centimeter water-bath should be imaged weekly, and the average value for water should be within _____ of 0. Furthermore, the uniformity across the image should not vary by more than _____ from center to periphery. Finally, the noise as determined by the built-in computational algorithm should not exceed _____.

Calculate the following problems on a separate sheet of paper.

21. Mark makes a photo-fluorospot image at 80 kVp in the 15-centimeter mode without a grid, as seen in Table 31-6 in your text. The measured ESE is 60 mR. What would be the ESE if the 30-centimeter mode was used?

22. Melissa makes a photo-fluorospot image at 90 kVp in the 20-centimeter mode without a grid, as seen in Table 31-6 in your text. The measured ESE is 55 mR. What would be the ESE if the 25-centimeter mode was used?

Answer each of the following on a separate sheet of paper.

23. List the ten steps involved in the JCAHO's "Ten-Step Monitoring and Evaluation Process" used for identifying and resolving problems with patient care in QA systems.

24. Suggest elements of a QC program for radiographic systems and the frequency with which each should be evaluated. Finally, what are the tolerance values selected for each?

25. Describe two accepted ways to evaluate exposure reproducibility.

26. Discuss the usefulness of photo-fluorospot images. What advantages do they offer?

27. You have been asked to monitor processor maintenance in your facility. (a) As a first step, identify everyday activities that tend to wear and corrode the mechanism of the transport system and contaminate processor chemistry. (b) What problems can these cause? (c) Outline preventive measures.

28. What is meant by (a) scheduled maintenance; (b) preventive maintenance; and (c) non-scheduled maintenance? What are the differences among them?

29. List steps to be done in processor monitoring.

CHALLENGE QUESTIONS
■ ■ ■ ■ ■ ■ ■ ■ ■ ■ ■ ■ ■ ■ ■ ■ ■ ■

1. Leslie is frustrated. She notices that the focal-spot sizes in several of the clinic's x-ray tubes do not match their advertised focal-spot sizes. Explain why vendors and manufacturers are permitted a substantial variance from their advertised focal-spot sizes. How great can these variations be?

2. A clinic calls on your expertise in establishing a system for evaluating automatic exposure systems. What will you include in your guidelines? Write these in a checklist format for display in the clinic office.

3. Your radiographic system proved so effective in question 2 that you are called back to provide guidelines for evaluation of each of the following in CT systems:
   • contrast resolution
   • slice thickness
   • couch incrementation
   • laser localizer
   • patient dose
   What will you include in each category?

4. Finally, as your last project for this clinic, list the scheduled processor monitoring program activities used to maintain QC. Include with each activity the procedures or items to be addressed and suggest a frequency for each activity.

Fill in the blanks below.

1. The three radiographic time periods in which artifacts occur are _____, _____, and _____.

2. The smoothness that occurs when cassettes do not have proper screen-film contact can _____ detail and is thus considered an artifact.

3. Foreshortening of a long bone on a radiographic image is an example of a _____ artifact caused by a warped cassette.

4. _____ buildup and _____ pickoff are caused by dirty or warped rollers. These artifacts usually appear as _____ areas of either increased or reduced optical density.

5. A dichroic stain appears as a _____ effect on the radiograph. Dichroic means _____ and can be applied to all chemical stains. These stains can appear in the following colors:

_____,

_____,

_____, or

_____.

6. Guide-shoe marks occur when the guide shoes in the _____ assembly of the processor are _____ or improperly positioned.

7. _____ leaks in the darkroom or within the cassette causes streak-like densities on the film.

8. A yellowish stain slowly appearing on the radiograph after storage time indicates a problem with _____ retention from the fixer. If _____ from the fixer solution remains after washing, silver sulfide slowly builds up, appearing yellow in the stored radiograph.

Answer each of the following on a separate sheet of paper.

9. How do artifacts interfere with the radiologist's diagnosis?

10. How did pi lines get their name?

11. Identify at least three ways fog can occur on a radiograph. Describe the appearance of each.

12. Name at least three examples (and the causes) of:

a. exposure artifacts

b. processing artifacts

c. static artifact patterns

CHALLENGE QUESTIONS
■ ■ ■ ■ ■ ■ ■ ■ ■ ■ ■ ■ ■ ■ ■

1. Create a matching exercise to quiz yourself on later. Mix types of artifacts and their causes in two lists, one with numbers, the other with letters. (Create the answer key as you go.) Later, this will make a thorough review for this test. Or, if you prefer, create a table of artifacts, sorted by types of causes (i.e., exposure, processing, and handling and storage artifacts). Then challenge yourself to fill in specific causes.

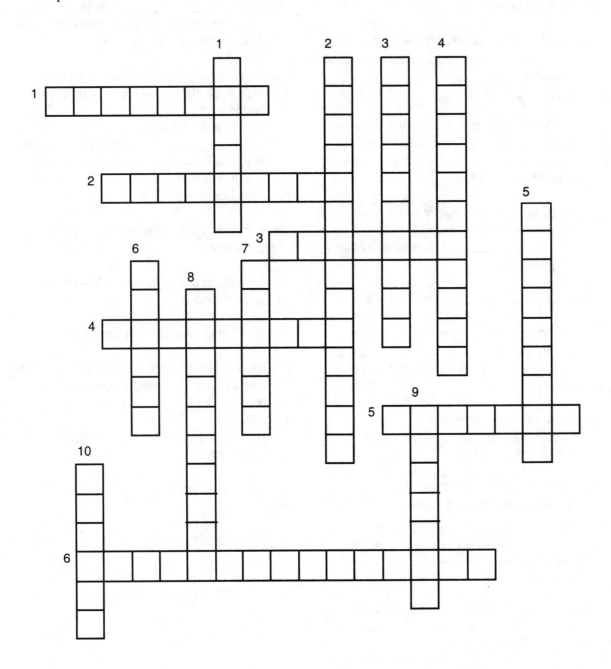

ACROSS

1. _____ fog looks like light or radiation fog and is usually a uniform, dull gray.
2. Warped cassettes cause _____ artifacts.
3. Dirt or chemical stain on a roller can cause _____ _____.
4. _____ fog and light fog look alike.
5. Chemistry not properly squeezed from the film creates a _____ effect.
6. When radiographers mix up cassettes, _____ _____ can occur.

DOWN

1. Dirty or _____ rollers can cause emulsion pickoff.
2. An artifact is any _____ on a radiograph that is not caused by superimposition of anatomy in the primary x-ray beam.
3. Cassettes that have not been checked for proper screen-film contact cause a _____ in the area of poor contact on the radiographic image.
4. _____-_____ sensitization is caused when irregular rollers cause pressure during development and produce small circular patterns.
5. Inadequate processing chemistry can result in a chemical fog called a _____ stain.
6. Crown, tree, and smudge, are three distinct patterns of _____.
7. If a patient is placed under the tube when the tube is not centered to the table or Bucky tray, _____ -_____ artifacts will occur.
8. Kinking or abrupt bending before processing can cause scratches that look like _____ marks.
9. A radiograph with patient motion appears blurred or _____.
10. Gelatin buildup can result in _____ deposits on the film.

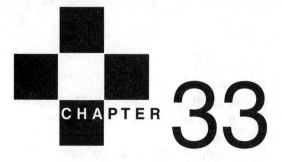

Human Biology

CHAPTER 33

1. Add a heading above each illustration below, indicating what process is being illustrated in each. Then, on a separate sheet of paper, describe these processes.

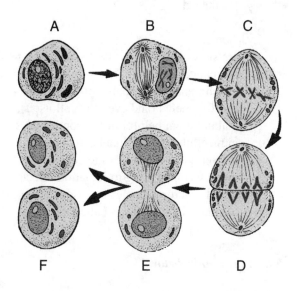

A   B   C

F   E   D

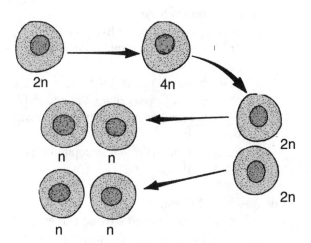

2n   4n   2n   2n
n   n   n   n

2. The list below shows some human responses to ionizing radiation. Identify each by writing E for early , F for fetal, and L for late effects.

_____ acute radiation syndrome

_____ childhood malignancy

_____ cytogenetic damage

_____ diminished growth and development

_____ extremity damage

_____ eye damage

_____ genetically significant dose

_____ hematologic syndrome

_____ leukemia

_____ life span shortening

_____ local tissue damage

_____ lung cancer

Circle the correct answer to each of the following.

3. Radiation hormesis suggests that:
   a. levels of radiation below 5 rad (50 mGy) provide a protective effect to the human body.
   b. moderate-to-high levels of radiation are needed to stimulate molecular repair mechanisms in the human body.
   c. levels of radiation below 7.5 rad (75 mGy) provide a protective effect.
   d. all of the above.

4. Robert Hooke:
   a. accurately described a living cell in 1673, based on his microscopic observations.
   b. first named the cell in 1665.
   c. showed conclusively that all plants and animals contain cells as their basic functional units.
   d. described the molecular structure of DNA in 1953.

5. Schneider and Schwann:
   a. accurately described a living cell in 1673, based on their microscopic observations.
   b. first named the cell in 1665.
   c. showed conclusively that all plants and animals contain cells as their basic functional units.
   d. described the molecular structure of DNA in 1953.

6. Watson and Crick:
   a. accurately described a living cell in 1673, based on their microscopic observations.
   b. first named the cell in 1665.
   c. showed conclusively that all plants and animals contain cells as their basic functional units.
   d. described the molecular structure of DNA in 1953.

7. Water:
   a. is the most abundant molecule in the body.
   b. is the simplest molecule in the human body.
   c. delivers energy to target molecules, thereby contributing to radiation effects.
   d. all of the above.

8. The mitochondria:
   a. digest macromolecules to produce energy for the cell.
   b. are called the workhorses of the cell.
   c. appear as large, bean-shaped structures inside the human cell.
   d. all of the above.

9. Ribosomes:
   a. are small pealike sacs capable of digesting cellular fragments, and even the cell itself.
   b. are helpful in the control of intracellular contaminants.
   c. are sites of protein synthesis, essential to normal cellular function.
   d. digest macromolecules to produce energy for the cell.

10. Lysosomes:
    a. are sites of protein synthesis, essential to normal cellular function.
    b. contain enzymes capable of digesting cell fragments (and even the cell itself), making them helpful in the control of intracellular contaminants.
    c. deliver energy to target molecules, thereby contributing to radiation effects.
    d. digest macromolecules to produce energy for the cell; sometimes called the workhorses of the cell.

Fill in the blanks below.

11. If radiation response occurs within minutes or days after the radiation exposure, it is classified as _____ effect of radiation, but if human injury is not observable for many months or years, it is called _____ effect of radiation.

12. Radiobiology is the study of the effects of _____ on _____ tissue.

13. Four types of macromolecules include _____, _____, _____, and _____.

14. Organic molecules are _____-supporting and contain _____.

15. The organic molecules include
_____,
_____, and
_____.

16. Water consists of _____ atom(s) of
_____ and _____
atom(s) of _____.

17. The chief function of carbohydrates in the
body is to _____.

18. RNA is found in the
_____ and in the
_____. There are two
types: _____ and
_____.

19. The two major segments of the cell are the
_____ and the
_____. The principal mol-
ecular component of the nucleus is
_____, which is the
genetic material of the cell. The nucleus also
contains some _____,
_____, and
_____.

20. A dose of approximately
_____ is required to pro-
duce a measurable change in any physical
characteristic of a molecule. The dose necessary to kill a human cell can be less than
_____.

21. In mitosis, during the synthesis portion of
interphase, the chromosomes replicate from a
_____ structure to a
_____ structure.

22. Mitosis is the phase of the cell cycle during
which the chromosomes
_____,
_____, and
_____.

23. Meiosis is the process of
_____ and
_____, and it occurs only
in _____ cells.

24. On the blanks below, enter a numerical percentage to show each item's percentage of
the atomic composition of the body.

_____ hydrogen

_____ oxygen

_____ carbon

_____ nitrogen

_____ calcium

_____ phosphorus

_____ sulfur

_____ trace elements

25. On the blanks below, assign a percentage to
each of these components in the molecular
composition of the body.

_____ water

_____ protein

_____ lipids

_____ carbohydrates

_____ nucleic acid

_____ other

Matching.

26. Match the following terms to their definitions.

_____ anabolism

_____ antibodies

_____ antigens

_____ catabolism

_____ enzymes

_____ homeostasis

_____ hormones

_____ metabolism

_____ proteins

a. constancy of internal environment in the human body

b. breaking down into smaller units

c. production of large molecules from small ones

d. the combined processes of breaking molecules into smaller units and producing large molecules from small ones

e. long-chain macromolecules that consist of a linear sequence of amino acids connected by peptide bonds

f. substances necessary in small quantities to allow a biochemical reaction to continue

g. substances that exercise regulatory control over some body functions such as growth and development; produced and secreted by the endocrine glands

h. substances that constitute a primary defense mechanism of the body against infection and disease

i. invasive or infectious agent

Labeling.

27. Label each of the components of the human cell shown in the illustration below.

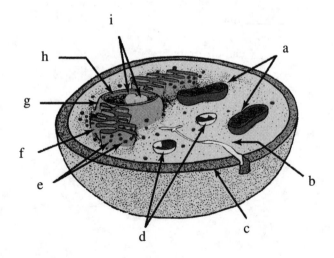

a. _____

b. _____

c. _____

d. _____

e. _____

f. _____

g. _____

h. _____

i. _____

Answer each of the following on a separate sheet of paper.

28. What happens when an atom is ionized?

29. What is the basis of the cell theory?

30. Write the generalized formulas for both a protein and a lipid.

31. Describe the structural composition of DNA and the manner in which the component molecules are joined. Be sure to include a discussion of the four organic bases and the double helix configuration.

32. How does RNA structure compare or contrast with DNA structure?

33. What is the difference between cell proliferation and cell division?

34. What is the difference between mitosis and meiosis?

35. Summarize the four subphases of mitosis and the four phases of the cell cycle seen in mitosis. What is the difference in how a cell biologist and a geneticist look at the cell cycle?

36. What is the purpose of meiosis? Describe the process. What is meant by "crossing over"?

37. Describe four types of tissue that can be classified according to structural or functional features that influence the degree of radiosensitivity of the tissue.

38. What are the two parts of an organ and of what is each composed?

CHALLENGE QUESTIONS

1. Create a table that compares the functions of proteins, lipids, water, carbohydrates, and nucleic acids (both DNA and RNA) in the body. Fill the table out partially, make a copy, and then complete both copies later as an excellent review for test preparation. Or, if you prefer, you may exchange one incomplete table with another student. This will make the required answers less predictable.

2. Create a diagram that shows the breakdown of an organ system into primary components and subcomponents.

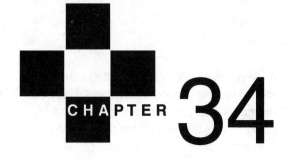

CHAPTER 34

Fundamental Principles of Radiobiology

1. Analyze the relationships represented by each curve in this illustration.

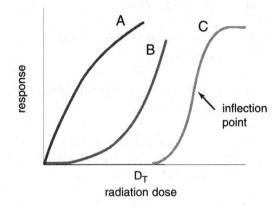

Circle the correct answer to each of the following.

2. Which of the following are true of radiosensitivity in living tissue?
   a. Stem cells themselves are not radiosensitive.
   b. The more mature a cell is, the less resistant it is to radiation.
   c. The younger the tissues and organs are, the more radiosensitive they are.
   d. As cell proliferation and tissue growth rate increase, radiosensitivity decreases.

3. When irradiating a biologic medium, the response (tissue damage) is determined by:
   a. the amount of energy deposited per unit mass.
   b. the MeV x-rays.
   c. heavy nuclei.
   d. neutron velocity.

4. Relative biologic effectiveness (RBE):
   a. represents radiosensitivity as a function of metabolic state.
   b. is the measure of the rate at which energy is transferred from ionizing radiation to soft tissue.
   c. is the ability of increased radiation LET to produce increased biologic damage.
   d. all of the above.

5. Dose protraction:
   a. represents a continuous and higher dose delivery rate.
   b. causes less effect because of the lower dose rate.
   c. causes greater effect because of the longer irradiation time.
   d. all of the above.

6. The OER:
   a. is the oxygen enhancement ratio.
   b. is greatest for low-LET radiation.
   c. decreases to approximately 1 for high-LET radiation.
   d. all of the above.

Fill in the blanks below.

7. The linear energy transfer (LET) is a measure of the rate at which energy is transferred from _____ to _____.

8. The LET of diagnostic x-rays is about _____, which is relatively low among all radiations.

9. The standard radiation, by convention, is orthovoltage x-radiation in the _____ range. Diagnostic x-rays have an RBE of _____.

10. It is suggested that the female can sustain approximately _____ more radiation than the male.

11. _____ are agents that enhance the effect of radiation. Examples include _____,

_____,

_____,

_____, and

_____.

12. _____ are compounds with molecules containing a sulfhydryl group such as cysteine and cysteamine.

Answer each of the following on a separate sheet of paper.

13. Summarize the Law of Bergonie and Tribondeau.

14. What are the differences between dose protraction and dose fractionation?

15. Define each of the following: (a) aerobic, (b) anoxic, and (c) hypoxic.

16. What is the principle behind the oxygen effect? Describe it. What is its numerical expression called? How is this calculated?

17. Under what level of oxygenation is tissue generally irradiated?

18. (a) What happens to an irradiated cell if the radiation dose is not sufficient to kill the cell before its next division (interphase death)? (b) How do you account for this? (c) What happens at the whole body level?

19. What is the difference in effectiveness ratio between the two types of chemical agents that can modify the response of cells, tissues, and organs to radiation?

20. Why haven't radioprotective agents found human application?

21. What is a dose-response relationship? How is it used in radiography?

22. What is meant by a linear, nonthreshold relationship? What is meant by a linear, threshold relationship?

23. Is the linear, nonthreshold dose-response relationship appropriate to use as a model for diagnostic imaging radiation protection guidelines? If no, explain why not. If yes, why?

CHALLENGE QUESTIONS

■ ■ ■ ■ ■ ■ ■ ■ ■ ■ ■ ■ ■ ■ ■ ■ ■

1. Create a chart that helps document the radiosensitivity of a biologic structure in terms of age over a lifetime.

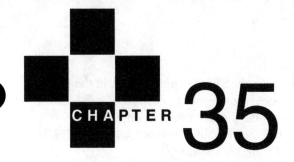

CHAPTER 35

Molecular and Cellular Radiobiology

1. What processes are illustrated in each of these figures? After identifying each process on the blanks below, describe each briefly on a separate sheet of paper.

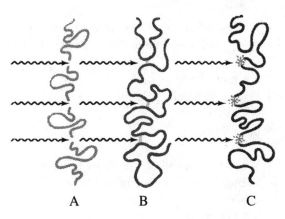

A   B   C

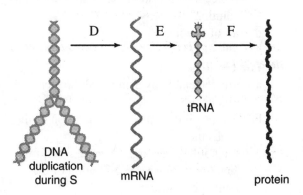

A. _____   D. _____

B. _____   E. _____

C. _____   F. _____

2. Match the following terms to their definitions.

_____ cross-linking

_____ free radicals

_____ in vitro

_____ main-chain scission

_____ point lesions

_____ in vivo

_____ point mutation

_____ viscosity

a. outside the body or cell

b. within the body or cell

c. breakage of the thread or backbone of the long-chain macromolecule

d. thick fluidity

e. process in which small, spurlike molecules extend off the main chain and attach to a neighboring macromolecule or to another segment of the same molecule

f. disruptions of single chemical bonds in a molecule that can result in minor modifications of the molecule

g. uncharged molecules containing a single unpaired electron in the valence or outermost shell

h. molecular lesions of the DNA that cause genetic mutations occurring as a result of radiation damage

Circle the correct answer to each of the following.

3. Main-chain scission:
   a. is the breakage of the thread or backbone of the long-chain macromolecule.
   b. results in the reduction of a long, single molecule into many smaller molecules.
   c. reduces not only the size of the macromolecule but also the viscosity of the the solution.
   d. all of the above.

4. Point lesions:
   a. are detectable by using analytic techniques.
   b. can result in a minor modification of the molecule.
   c. are not large enough to cause a cell malfunction—hence the derivation of the name point lesion.
   d. at high radiation doses, represent the cellular radiation damage process that results in the late radiation effects observed at the whole-body level.

5. Radiolysis of water results in the formation of:
   a. ions and free radicals.
   b. electrolytes.
   c. mineral waters.
   d. Na+ and Cl– ions.

6. Free radicals:
   a. recombine and therefore produce no biologic damage.
   b. can produce point lesions at some distance from the initial ionizing event.
   c. exist with a lifetime of less than 1 millisecond and therefore produce no biologic damage.
   d. are relatively unstable and can dissociate into smaller molecules.

7. According to target theory, cell death occurs only if the target molecule is:
   a. a free radical.
   b. ionized.
   c. inactivated.
   d. amplified.

8. According to the target theory, in the presence of oxygen:
   a. the indirect effect is amplified.
   b. the volume of action for low-LET radiation is unchanged.
   c. the effective volume of action for high-LET radiation is enlarged.
   d. minimum injury will be inflicted by either direct or indirect effect.

9. Fibroblasts are most radiosensitive during _____ and most radioresistant during the late _____.
   a. meiosis; M
   b. mitosis; cell cycle time
   c. mitosis; S
   d. mitosis; M

10. When human cells replicate by mitosis, the average time from one mitosis to another is called the:
   a. G1 phase.
   b. M phase.
   c. age-response time.
   d. cell cycle time.

11. At very high-LET values, even with mammalian cells, the cell survival kinetics follow the _____ model.
   a. multitarget, multi-hit
   b. single-target, single-hit
   c. single-target, multi-hit
   d. multitarget, single-hit

Fill in the blanks below.

12. It is believed that observable human radiation injury results from change at the _____ level. The occurrence of molecular lesions is categorized into effects on _____ and effects on _____.

13. Since the human body is an aqueous solution containing 80% _____ molecules, radiation interaction with _____ is the principal radiation interaction in the body.

14. When macromolecules are irradiated _____, a larger radiation dose is required to produce a measurable effect than with in vivo irradiation.

15. Proteins are manufactured by _____ of the genetic code from tRNA, which in turn is _____ from mRNA. The information carried by the mRNA is in turn _____ from the DNA.

16. _____ is the most important molecule in the human body because it contains the _____ information for each cell. _____ control the growth and development of the cell.

17. The three principal observable effects from irradiation of DNA are:
_____,
_____, and
_____. The latter two effects at the molecular level conform to the _____ relationship (any dose is expected to produce a tissue or cellular response).

18. When water is irradiated, it _____ into other molecular products. This action is termed the _____ of water.

19. When biologic material is irradiated in vivo, if the initial ionizing event occurs on a molecule, the effect is said to be _____. If the initial ionizing event occurs on a distant, noncritical molecule that transfers energy of ionization to the target molecule, the _____ effect has occurred. _____, with their excess energy of reaction, are the intermediate molecules.

20. When an interaction occurs between radiation and the target, a _____ is said to have occurred. When it occurs through indirect effect, the size of the target appears consider-

ably _____ because of the mobility of the _____.

21. In the presence of oxygen, the effect of low-LET radiation is _____.

Answer each of the following on a separate sheet of paper.

22. In what way is DNA synthesized differently than proteins?

23. Describe the five types of radiation damage that can occur in the DNA molecule.

24. Write (a) the equation for when an atom of water is irradiated and ionized. What happens to it then? (b) Write the formula for the action occurring when a negative ion (electron) attaches to another water molecule, and the formula that shows the HOH+ and HOH– ions dissociating into smaller molecules.

25. What is the final result of the radiolysis of water? How do the ion pairs and free radicals differ?

26. After radiolysis of water, how is hydrogen peroxide formed? Write and explain two equations for the formation of hydrogen peroxide.

27. Explain the role of a sensitive key molecule in the target theory. What role is DNA supposed to play?

28. When discussing the interaction between radiation and cellular components, what do we mean by the expression "a hit has occurred"?

29. Describe a threshold phenomenon.

30. When the multi-target, single-hit model was first applied to human cells, what was the observed extrapolation number? What hypothesis did that support? How has the concept of threshold dose affected this theory?

31. Explain the purpose of a split-dose technique. What do related experiments show?

32. Describe the age-response function.

33. Write the equation for the RBE of neutrons relative to x-rays.

CHALLENGE QUESTIONS
■ ■ ■ ■ ■ ■ ■ ■ ■ ■ ■ ■ ■ ■ ■ ■ ■

1. Create an illustration of point mutations of DNA that transfer the incorrect genetic code to one of the two daughter cells. Later, come back and write an explanation of your own diagram.

2. Using the target theory, create a model that aids in discussion and comprehension of the relationships among LET, the oxygen effect, and direct/indirect effect.

3. Summarize the two models for the radiation dose-response relationships for the cell. Write and explain the equation for each. Label each component in the equation.

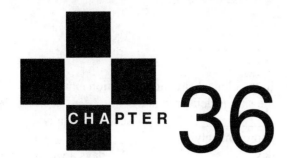

Early Effects of Radiation

CHAPTER 36

Circle the correct answer to each of the following.

1. The acute radiation syndrome:
   a. is the sequence of events that occur after low-level radiation exposure.
   b. leads to death within days or weeks.
   c. is completely reversible.
   d. all of the above.

2. The prodromal syndrome:
   a. consists of acute clinical symptoms that occur within hours of the exposure.
   b. is that time when the subject is free of visible effects.
   c. can be classified into three groups—hematologic, gastrointestinal, and neuromuscular.
   d. all of the above.

3. The manifest illness stage of acute radiation lethality:
   a. is characterized by malaise, lethargy, and fever.
   b. is characterized by possible vomiting and mild diarrhea.
   c. can be classified into three groups—hematologic, gastrointestinal, and neuromuscular.
   d. all of the above.

4. As the radiation dose increases from 200 to 1000 rad:
   a. the mean survival time decreases from approximately 60 to 4 days.
   b. death can result from the hematologic syndrome.
   c. mean survival time is dose dependent.
   d. all of the above.

5. In the GI syndrome, mean survival time:
   a. remains relatively constant at 4 days.
   b. is dose dependent.

   c. varies from approximately 3 days to a matter of hours.
   d. none of the above.

6. The skin erythema dose required to affect 50% of persons irradiated:
   a. is achieved only through grenz rays.
   b. is about 400 rad.
   c. is expressed as SED50.
   d. all of the above.

7. Grenz rays:
   a. are soft x-rays of 10 to 20 kVp.
   b. cause reversible epilation at high doses.
   c. are still the treatment of choice for ringworm.
   d. all of the above.

8. The principal effect of radiation on the hemopoietic system is:
   a. not affected by growth or maturation of the affected cells.
   b. called the pluripotential effect.
   c. depression of the number of blood cells in the peripheral circulation.
   d. all of the above.

9. A pluripotential stem call:
   a. produces granulocytopenia.
   b. can develop into several different types of mature cells.
   c. can destroy lymphocytes, granulocytes, thrombocytes, and erythrocytes.
   d. all of the above.

10. Cytogenetic damage to the stem cells:
    a. will be sustained immediately with high doses of radiation.
    b. may not be manifested for the time required for the stem cell to reach maturity as a circulating lymphocyte.
    c. causes immediate chromosome damage.
    d. all of the above.

11. Chromosome damage results in:
    a. chromatid deletion.
    b. ring chromosome aberration.
    c. reciprocal translocations.
    d. all of the above.

Fill in the blanks below.

12. At radiation doses above approximately _____ delivered to the total body, the signs and symptoms of radiation sickness may appear within a matter of minutes to hours.

13. Radiation doses in the range of approximately _____ produce the hematologic syndrome.

14. At a dose of _____, death is not expected, whereas above approximately _____, all those so irradiated would die unless vigorous medical support was available. Above _____, even vigorous medical support will not prevent death.

15. Acute lethality is measured quantitatively by the _____, the dose of radiation to the whole body that will result in death within _____ to 50% of the subjects so irradiated. For humans, this is estimated to be a dose of approximately _____.

16. Radiation-induced death in humans follows a _____, _____ dose-response relationship.

17. If death occurs because of _____ or _____ effects, the mean survival time will depend on the dose. If _____ cause death, it occurs in approximately 4 days.

18. In the clinical situation, radiation exposure of the skin is delivered in a _____ scheme, usually approximately _____ per day, _____ days a week.

19. The _____ and the _____ are considered to be the most radiosensitive cells in the body. Because their response is so immediate, the radiation effect is apparently a _____ one on the _____ themselves, rather than on the _____ cells.

20. Multihit chromosome aberrations after irradiation in G1 phase result in _____ and _____ chromosomes in addition to _____ fragments.

21. The skin erythema dose or _____, is _____ rad. A dose of _____ produces temporary infertility. A dose of _____ to the testes results in permanent sterility.

From Figure 36-1, shown here, estimate the doses in questions 22 through 24.

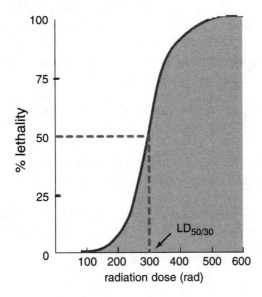

22. Estimate the radiation dose that will produce 75% lethality in humans within 30 days.

23. Estimate the radiation dose that will produce 8% lethality in humans within 30 days.

24. Estimate the radiation dose that will produce 91% lethality in humans within 30 days.

Answer each of the following on a separate sheet of paper.

25. Describe the three stages of the gastrointestinal (GI) syndrome. What is the cause of death in this syndrome?

26. A patient assigned to you has received acute radiation at a single dose of about 500 rad. When you ask if this is an accurate measure of the dose, no one knows for sure. It is estimated that it could have been as low as 300 rad and as high as 1000 rad. (a) Is there any predictable level of skin damage you can expect to encounter in this patient? If not, why not? If so, what might you expect to see? (b) What would change at higher doses?

27. Sketch and describe the progression of germ cells in both ovaries and testes, from the stem cell phase to the mature cell.

28. Create a chart that shows how radiation effects on the ovaries are somewhat age-dependent. When are the ovaries especially radiosensitive?

29. Summarize testicular damage from radiation. When are the spermatogonial stem cells most sensitive?

30. What doses can result in a reduction in the number of spermatozoa? How does this change with increased doses?

31. What are the first cells to become affected after exposure?

32. Compare the responses of granulocytes, platelets, and erythrocytes to irradiation.

33. Describe and illustrate single-hit effects produced by radiation during the G1 phase of the cell cycle. Then do the same for multihit chromosome aberrations.

34. Write the approximate equations for both single-hit aberrations and multi-hit aberrations? What kind of dose-response relationship is each associated with?

CHALLENGE QUESTIONS

■ ■ ■ ■ ■ ■ ■ ■ ■ ■ ■ ■ ■ ■ ■ ■ ■ ■

1. You are notified that a patient is being brought into the ER who is suspected to have the hematologic syndrome of acute radiation. This patient is not expected to live. (a) As a radiation expert in your hospital, you are asked to describe for ER personnel symptoms they may expect to have to treat. What will you include? (b) Personnel ask you to describe death in the hematologic syndrome. What will you add?

2. Partially recreate Table 36-2. Exchange with a colleague or wait several days before returning to your own table. Complete the missing entries.

3. Make a table comparing related doses and each of the three stages of the three syndromes associated with specific doses. Then add a fourth column, comparing the cause of death in each.

4. Jeff, 23, has received acute testicular irradiation of doses above approximately 10 rad (100 mGy). He is told to refrain for a while from procreation. Jeff asks why. What would you say? For how long should Jeff refrain? Will this eliminate risk?

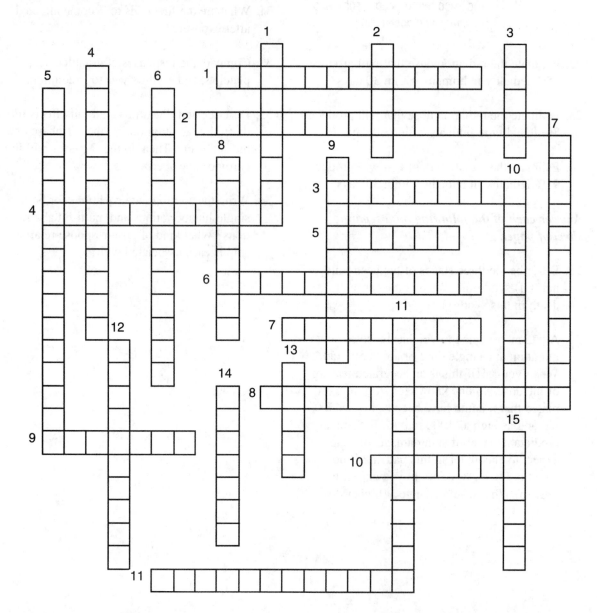

ACROSS

1. Platelets involved in blood clotting.
2. Syndrome produced by radiation doses extending from approximately 1000 to 5000 rad.
3. Syndrome of acute clinical symptoms that occur within hours of exposure and continue for up to a day or two.
4. Reduction in the number of immune response cells.
5. Intermediate layer of connective tissue in the skin.
6. Red blood cells that are the transportation agents for oxygen.
7. Loss of hair.
8. Rapid rise in scavenger cells.
9. Effect of cell death, resulting in a shrinkage, or reduction in size of tissue or organ.
10. Stem cells of the ovaries.
11. Scavenger cells used to fight bacteria.

DOWN

1. Sunburnlike reddening of the skin.
2. Syndrome represented by the sequence of events after high-level radiation exposure that leads to death within days or weeks.
3. Stem cells in the lowest layer of the skin that mature as they slowly migrate to the surface of the epidermis.
4. Ulceration and denudation of the skin.
5. Rapid decrease then slower decrease in scavenger cells.
6. Development of germ cells by both ovaries and testes, occurring at varying rates and times.
7. Study of the genetics of cells.
8. _____ illness refers to acute radiation lethality stage demonstrating hematologic, gastrointestinal, and neuromuscular symptoms.
9. Outer layer of the skin.
10. White cells.
11. Platelets.
12. Reduction in the white cells of the peripheral blood.
13. Soft x-rays once used to treat skin diseases such as ringworm.
14. Ovarian stem cells encapsulated by primordial follicles during late fetal life.
15. Period during which a subject exposed to radiation is free of visible effects.

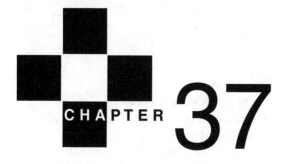

Late Effects of Radiation

1. The figure on the left shows the absolute age-response risk relationship model for radiation-induced cancer; the figure on the right shows the relative age-response relationship risk model. Label each of these illustrations; then use them to compare what these two models are asserting. Which one, if either, is more widely accepted?

Absolute Risk Model

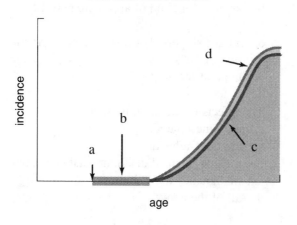

Relative Risk Model

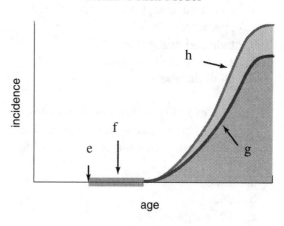

Absolute Risk Model

a. _____

b. _____

c. _____

d. _____

Relative Risk Model

e. _____

f. _____

g. _____

h. _____

i. Compare and contrast these models:

Circle the correct answer to each of the following.

2. Early effects of radiation exposure:
   a. are produced by high radiation doses.
   b. are the result of low doses delivered over a long time period.
   c. are experienced regularly by personnel in diagnostic imaging.
   d. none of the above.

3. Chronic irradiation of the skin can result in:
   a. calloused, discolored, and weathered appearance.
   b. tight and brittle skin.
   c. severe cracking or flaking.
   d. all of the above.

4. The risk of life-span shortening as a consequence of being a radiation worker produces how many expected number of days of life lost?
   a. 2100
   b. 980
   c. 12
   d. 1

5. Radiation-induced like-span shortening:
   a. is nonspecific.
   b. has no characteristic disease entities associated with it.
   c. does not include late malignant effects.
   d. all of the above.

6. Relative risk:
   a. involves estimating early radiation effects in large populations without having any precise knowledge of their radiation dose.
   b. is computed by comparing the number of persons in the exposed population showing a given late effect with the number of persons who developed the same late effect in an unexposed population.
   c. of 1 would indicate a risk of 50% higher in the irradiated group compared with the nonirradiated group.
   d. factors for radiation-induced late effects in humans range from 1 to 2.

7. The relative risk:
   a. is a dimensionless ratio.
   b. has units of number of cases/106 persons/rad/year.
   c. values range from approximately 1 to 10 cases/106 persons/rad/year.
   d. assumes a linear dose-response relationship.

8. Radiation-induced leukemia is considered to have:
   a. a latent period of 4 to 7 years.
   b. an at-risk period of approximately 12 years.
   c. an at-risk period occurring before irradiation of 10%.
   d. none of the above.

9. The effects of radiation in utero:
   a. are time-related.
   b. are dose-related.
   c. include prenatal death, neontal death, and malignancy induction.
   d. all of the above.

10. During the period of major organogenesis:
    a. skeletal and organ abnormalities can be induced.
    b. congenital abnormalities of the central nervous system can be observed.
    c. the result can be neonatal death.
    d. all of the above.

Fill in the blanks below.

11. The radiation exposures experienced by personnel in diagnostic imaging are low-_____ and low-_____.

12. At the time of the atomic bombings of Hiroshima and Nagasaki, approximately _____ persons were living in those two cities. Nearly _____ were killed from the blast and early effects of radiation. Another _____ persons received significant doses of radiation and survived. The remainder were unaffected because their radiation exposure was less than _____. The spontaneous incidence of leukemia in this population after high doses was _____ times that in the nonirradiated population. This suggests that the response is _____, _____.

13. Within 2 weeks of fertilization, the most pronounced effect of a high-radiation dose is _____, which is manifested as a _____.

14. Muller's studies show that the dose-response relationship for radiation-induced genetic damage is unmistakably _____, _____. They also showed that radiation does not alter the _____ of mutations but rather increases the _____ of those mutations that are observed spontaneously.

Indicate whether the following are true or false.

15. T F The relationship between life-span shortening and dose is apparently linear, nonthreshold.

16. T F The age at death in radiologists in the past has been less than that of the general population, but this difference has disappeared.

17. T F Contrary to popular belief, skin cancer does not begin with the development of a radiodermatitis.

18. T F The latent period in skin cancer is approximately 3 to 5 years and follows a nonthreshold dose-response relationship.

19. T F Exposure at an early age can result in an excess increase of cancer cases after a latent period.

20. T F The absolute risk model predicts that excess radiation-induced cancer is exponential, whereas the relative risk model predicts that it is proportional to the natural incidence.

21. T F Any dose of radiation, however small, to a germ cell results in some genetic risk.

22. T F Most radiation-induced mutations are dominant.

Calculate the following problems on a separate sheet of paper.

23. In a study of radiation-induced leukemia after receiving diagnostic levels of radiation, 300 cases were observed in 100,000 persons so irradiated. The normal incidence of leukemia in the United States is 150 cases per 100,000. If this normal incidence was assumed to occur in a completely nonirradiated population, what would be the relative risk of radiation-induced leukemia?

24. In a similar study to that described in the previous problem, 250 cases were observed in 100,000 persons. What would be the relative risk of radiation-induced leukemia in this case?

25. Thirty cases of skin cancer were observed in a certain population of 1000 persons. The incidence in the general population is 0.5/100,000. How many excess skin cancers where produced in the special study population?

26. The absolute risk for radiation-induced breast cancer is six cases/106 persons/rad/year for a 20-year at-risk period. If 100,000 women receive 150 mrad during mammography, what total number of cancers would be expected to be induced?

27. There are approximately 300,000 American radiographers, and they receive an annual effective dose of less than 10 mrem. What is the expected number of annual deaths because of this occupational exposure?

Answer each of the following on a separate sheet of paper.

28. Why are epidemiologic studies of people exposed to radiation difficult?

29. What conclusions can be drawn regarding radiation-induced cataracts? Include in your answering the following issues: (a) radiosensitivity of the lens of the eye; (b) latent periods; and (c) the dose-response relationship for radiation-induced cataracts.

30. How does the need for eye protection differ for radiographers as opposed to patients?

31. What is the unit of absolute risk? How does this differ from that of relative risk?

32. What might explain the difference in radiation experiences between American and British radiologists?

33. What kind of dose-response relationship was suggested in the British studies of leukemia in ankylosing spondylitis patients treated with x-ray therapy?

34. Why is analysis of radiation-induced leukemia easier than analysis of radiation-induced cancer?

35. Describe two population groups who have contributed an enormous amount of data showing that radiation causes bone cancer. Summarize findings.

36. Exactly what causes radiation exposure in uranium miners? How does smoking affect their relative risk?

37. Summarize the three situations the BEIR committee examined.

CHALLENGE QUESTIONS
■ ■ ■ ■ ■ ■ ■ ■ ■ ■ ■ ■ ■ ■ ■ ■ ■ ■

1. Give a brief history of thyroid radiation exposure in three patient groups. How were their situations different? similar? Summarize the results.

2. Describe the continuing controversy regarding the risk of radiation-induced breast cancer, and the implications of this controversy for mammography. What does tuberculosis treatment have to do with this controversy?

3. Discuss the following issues: (a) Which effects of irradiation in utero are the responses of greatest concern to diagnostic imaging? (b) When are radioisotope examinations of greatest concern in fetal development and well-being.

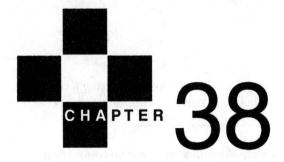

Health Physics

CHAPTER 38

Circle the correct answer to each of the following.

1. The first American fatality from radiation exposure was:
   a. Thomas Edison.
   b. Clarence Dally.
   c. Neils Bohr.
   d. Wilhelm Roentgen.

2. Maximum permissible dose (MPD):
   a. is the maximum dose of radiation that, in light of current knowledge, would be expected to produce no significant radiation effects.
   b. is the dose level at which the risk is zero.
   c. indicates the level at which the associated risks are higher than with other occupations, but reasonable in light of the benefits derived.
   d. all of the above.

3. Current DLs (dose limits) are:
   a. based on a linear, nonthreshold dose-response relationship.
   b. considered the level of exposure acceptable as an occupational hazard.
   c. are dose limits prescribed for various organs, as well as the whole body, and for various working conditions so that the lifetime risk from each year's occupational radiation exposure does not exceed 10–4 year –1.
   d. all of the above.

4. Effective dose (E):
   a. is expressed as "the weighting factor" and is LET dependent.
   b. is the basis for our dose limits.
   c. accounts for the relative radiosensitivity of various tissues and organs.
   d. all of the above.

5. Individuals in the general population are limited to:
   a. 1 mSv per year (100 mrem per year).
   b. 2.5 mSv per year (250 mrem per year).
   c. 5 mSv per year (500 mrem per year).
   d. the current DL.

6. If a barrier separates an x-ray examining room from an area occupied by the general public, then the shielding is designed so that the annual exposure in the adjacent area cannot exceed:
   a. 10 mSv per year.
   b. 5 mSv per year.
   c. 1 mSv per year .
   d. 0.25 mSv per year.

7. The severe potential response to radiation exposure in utero is:
   a. both time-related and dose-related.
   b. as low as reasonably achievable.
   c. the same as that for children and young adults of childbearing age.
   d. all of the above.

8. The biologic response to irradiation during the first 2 weeks of pregnancy is:
   a. congenital abnormalities.
   b. neurologic deficits.
   c. resorption of the embryo.
   d. all of the above.

9. During the period of major organogenesis:
   a. spontaneous abortion is no longer the major biologic response to irradiation.
   b. congenital abnormalities are associated with skeletal deformities early on.
   c. neurologic deficiencies are more likely to occur later in this period.
   d. all of the above.

10. When a radiographer's pregnancy becomes declared:
    a. the DL becomes 0.5 mSv per month.
    b. the supervisor should review the radiographer's previous radiation exposure history.
    c. the radiographer's dose must not exceed 5 mSv for the period of the pregnancy.
    d. all of the above.

Fill in the blanks below.

11. Three cardinal principles of radiation protection are _____, _____, and _____.

12. During radiography, the time of exposure is kept to a minimum to reduce _____. During fluoroscopy, the time of exposure should also be kept to a minimum to reduce _____.

13. As the distance between the source of radiation and a person increases, the radiation exposure _____ rapidly. This is calculated using the _____.

14. One TVL is the thickness of material that will _____ the radiation intensity to _____ its original value.

15. The value _____ is the approximate risk of death to those working in safe industries. The _____ are set to ensure that radiation workers have the same risk as those in safe industries.

16. The DL is specified only for _____ exposure. The current DL is _____ per week. Through the years there has been a _____ revision of the DL.

17. The effective DL is _____ of that for the radiation worker.

18. ALARA is an acronym indicating a concept to maintain radiation exposures _____.

Calculate the following problems on a separate sheet of paper.

19. A radiation source has an exposure rate of 300 mR per hour at a position occupied by a radiation worker. If the worker remains at that position for 40 minutes, what will the total occupational exposure be?

20. A nuclear power plant worker is assigned a task in an area where the radiation exposure level is 500 mR per hour. If the allowable daily exposure is 40 mR, how long may the worker remain?

21. A fluoroscope emits 5 R per minute at the tabletop for every milliampere of operation (5 mR/mA-minute). What is the patient exposure in a barium enema examination that is conducted at 2.2 mA and requires 3 minutes of fluoroscopic time?

22. An x-ray tube has an output intensity of 2.4 mR/mAs when operated at 70 kVp at 100-cm SID. What would be the radiation exposure 400 cm from the target?

23. A radiographer stands at the head of a patient and holds a barium cup for the patient to drink during a fluoroscopy examination which lasts 3 minutes. What is the radiographer's exposure during this procedure?

24. Suppose 400,000 radiation workers receive the dose limit (5000 mrem) this year. How many would be expected to die prematurely?

Answer each of the following on a separate sheet of paper.

25. Write the equation that shows the relationship between HVL and TVL.

26. Using Table 38-3, summarize how dose limits for occupational exposure have changed since 1902.

27. Jackie is a nuclear medicine technologist concerned with exposure to her hands. She often has her hands near a radiation source. How can she monitor this?

28. During an in-service training program, you are asked to discuss:
    a. the effective DL for staff members;
    b. environmental background radiation;
    c. which of the two above (a or b) is closer to realistic occupational exposure.

    What will you say about each?

29. Explain what is meant by "elective booking."

30. A pregnant patient undergoing KUB escapes detection and is irradiated. (a) What is the subsequent responsibility of the diagnostic imaging service? What follow-up should be in place? (b) What is the estimated fetal dose in this particular case? (c) Once this fetal dose is known—in any case—what should the referring physician and radiologist do?

CHALLENGE QUESTIONS

1. Make a chart of significant DL values, inserting headings to identify each, but omitting some values. Exchange charts with another student and complete each other's for a quick review. DL values you might want to include are:
   a. basic annual DL
   b. DL for the lens of the eye
   c. DL for other organs
   d. cumulative whole-body DL
   e. DL during pregnancy
   f. DL for the skin
   g. DL for extremities

2. Frank is using a collar-positioned monitor. Erica tells him he needs a change in procedure to estimate effective dose (E). (a) Why? (b) What should he do differently? (c) How would this change if he did no fluoroscopy?

3. A fellow student makes the following statement: "When normal protective measures are taken, it is nearly impossible for a pregnant radiographer to approach the fetal DL." Do you agree or disagree? Why?

4. Pete is the director of diagnostic imaging in a new facility. Suggest steps he should incorporate into the radiation protection program. Outline issues to be covered in each category.

5. Write a problem, including questions, in which another student must determine responses, effects of irradiation in utero, or protective measures for the pregnant radiographer. Examples of specific kinds of questions include the following:
   a. genetic effects of low-level x-ray exposure
   b. risks for cataracts or cancer
   c. effects of irradiation in utero at various, specific periods during the pregnancy

   Make your questions very specific, focusing on only one issue. Then exchange questions with another student and solve.

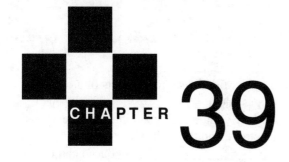

CHAPTER 39

Designing for Radiation Protection

Circle the correct answer to each of the following.

1. The total filtration of the fluoroscope:
   a. must be at least 2.5-millimeters aluminum equivalent.
   b. includes table top, patient cradle, or other material positioned between the x-ray tube and table top.
   c. can be estimated as adequate or not by measuring the HVL, if filtration is unknown.
   d. all of the above.

2. A primary protective barrier:
   a. is a wall to which the useful beam can be directed.
   b. must be lead that is not bonded to other materials (such as the sheet rock or wood used in the past).
   c. must have a lead shielding only in excess of 4 lb/ft2.
   d. all of the above.

3. Factors affecting barrier thickness include:
   a. distance between the source of radiation and the barrier.
   b. the use of the area being protected.
   c. the level of radiation activity and the pentrability of the x-ray beam.
   d. all of the above.

4. Dosimetry instruments designed for radiation detection can operate in the:
   a. pulse mode.
   b. rate mode
   c. integrate mode.
   d. all of the above.

5. Types of gas-filled radiation detectors include:
   a. thermoluminescence dosimeters.
   b. Geiger-Muller detectors.
   c. scintillation detectors.
   d. all of the above.

6. Ionization chambers are the only radiation detection devices used for:
   a. personnel monitoring.
   b. imaging film.
   c. survey for fields greater than 1 mR per hour.
   d. portable instruments.

7. Proportional counters are the only radiation detection devices used for:
   a. stationary instrument monitoring.
   b. assay of radionuclides.
   c. photospectroscopy.
   d. imaging.

Fill in the blanks below.

8. Complete the following table to show the minimum total filtration required for general-purpose diagnostic x-ray beams.

kVp Used	Required Filtration
70 (general)	a. _____ mm aluminum
50–70 kVp (x-ray tube)	b. _____ mm aluminum
below 50 kVp	c. _____ mm aluminum

9. In fluoroscopy, the Bucky slot cover must have at least _____ lead equivalent, and a protective curtain or panel should have at least _____ lead equivalent between the fluoroscopist and the patient.

10. In fluoroscopy, a cumulative timer interrupts the x-ray beam when the fluoroscopic time has exceeded _____ minutes.

11. The intensity of the x-ray beam at the table-top of a fluoroscope should not exceed _____ per minute for each mA of operation at 80 kVp. If there is no optional high level control, the intensity must not exceed _____ per minute. If an optional high level control is provided, the maximum table top intensity allowed is _____ per minute.

12. In designing a primary barrier, an adequate thickness for lead shielding would be _____ in a diagnostic room. As a rule of thumb, _____ of masonry is equivalent to 1/16 inch of lead.

13. Never direct the useful beam toward the control booth because it is _____.

14. Radiographers get most of their exposure during _____.

15. An area occupied primarily by diagnostic imaging personnel and patients is called a _____. The design limits for this area require that the barrier reduce the exposure rate in the area to _____ per week. An _____ area can be occupied by anyone, and therefore the maximum exposure rate allowed in such an area is _____. Consequently, a wall protecting an uncontrolled area must have nearly _____ more lead than one protecting a controlled area.

16. The greater the number of exams performed each week, the _____ the shielding required. This characteristic is called _____ and has a unit of _____ per week, which is abbreviated as _____.

17. The percentage of time during which the x-ray beam is on and directed toward a particular wall is called the _____ for that wall. The NCRP-recommended value for this unit of measure for walls is _____ and _____ for floors.

18. The gas-filled detector consists of a cylinder of gas and a _____ electrode. By maintaining a voltage between this electrode and the wall of the chamber, _____ produced can be collected and measured. The intensity of the signal from this gas-filled detector _____ in stages as the voltage across the chamber _____.

19. The overall result of scintillation detection is that a single _____ interaction produces a burst of _____, which produces a _____ emission, which is amplified to produce a large _____ pulse. The size of this pulse is proportional to the _____.

Indicate whether the following are true or false.

20. T F Every x-ray tube must be contained within a protective housing that reduces the leakage radiation to less than 75 mR per hour at a distance of 1 meter from the housing.

21. T F The source-to-image receptor distance (SID) must be accurate to within 2% of the indicated SID.

22. T F The average variation in radiation intensity for any given radiographic technique should not exceed 7.5%.

23. T F The radiation intensity is expressed in units of mR/mAs and has a maximum acceptable variation of 10%.

24. T F In fluoroscopy, the source-to-skin distance must be not less than 36 cm on stationary fluoroscopes and not less than 30 cm on mobile fluoroscopes.

25. T F Increasing the distance between the fluoroscopic tube and the patient results in increased patient dose.

26. T F Leakage radiation results when the useful beam intercepts any object so that some x-rays are scattered.

27. T F During both radiography and fluoroscopy, the table top is the single most important scattering object.

28. T F Dosimeters operate in the integrate mode and accumulate the signal, responding with a total exposure of mR or R.

29. T F The earliest radiation detection device was the photographic emulsion, which is still the primary means of radiation detection and measurement.

30. T F Geiger-Muller counters are limited to less than 100 mR per hour.

31. T F Scintillation detection devices are used for photo spectroscopy.

Calculate the following problems on a separate sheet of paper.

32. The output intensity of a radiographic unit at patient position is 250 mR for a specific examination. What will be the approximate radiation exposure 1 meter from the patient? 3 meters from the patient?

33. What percentage of the dose limit (100 mR per week) will be incident on a control booth barrier located 3 meters from the x-ray tube and patient? Assume the x-ray output is 6 mR/mAs and that the weekly beam-on time is 4 minutes at an average 100 mA.

Answer each of the following on a separate sheet of paper.

34. List radiation-protection designs mandated for x-ray equipment. How do these compare with those for fluoroscopic equipment?

35. List the nine radiation protection features of fluoroscopic equipment with a concise statement summing up each one.

36. Bill starts a company that will focus on designing protective barriers. What three types of radiation will he need to consider?

37. Why is lead rarely required for secondary protective barriers? What other materials are used instead?

38. Why is it usually desirable to position the x-ray machine in the middle of the room?

39. (a) List the three types of radiation detection devices other than film badges, briefly summing up their uses. (b) Next, list the three types of gas-filled detectors.

40. Label the figure below and use it as an aid as you explain the function of each component of a scintillation detector and summarize its use in general.

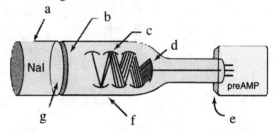

41. What are the uses of thermoluminescence dosimetry? Describe the basic steps involved.

42. What is a glow curve?

CHALLENGE QUESTIONS
■ ■ ■ ■ ■ ■ ■ ■ ■ ■ ■ ■ ■ ■ ■ ■ ■ ■

1. Why is the use of the area being protected of such principal importance in calculating the required protective barrier thickness? What is this factor called? Suggest guidelines for determining levels of occupancy of areas that may be adjacent to x-ray rooms.

2. Use the figure below to explain the principle of operation behind gas-filled detectors. In particular, describe the role of each of the following:
   - central electrode
   - region of recombination
   - ionization and proportion regions
   - Geiger-Muller region
   - region of continuous discharge

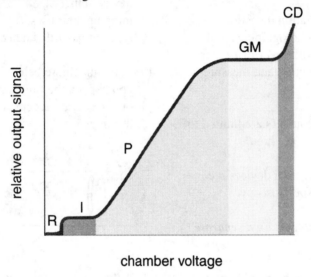

chamber voltage

3. You are a sales representative for a company that makes scintillation detectors. Answer the following questions about the scintillation process:
   - What kinds of diagnostic imaging equipment use these detectors?
   - What would happen if a 50-keV photon underwent photoelectric absorption in the crystal? What would happen if the photon underwent Compton scattering and 30 keV of the energy was absorbed?
   - What are the most widely used scintillation phosphors?
   - When used as a radiation detector, why are scintillation crystals enclosed in aluminum?
   - Why are scintillation detectors so useful as portable radiation detectors to monitor the presence of contamination and low levels of radiation?

4. Create a table to help you summarize, at a glance, each of the major aspects of radiation protection requirements for radiographic equipment. Then create a similar table to summarize radiographic protection requirements for each of the major aspects of fluoroscopic equipment as well. To make this more challenging, however, take the following steps: (1) Only partially fill in each table. Exchange these with another student. (2) With these new tables, give each a title to indicate which topic is being covered. (3) Complete each table and return to its original owner. (4) Check your partner's work, correcting and completing your original tables. (pp. 520–521)

CHAPTER 40

Radiation Protection Procedures

Fill in the blanks below.

1. The dose limit for imaging personnel is
   _____, but the actual
   occupational exposure of imaging personnel
   engaged in general x-ray activity should not
   normally exceed about
   _____.

2. _____ generally receive
   slightly higher exposures than
   _____ because the
   _____ receives most of his
   or her exposure during fluoroscopy and is
   usually closer to the radiation source and the
   patient during such procedures.

3. The highest occuaptional exposure of diagnostic x-ray personnel occurs during
   _____ and
   _____.

4. For the average fluoroscopic exam, one can
   assume an ESE of _____.

5. The estimate for GSD reported by the U.S.
   Public Health Service is
   _____.

6. In mammography, the use of grids increases
   patient dose by approximately
   _____.

7. Total glandular dose should not exceed
   _____ per view with non-
   grid screen film mammography, and it should
   not exceed
   _____ per
   view with a grid.

8. Two mammographic exposures result in a
   total glandular dose that is the sum of the
   _____ doses.

9. The exposure cord on a portable x-ray unit
   must have a length of at least
   _____.

10. Personnel monitoring is required when there
    is any likelihood that an individual will
    receive more than _____
    of the dose limit.

11. The personnel monitor offers
    _____ protection against
    radiation exposure.

12. The normal thicknesses for protective apparel
    are _____, _____, and
    _____ millimeter of lead equivalent.

13. Protective aprons for angiointerventional
    suites should be of the
    _____ type.

***Calculate the following problems on a separate
sheet of paper.***

14. An examination requires 1.5 minutes of fluo-
    roscopic x-ray beam time. If the radiographer
    is exposed to 300 mR per hour, what will be
    her occupational exposure?

15. A radiographer remains in the CT room at
    midtable position during a 25-scan examina-
    tion. Use Figure 40-2 to help you answer the
    following question. Assuming an exposure of
    0.1 mR per scan, what would be the occupa-
    tional exposure if no protective apron were
    worn?

16. With reference to Figure 40-3, estimate the
    skin dose from a lateral skull film taken at 70
    kVp, 20 mAs, with a radiographic unit hav-
    ing 3 millimeters aluminum total filtration.

17. The output intensity of a radiographic unit is reported as 3.2 mR/mAs at 100 centimeters SID. What is the intensity at 80 centimeters SSD?

18. The output intensity at 72 kVp and 75-cm SSD is 7.1 mR/mAs. What is the output intensity of 80 kVp?

19. The output intensity for a radiographic unit is 5 mR/mAs at 70 kVp and 80 centimeters. If a film is taken at 63 kVp, 200 mAs, what will the skin dose be at an 80-centimeters SSD? What would the skin dose be at a 90-centimeters SSD?

20. A fluoroscopic procedure requires 3 minutes at 90 kVp, 2 mA. What is the approximate ESE?

21. A fluoroscopic procedure requires 1.5 minutes at 90 kVp, 2 mA. What is the approximate ESE?

22. A radiograph is obtained at 70 kVp, 90 mAs and results in an ESE of 420 mR. If the tube potential is increased to 74 kVp and the mAs reduced to 45 mAs, the optical density will remain the same. What will the new skin dose be?

Answer each of the following on a separate sheet of paper.

23. During a class presentation, you claim that "the highest occupational exposure of diagnostic x-ray personnel occurs during fluoroscopy." A second student challenges you, saying that he believes the highest occupational exposure occurs during portable radiography. Who is right and why?

24. You become part of a committee assigned to review your facility's radiation protection procedures. One of the things you are warned about is that personnel engaged in angiointerventional procedures often receive higher exposrues than do those in general imaging practice. Why would that be?

25. At your next protection procedures review committee meeting, a representative from the mammography staff claims that personnel exposures associated with mammography are quite low. A radiographer who works in computed tomography challenges her, saying, "Personnel exposures in our part of the facility are the ones that are low." With whom do you agree? Why?

26. Why is the exposure of patients to medical x-rays commanding increasing attention?

27. Identify and discuss the usefulness of each method of estimating and reporting patient dose from diagnostic x-rays.

28. Describe several straightforward methods for estimating ESE in the absence of patient measurements.

29. What is the genetically significant dose (GSD)? What is the estimated GSD reported by the U.S. Public Health Service?

30. Your patient receives a chest exam at 110/3 kVp/mAs technique. What is this patient's ESE? mean marrow dose? gonad dose?

31. Write the expression for calculating GSD; identify each symbol.

32. Mrs. Wren has a mammogram. Why can the radiographer omit ESE when announcing values stated for patient dose? Why would adverse reactions in mammography be more closely related? Finally, how can the values stated for patient dose in mammography be misleading?

33. On the basis of skin dose, how does CT compare with other diagnosis procedures? How is the difference in delivery?

34. Write the formula for patient dose. Then explain what each component represents.

35. Describe a film badge. How does each component work? Why is it so important for pregnant workers?

36. Discuss advantages and disadvantages of a TLD monitoring device over film.

37. Describe pocket ionization chambers. How are they used? What are some disadvantages of using these items?

38. List data that must be included in a personnel radiation monitoring report.

39. A patient referred for an x-ray exam is not physically able to support himself. What will you do?

40. An unnecessary examination is selected. What can the radiographer and radiologist do? Identify examples of routine, unnecessary x-ray exams.

41. List the four concepts of patient shielding during x-ray examinations.

CHALLENGE QUESTIONS
▪ ▪ ▪ ▪ ▪ ▪ ▪ ▪ ▪ ▪ ▪ ▪ ▪ ▪ ▪ ▪ ▪ ▪

1. In your clinic, some staff members seem to find it necessary to wear more than one personnel monitor. Identify the only two times there might be a rationale for wearing two monitors.

2. Create a comprehensive list to be displayed in an exam room to aid in reduction of occupational exposure. Include and elaborate on each of the following:
   a. required length of exposure cord on a mobile radiographic unit
   b. personnel radiation monitor
   c. exposure data included in a personnel monitoring report
   d. thickness of protective apparel
   e. procedure for holding patients during an x-ray exam

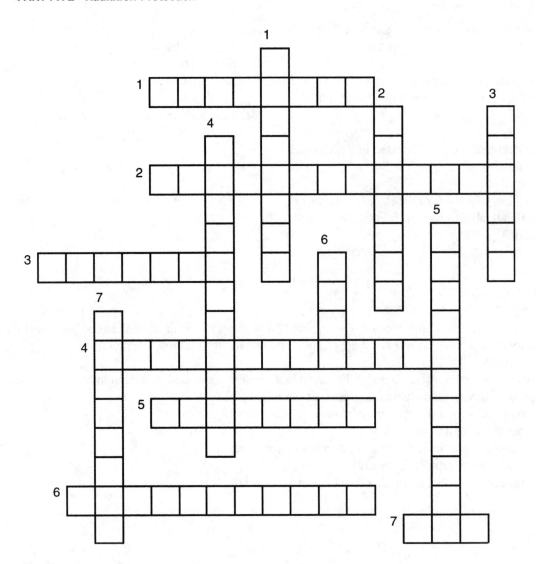

ACROSS

1. Proper unit for measuring exposure of occupational workers.
2. Proper unit for measuring radiation exposure.
3. Monitoring periods and associated exposure records must not exceed a calendar _____.
4. Biologic effectiveness of radiation energy absorbed. (2 words)
5. Term referring to radiation intensity in air.
6. The population gonad dose of importance is the _____ significant dose.
7. Unit of effective dose, used for radiation protection purposes; usually applied to occupationally exposed persons.

DOWN

1. Proper unit for measuring radiation dose.
2. The _____ monitor is used to measure the background exposure during transportation, handling, and storage.
3. One of the factors considered when computing GSD.
4. Procedure that gives diagnostic x-ray personnel one of the highest occupational exposures.
5. Exposure to the skin (ESE). (2 words)
6. Measures radiation energy absorbed as a result of a radiation exposure during patient examinations.
7. The GSD is a _____-average gonad dose.

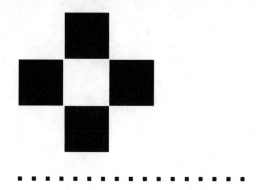

Math Tutor

Contributed by Quinn B. Carroll

Name_____

EXERCISE   1

Date_____

Working with Decimal Timers

CALCULATING TOTAL mAs VALUES

One of the first things you will learn in any radiographic imaging course is the relationship between milliamperage (mA) and exposure time (s) in producing a total mAs. The total mAs value is very important, because it directly relates to how dark the radiograph will turn out. The exposure time cannot be considered alone, nor can the mA, in controlling the *total* density of the resulting image.

A key point to remember is that mA is a *rate*. It tells us how many x rays are emitted from the x-ray tube per second, or how "fast" they are coming out.

The speedometer in your car measures a *rate* as well. It does not tell you what the end result of your trip will be, however. To determine when you will arrive in, for example, Dallas, you must also known how long you will be driving at that rate. That is, you must multiply the miles per hour (the rate) by the number of hours (the time) to find the total miles you will travel. It makes no difference whether you go 50 mph for 2 hours or 25 mph for 4 hours—the end result will be the same distance covered.

Likewise, whether the x-ray tube emits 1 million x rays per second for 1 second, or 0.5 million x rays per second for 2 seconds, the resulting total exposure to the film will be the same. As a radiologic technologist, your first concern is to produce adequate density on the film for a visible image. This depends on how "fast" the x rays are being emitted *and* how long the tube is left on. It depends on the mA multiplied by the time, or the *total mAs.*

Since many combinations of mA and time can be used to achieve the same total mAs, radiologic technologists must become skilled at computing these numbers, so they can adapt to different equipment and different situations. Some would argue that mAs conversion charts are often available on the wall in the control booth—all you need to do is look it up; but such charts are almost never found on mobile (portable) machines or in surgery, and often they do not match the equipment in the department.

Suppose you normally use 400 mA and 1/80 second for an ankle radiograph in the department and you are called to do a portable ankle radiograph using a mobile unit with a maximum of 300 mA available. It is a time-saving and repeat-avoiding skill to be able to quickly, mentally convert the total mAs value as 5 mAs, to be obtained at 300 mA, yielding a needed time of 1/60 second.

Such mental math should be second nature to every radiologic technologist. It is not as hard as you might think; it just requires practice. The drills that follow are designed to provide the practice needed to develop that skill.

This section first focuses on total mAs conversions using decimals (since most modern equipment uses decimal timers), followed by several drills on conversions using fractional times. Next, conversion of fractions to decimals and vice versa are reviewed. This is helpful because radiologic technologists often must adjust from equipment using decimal timers to equipment with fractional timers, and back.

On x-ray machines the most used mA stations are in multiples of 100. On the exposure timers the most used decimal times consist of two digits after the decimal, that is, they are "hundredths" (e.g., 0.25, 0.05). This provides an easy starting point for practicing decimal conversions:

all you must do to figure the total mAs is to get into the habit of moving the decimal point on the exposure time two places to the right in your mind's eye; then ignore the two zeros on the mA station while multiplying. You are simply cancelling the hundreds with hundredths.

For example, find the total mAs for the following:

200 mA at 0.05 s

Moving the time decimal two places to the right, you have 5. Ignoring the two zeros on the mA, you have 2. This is simply 2 x 5, or 10 mAs.

Think of 300 mA at 0.080 seconds (ignore the last zero) as simply 3 x 8, or 24 mAs; and 100 mA at 0.025 seconds is 1 x 2.5, or 2.5 mAs. Examine these three examples carefully before going on.

If three digits follow the decimal, as in 0.008 seconds, you will use the same method but will still be dealing with a decimal in multiplying. For example, 200 mA at 0.008 seconds should be thought of as 2 x 0.8, for a total of 1.6 mAs. There are relatively few time settings on x-ray machines in the thousandths like this.

If there is only one digit behind the decimal point, such as 0.4 seconds, again move the decimal two places over. This time it will add a zero to your time number, so you will consider 0.4 as 40. Hence, 200 mA at 0.4 seconds will be thought of as 2 x 40, for a total of 80 mAs. Think of 100 mA at 0.2 seconds as 1 x 20; and 500 at 0.8 is 5 x 80, or 400 mAs.

If there are two nonzero numbers after the decimal, you will simply ignore the decimal. That is, 0.16 will be thought of as 16. Three positive numbers after the decimal keep the decimal in the problem: 300 mA at 0.125 is thought of as 3 x 12.5. Multiply 3 x 12 first for 36; then add 3 halves for a total of 37.5 mAs.

On most x-ray machines a repeating pattern is available in the time settings. Note for example the following times from one common brand of equipment, in order: .002 s, .003, .004, .005, .007, .01, .015, .02, .025, .03, .035, .05, .07, .1, .15, .2, .25, .3, .35, .5, .7, 1, 2, and 4. One pattern you will see is that between a 5 and a 1 there is always a 7. Table MT-1 simply reorganizes these numbers so you can see the repetition.

Consider the recurring sevens on this machine: .007, .07, and .7. Once you become familiar with mAs values at, say, the .07 time, you can easily do figuring with the other two "seven" times by simply moving the decimal point in your answer:

As previously discussed, you should be thinking of 200 mA at 0.07 seconds as 2 x 7, for 14 mAs total.

Think of 200 mA at 0.007 also as 2 x 7, only with a decimal added in the answer: 1.4 mAs.

Think of 200 mA at 0.7 seconds as 2 x 7 with a zero added, or 2 x 70, for 140 mAs.

TABLE MT-1 Decimal exposure times available on typical x-ray machine

	.01	.1	1
	.015	.15	
.002	.02	.2	2
	.025	.25	
.003	.03	.3	
	.035	.35	
.004			4
.005	.05	.5	
.007	.07	.7	

The act of writing down something helps you to remember it, even if you never refer again to your note. An excellent exercise for memorizing mAs values on a particular machine is to jot down the available times in just the format shown in Table MT-1. Write at the top the mA station you use most, perhaps 200 or 300 mA, and then write to the side of each time setting the total mAs produced at that mA station. When you are through, look at the pattern of mAs values. Note the repeating patterns.

Do the following part of this exercise on your own, calculating total mAs values mentally. If you get stuck on one, review the instructions above for help. Do not check your answers after each question; do the whole exercise first, figuring the problems in your head and then writing the answer down. When completed, check your answers and correct those you missed.

To benefit from this drill, *do not figure your calculations on paper—do them mentally*, and then write your answer in. Do not look at the answers after trying each question; try the entire exercise, writing your answers down, and then check all your answers with the Math Tutor Answer Key.

	mA	x	Time(s)	=	mAs
1	100	@	0.05	=	
2	100	@	0.064	=	
3	100	@	0.019	=	
4	100	@	0.125	=	
5	100	@	0.8	=	
6	200	@	0.02	=	
7	200	@	0.05	=	
8	200	@	0.064	=	
9	200	@	0.15	=	
10	200	@	0.015	=	
11	200	@	0.125	=	
12	200	@	0.3	=	
13	200	@	0.4	=	
14	200	@	0.008	=	
15	200	@	0.003	=	

	mA	x	Time(s)	=	mAs		mA	x	Time(s)	=	mAs
16	200	@	0.035	=		36	400	@	0.07	=	
17	300	@	0.03	=		37	400	@	0.16	=	
18	300	@	0.07	=		38	400	@	0.016	=	
19	300	@	0.7	=		39	400	@	0.33	=	
20	600	@	0.05	=		40	400	@	0.8	=	
21	600	@	0.25	=		41	400	@	0.7	=	
22	600	@	0.8	=		42	400	@	0.007	=	
23	600	@	0.006	=		43	500	@	0.08	=	
24	600	@	0.008	=		44	500	@	0.03	=	
25	300	@	0.1	=		45	500	@	0.2	=	
26	300	@	0.3	=		46	500	@	0.7	=	
27	300	@	0.04	=		47	500	@	0.007	=	
28	300	@	0.015	=		48	500	@	0.125	=	
29	300	@	0.25	=							
30	300	@	0.025	=							
31	300	@	0.15	=							
32	300	@	0.006	=							
33	300	@	0.004	=							
34	400	@	0.01	=							
35	400	@	0.04	=							

Be sure to review those problems you answered incorrectly, going back to the instructions just given.

EXERCISE   2

Working with Fractional Timers

THE 100 mA STATION

....

Exposure timers reading in fractions are somewhat more difficult than decimals to work mentally, yet they also tend to follow patterned sequences, and with just a few memorized pairs of numbers you can do most of them.

For this unit we will practice drills for each mA station separately. At each mA station, certain pairs of numbers always go together. For example, at the 100 mA station, fives and twos always go together:

100 mA at 1/2 s = 50 mAs
100 mA at 1/5 s = 20 mAs
100 mA at 1/50 s = 2 mAs
100 mA at 1/20 s = 5 mAs

and so on. Zeros may be added or decimal points moved, but a time fraction using a 5 will always result in a total mAs involving a 2 and vice versa.

At the 100 mA station, the following pairs of numbers always go together—commit them to memory before you go on. The best way to memorize them is to get a study partner to drill you as if it were an oral test.

3 and 33
4 and 25
5 and 2
6 and 16
7 and 15
8 and 12

Note that these numbers are rounded up or down to make it easier to memorize them. For example, 100 mA

at 1/6 second is actually 16.67 mAs and would normally round up to 17. However, it is easier to remember 16, because the mind associates the sixes in 1/6 and 16 together. The results are close enough for any radiographic technique. Likewise, 1/8 of 100 is actually 12.5, and 1/12 of 100 is actually 8.33. In these units on fractions, all answers will be rounded out. The goal is for you to *mentally* derive a good estimated technique, not an exact answer.

Memorizing the pairs of numbers will not tell you where to put any decimal points—you will have to learn that by practice.

It is important to solve these problems mentally, not on paper. After you have completed this entire exercise, check your answers and review those you missed.

	mA	x	Time(s)	=	mAs
1	100	@	1/2	=	
2	100	@	1/20	=	
3	100	@	1/50	=	
4	100	@	1/5	=	
5	100	@	1/8	=	
6	100	@	1/80	=	
7	100	@	1/12	=	
8	100	@	1/120	=	
9	100	@	1/7	=	
10	100	@	1/15	=	
11	100	@	1/40	=	
12	100	@	1/3	=	
13	100	@	1/30	=	
14	100	@	1/6	=	
15	100	@	1/60	=	
16	100	@	2/3	=	

EXERCISE   3

Working with Fractional Timers

THE 200 mA AND 50 mA STATIONS

....

    Having memorized the number pairs for the 100 mA station, you can figure the total mAs for most time settings at the 200 mA station simply by doubling the answer you would get at 100 mA. For example, once it becomes second nature to you that 100 mA at 1/60 second is 1.7 mAs, whenever you see 200 mA at 1/60 second you can simply double 1.7 in your mind for a total of 3.4 mAs.

    In a similar fashion you can cope with the 50 mA station: simply cut the answer you would get at the 100 mA station in half. If 100 mA at 1/30 second is 3.3 mAs, 50 mA at 1/30 second will be approximately 1.6 or 1.7 mAs.

    Practice these conversions for typical fractions in this exercise. Carefully correct and review your answers with the Math Tutor Answer Key after completing the entire exercise.

	mA	x	Time(s)	=	mAs
1	200	@	1/8	=	
2	50	@	1/20	=	
3	200	@	1/5	=	
4	200	@	1/50	=	
5	50	@	1/8	=	
6	200	@	1/80	=	
7	200	@	1/12	=	
8	200	@	1/120	=	
9	50	@	1/12	=	
10	50	@	1/120	=	
11	50	@	1/7	=	
12	200	@	1/15	=	
13	200	@	1/40	=	
14	50	@	1/3	=	
15	50	@	1/30	=	
16	200	@	1/3	=	
17	200	@	1/30	=	
18	200	@	1/6	=	
19	200	@	1/60	=	
20	200	@	2/3	=	
21	50	@	1/6	=	
22	50	@	1/60	=	
23	50	@	1/80	=	
24	200	@	1/7	=	

Working with Fractional Timers

THE 300 mA STATION

The 300 mA station is an odd number and produces its own unique number pairs when a fractional timer is used. For example, at the 300 mA station, fives and sixes always go together: 1/5 second yields 60 mAs total, whereas 1/6 second produces 50 mAs. The following pairs of numbers always go together when using 300 mA. Commit these to memory, drilling with a study partner if you can:

5 and 6
15 and 20
12 and 25

Other combinations can be made, but these three pairs are very common. For other times, such as 1/8 second or 1/7 second, it is easier to simply use the paired number you memorized for the 100 mA station and then triple that number. Here are some examples:

300 mA at 1/7 s   Remember that at the 100 mA station, sevens always pair with fifteens. One seventh of 100 is about 15. So think of this as:

= 3 sets of 15
= approx. 45 mAs

300 mA at 1/8 s   Remember that at the 100 mA station, eights always pair with twelves. So think of this as:

= 3 sets of 12
= approx. 36 mAs

With these tips and with the previous exercises completed, you should be able to figure most mAs values for the 300 mA station in your head.

Proceed to solve the following problems mentally and write only your answer down. Then check and review your answers using the answers in the Math Tutor Answer Key.

	mA	x	Time(s)	=	mAs
1	300	@	1/5	=	
2	300	@	1/6	=	
3	300	@	1/50	=	
4	300	@	1/60	=	
5	300	@	1/20	=	
6	300	@	1/2	=	
7	300	@	1/15	=	
8	300	@	1/12	=	
9	300	@	1/120	=	
10	300	@	1/25	=	
11	300	@	1/4	=	
12	300	@	1/40	=	
13	300	@	1/8	=	
14	300	@	1/80	=	
15	300	@	1/7	=	
16	300	@	1/30	=	

Name_____

Date_____

Working with Fractional Timers

THE 400, 500, AND 600 mA STATIONS

....

Number pairs can also be made for these higher (400, 500, and 600) mA stations, but once you become comfortable with fractions at those stations up to 300 mA, it would be unnecessary. For the 600 mA station, the total mAs values learned at the 300 mA station can simply be doubled. The same thing can be done with the 400 mA station, doubling the results from the 200 mA station.

Further, any of these can be solved by going back to the number pairs you memorized for the 100 mA station. Whenever you get stuck, use this approach of solving for the 100 mA station and then multiplying the result by the first digit of the mA. As an example, when you see:

500 mA at 1/20 s   You may recognize right away that the answer is 25 mAs. Or, you may mentally remove a zero from both the mA and the time, yielding

    = 50 at 1/2 s

    = 25 mAs

        But *if you are not comfortable* with these other approaches, *go back to the 100 mA number pairs* you memorized. Remembering that 2 and 5 always go together and that 1/20 of 100 is 5, think of this problem as:

500 mA at 1/20 s

    = 5 *sets* of 5

    = 25 mAs

Proceed to the following questions, and then check and review your answers using the Math Tutor Answer Key.

	mA	x	Time(s)	=	mAs
1	400	@	1/20	=	
2	500	@	1/20	=	
3	600	@	1/20	=	
4	400	@	1/5	=	
5	600	@	1/5	=	
6	400	@	1/50	=	
7	600	@	1/50	=	
8	500	@	1/4	=	
9	600	@	1/4	=	
10	500	@	1/40	=	
11	600	@	1/40	=	
12	600	@	1/30	=	
13	400	@	1/30	=	
14	400	@	1/60	=	
15	400	@	1/7	=	
16	400	@	1/8	=	
17	400	@	1/80	=	
18	500	@	1/8	=	
19	600	@	1/12	=	
20	600	@	1/120	=	
21	500	@	1/12	=	
22	400	@	1/120	=	
23	400	@	1/15	=	
24	500	@	1/15	=	
25	400	@	1/25	=	
26	500	@	1/25	=	
27	600	@	1/25	=	
28	400	@	1/3	=	

EXERCISE   6

Working with Fractional Timers

COMPLEX FRACTIONS

....

If you have completed all of the previous sections, you are ready to move on to fractional times that involve numerators other than "1" on the top, such as 2/5 or 7/20. These are not as hard as they might seem at a glance. You must do them in two steps, dividing the bottom (denominator) into the mA station first and then thinking of the top number as "sets."

For example, to solve:

200 mA at 2/5 s

first, ignore the top (numerator) in the fraction, considering it as a " l "; in other words, find 1/5 of 200. When you have this number, multiply it by the top of the fraction, thinking in "sets," as follows:

1/5 of 200 = 40
2 sets of 40 = 80 mAs

Think of 200 mA at 7/20 second as 7 sets of 10, and think of 300 mA at 3/15 second as 3 sets of 20. Using this approach, solve all of the following problems mentally, and then check and review your answers.

	mA	x	Time(s)	=	mAs
1	100	@	2/5	=	
2	100	@	2/15	=	
3	100	@	3/15	=	
4	100	@	3/20	=	
5	100	@	7/20	=	
6	200	@	3/4	=	
7	200	@	2/5	=	
8	200	@	3/5	=	
9	200	@	4/5	=	

	mA	x	Time(s)	=	mAs
10	200	@	3/10	=	
11	200	@	7/10	=	
12	200	@	2/15	=	
13	200	@	3/15	=	
14	200	@	3/20	=	
15	200	@	7/20	=	
16	400	@	2/5	=	
17	400	@	3/5	=	
18	400	@	4/5	=	
19	400	@	3/10	=	
20	400	@	7/10	=	
21	300	@	2/3	=	
22	300	@	2/5	=	
23	300	@	3/5	=	
24	300	@	4/5	=	
25	300	@	3/10	=	
26	300	@	7/10	=	
27	300	@	2/15	=	
28	300	@	3/15	=	
29	300	@	3/20	=	
30	400	@	3/20	=	
31	400	@	7/20	=	
32	500	@	2/5	=	
33	500	@	3/10	=	
34	500	@	7/10	=	
35	500	@	3/20	=	
36	600	@	2/5	=	
37	600	@	3/5	=	
38	600	@	3/10	=	
39	600	@	3/20	=	
40	600	@	3/15	=	

EXERCISE   7

Timers: Converting Fractions into Decimals and Vice Versa

CONVERTING FRACTIONS INTO DECIMALS

A radiologic technologist who is used to working with decimal timers should be able to quickly adapt to an x-ray machine employing a fractional timer. The reverse is also true, and both types of machines are commonly found. It turns out that the mathematics for doing this is very similar to the mathematics used for mAs conversions.

For example, to convert the fraction 1/6 into a decimal number, 6 is simply divided into 1.00 for an answer of 0.16. Note how similar this operation is to taking 1/6 second at 100 mA to obtain 16 mAs. The only difference is the placement of the decimal point.

Further, you should recall from "Working with Fractional Timers" that certain number pairs always go together; one of these pairs was 6 and 16. In converting fractions to decimals and back, these number pairs always apply: 1/6 = 0.16, 1/16 = 0.6. (Although the sixteens are actually 16.6666, we are rounding down rather than up because it results in an easy memory device, associating the sixes.) Once again, the list of number pairs that always go together is as follows:

3 and 33
4 and 25
5 and 2
6 and 16
7 and 15
8 and 12

Committing these number pairs to memory will be of great help in solving technique problems in your head.

To change a fraction into a decimal, simply divide the numerator (top) by the denominator (bottom), but first place a decimal point to the right of the numerator and add as many zeros as needed to complete the division. For example, to find the decimal equivalent for 3/20:

$\dfrac{3.0}{20}$ Temporarily remove the decimal:

$\dfrac{30}{20}$ Remove the extra zeros:

$\dfrac{3}{2} = 1.5$ Now, "replacing" the decimal moves it one place to the left in the answer:

$\dfrac{3.0}{20} = 0.15$

If you are comfortable with the mA station exercises in "Working with Decimal Timers" and "Working with Fractional Timers," you will find it even easier to pretend that the numerator is an mA station, in multiples of 100. To illustrate:

$\dfrac{3.0}{20}$ Think of the numerator (3.0) as the 300 mA station:

$\dfrac{300}{20}$ Recall from "Working with Fractional Timers" that at 300 mA, the number pair 15 and 20 always go together:

$\dfrac{300}{20} = 15$ Now, since you added two zeros to the numerator above, you must move the decimal two places to the left in your answer:

$\dfrac{3.00}{20} = 0.15$

In this exercise, convert each fraction listed into its decimal equivalent. Rely as much as you can on the skills developed in "Working with Decimal Timers" and "Working with Fractional Timers." For unusual fractions or where these skills do not apply, simply divide the numerator by the denominator. Do the entire exercise, and then review your answers using the Math Tutor Answer Key.

	Fraction	Decimal		Fraction	Decimal
1	3/4	=	16	1/80	=
2	2/3	=	17	1/100	=
3	1/4	=	18	1/200	=
4	1/5	=	19	7/10	=
5	1/6	=	20	2/15	=
6	1/7	=	21	3/20	=
7	1/8	=	22	2/5	=
8	1/12	=	23	3/5	=
9	1/15	=	24	4/5	=
10	1/20	=	25	1/3	=
11	1/25	=	26	3/15	=
12	1/30	=	27	7/20	=
13	1/40	=	28	1/150	=
14	1/50	=	29	3/8	=
15	1/60	=	30	5/16	=

EXERCISE 8

Timers: Converting Fractions into Decimals and Vice Versa

CONVERTING DECIMALS INTO FRACTIONS

To convert a decimal number into a fraction requires three steps. First, find the numerator (top of the fraction) by simply writing out all of the nonzero figures to the right of the decimal point. Then, to find the denominator (bottom of the fraction), write 1 for the decimal point and a zero for each decimal place after it. For example, find the fractional equivalent for 0.0125:

0.0125   For the numerator, write out nonzero figures to the right of the decimal point: 125 is the numerator.
For the denominator, write a 1 in place of the decimal point There are four figures or decimal places to the right of the decimal point (0.0125), so you will write four zeros after the 1: 10,000 is the denominator. The fraction is:

$$\frac{125}{10,000}$$

Finally, reduce the fraction if possible to its lowest common denominator. In the preceding example, 125 and 10,000 do not have a lower common denominator, and the fraction cannot be reduced. Following is an example of a decimal number that can be reduced after converting it into a fraction:

0.6   For the numerator, write the nonzero figures to the right of the decimal point: 6 is the numerator. For the denominator, write a 1 for the decimal point and a zero for each place after it: 10 is the denominator. The fraction is:

$$\frac{6}{10}$$

Six and ten share a common : they are both divisible by 2. Reduce the fmction by dividing both numbers by 2:

$$\frac{6/2}{10/2}$$

$$\frac{3}{5}$$ This fraction cannot be further reduced, and it is the answer.

In this exercise, convert the decimal numbers listed into equivalent fractions. Some of these problems are easily solved by computing them, whereas *others are better solved by simply recognizing the number pairs listed in Exercise 2.* Do the entire exercise; then check and review your answers using the Math Tutor Answer Key.

	Decimal		Fraction
1	0.05	=	
2	0.0333	=	
3	0.2	=	
4	0.75	=	
5	0.025	=	
6	0.6667	=	
7	0.143	=	
8	0.002	=	
9	0.08	=	
10	0.167	=	
11	0.125	=	
12	0.6	=	
13	0.0625	=	
14	0.00833	=	

Name_____

EXERCISE   9

Date_____

Finding mA and Time Combinations for a Desired mAs

WARM-UP CALCULATIONS

....

Common mathematics problems each radiologic technologist faces in daily practice include (1) having a desired total mAs in mind and trying to mentally determine an mA-time combination that will yield that total, (2) mentally applying the 15% rule for kVp to adjust techniques, and (3) mentally applying the inverse square law for distance changes.

The following exercises will help you to develop the ability to do all three of these types of problems in your head. If you have trouble following the instructions on any of these, you may wish to review Part One.

Probably the most common mathematics problem a radiologic technologist faces every day is that of having a desired total mAs in mind and trying to mentally determine an mA-time combination that will yield that total.

This is exactly the reverse of the exercises in Part One, yet if you have completed those previous exercises, you will see how they help you in this one. The same number pairs are used. The only difference is that now you must decide what mA station your desired total mAs will divide into easily. With a little practice the correct time fraction will then come to mind.

One unique thing about fractions (which you will not find in working with decimals) is that some of the answers can only be found in "complex fractions" as we have defined them. To solve these, you must again learn to think in "sets," such as using two sets of 20 mAs to obtain 40 mAs.

For example, how would you obtain 80 mAs using the 200 mA station? Since 80 does not divide *evenly* into 200, no usable fraction with a "1" on top as the numerator can be found (that is, to simply divide it out, you will get 2.5 as the denominator, resulting in a fraction of 1/2.5; this is a complex fraction that will not be found on the timer knob). However, if you learn to recognize that 80 is 2 sets of 40, you can find a usable time:

First, divide 40 mAs into 200 mA = 5.
5 is the denominator of your fraction.
In other words, the fraction used to obtain 40 mAs is 1/5.
Now, simply go back and take 2 *sets* of 1/5 by changing the numerator to 2.
The answer is 2/5 second.
80 mAs = 200 mA at 2/5 second
(80 mAs = 2 sets of 40 mAs)

This exercise will "warm you up" to finding these sets of numbers. For each total mAs listed, express it as so many sets of a smaller number that will easily divide into one of the typical mA stations. There are *one* or *two* answers to each problem but no more, because, for that smaller number, you must choose a number that does not require further reduction. For example:

120 mAs can be expressed as _____ sets of _____.
If you use 6 sets of 20, this ratio can then be reduced to 3 sets (of 40). It is not a good answer.

One good answer is *3 sets of 40*, since this number of sets cannot be further reduced.

Another good answer is *2 sets of 60*, since, again, this number of sets cannot be further reduced. (One set of 120 is absurd, because there is no 120 mA station available.)

Note that sets of 40 will be evenly divisible into the 200 mA station, whereas sets of 60 will be divisible into the 300 mA station.

It sounds complicated at first, but try the following part of this exercise and you will find it is not as hard as you might have expected:

1 80 mAs can be expressed as ____ sets of ____.
2 45 mAs can be expressed as ____ sets of ____.
3 66 mAs can be expressed as ____ sets of ____.
4 75 mAs can be expressed as ____ sets of ____.
5 180 mAs can be expressed as ____sets of ____.
6 120 mAs can be expressed as ____ sets of ____
                    or as ____ sets of ____.

7 160 mAs can be expressed as ____ sets of ____
                    or as ____ sets of ____.
8 240 mAs can be expressed as ____ sets of ____
                    or as ____ sets of ____.
9 90 mAs can be expressed as ____ sets of ____.
10 320 mAs can be expressed as ____ sets of ____.
Check your answers in the Math Tutor Answer Key.

In Exercises 10 and 11 the total mAs desired is given along with the mA station to be used. You must mentally decide which time to use. Use only those times that are available on most x-ray machines. In Exercise 10 your times must be expressed as fractions. In Exercise 11 use decimals. Do the exercises mentally, and then check your answers.

EXERCISE   10

Finding mA and Time Combinations
for a Desired mAs

CALCULATIONS USING FRACTIONS

	Total mAs	= mA	x seconds
1	4 mAs	= 100 mA	x _____
2	2.5 mAs	= 100 mA	x _____
3	66 mAs	= 100 mA	x _____
4	7 mAs	= 100 mA	x _____
5	17 mAs	= 100 mA	x _____
6	8 mAs	= 100 mA	x _____
7	3.3 mAs	= 100 mA	x _____
8	1.7 mAs	= 100 mA	x _____
9	1.25 mAs	= 100 mA	x _____
10	0.8 mAs	= 100 mA	x _____
11	40 mAs	= 100 mA	x _____
12	5 mAs	= 150 mA	x _____
13	2.5 mAs	= 50 mA	x _____
14	25 mAs	= 50 mA	x _____
15	25 mAs	= 200 mA	x _____
16	40 mAs	= 200 mA	x _____
17	120 mAs	= 200 mA	x _____
18	5 mAs	= 200 mA	x _____
19	2.5 mAs	= 200 mA	x _____
20	14 mAs	= 200 mA	x _____
21	50 mAs	= 300 mA	x _____
22	6 mAs	= 300 mA	x _____
23	20 mAs	= 300 mA	x _____
24	2.5 mAs	= 300 mA	x _____
25	45 mAs	= 300 mA	x _____
26	180 mAs	= 300 mA	x _____
27	240 mAs	= 300 mA	x _____
28	75 mAs	= 300 mA	x _____
29	80 mAs	= 400 mA	x _____
30	240 mAs	= 400 mA	x _____

Name_____

Date_____

Finding mA and Time Combinations for a Desired mAs

CALCULATIONS USING DECIMALS

	Total mAs	= mA	x seconds
1	4 mAs	= 100 mA	x _____
2	2.5 mAs	= 100 mA	x _____
3	66 mAs	= 100 mA	x _____
4	7 mAs	= 100 mA	x _____
5	16 mAs	= 100 mA	x _____
6	8 mAs	= 100 mA	x _____
7	3.3 mAs	= 100 mA	x _____
8	1.7 mAs	= 100 mA	x _____
9	40 mAs	= 100 mA	x _____
10	2.5 mAs	= 50 mA	x _____
11	1.25 mAs	= 50 mA	x _____
12	25 mAs	= 200 mA	x _____
13	40 mAs	= 200 mA	x _____
14	120 mAs	= 200 mA	x _____
15	5 mAs	= 200 mA	x _____
16	2.5 mAs	= 200 mA	x _____
17	14 mAs	= 200 mA	x _____
18	50 mAs	= 300 mA	x _____
19	6 mAs	= 300 mA	x _____
20	21 mAs	= 300 mA	x _____
21	180 mAs	= 300 mA	x _____
22	75 mAs	= 300 mA	x _____
23	80 mAs	= 400 mA	x _____
24	240 mAs	= 400 mA	x _____

EXERCISE   12

Technique Adjustments

APPLYING THE 15% RULE FOR kVp

....

APPLYING THE RULE IN STEPS

....

APPLYING THE RULE IN PORTIONS

....

Radiologic technologists must often adjust techniques using the 15% rule for kVp in order to increase penetration or change the contrast on the radiograph while maintaining overall density. The ability to make these adjustments mentally should be second nature to the radiologic technologist. It is not very difficult to develop this ability, but it does require practice and repetition. The following drills will help you develop this ability.

The rule states that a 15% adjustment in kVp will change the resulting image density by a *factor of 2*. A 15% increase will double the film density, and a 15% reduction will cut the image density to one half the original. This is an approximation, but it works very well and is the only practical rule of thumb for predicting the effects of kVp on the ultimate darkness of the radiograph.

To find 15% of the original kVp mentally, think of the operation as taking 10% first and then adding half as much again. For example, to find 15% of 80 kVp:

80 x 10% = 8	Take 10% of the kVp.
8/2 = 4	Figure one half of 8.
8 + 4 = 12	Add these two numbers.
80 x 15% = 12	

Fifteen percent of 60 kVp would be 6 + 3 = 9. Fifteen percent of 120 would be 12 + 6 = 18.

This number is added to the original kVp to double film density, and it is subtracted to obtain one half of the original density. In the above example using 80 kVp, what new total kVp would compensate for cutting the mAs to one half? The answer is 92 kVp (80 + 12). What-

would the new kVp be if, because of overpenetration, a radiograph turned out twice too dark and you wished to cut the density in half? The answer is 68 kVp.

You should also become comfortable with applying the 15% rule in steps and in portions.

A common misconception is that an adjustment of 10 kVp changes density by a factor of 2. This stems from the fact that 15% of 70 is 10.5, and 70 may be considered an "average" kVp for radiographic procedures. However, a 10 kVp change in the range of 40 kVp will almost double the density *twice*, whereas a 10 kVp change in the range of 100 kVp is only two thirds of the change needed to double or halve the density. For accuracy it is important to use the 15% rule as prescribed rather than the "10 kVp rule."

Sometimes the desired adjustment in image density is much greater than a doubling or halving. Suppose you need to repeat an extremely light radiograph caused by underpenetration, and the density needs to be increased fourfold. Always translate the desired changes into terms of doublings (factors of two), and you can apply the rule.

To produce a radiograph four times darker, think of this change as two doublings. To obtain two doublings, you will need to increase 15% kVp *in two steps*. (It is not as accurate to simply make a 30% change, and the greater the change, the less accurate this approach is.) For example, if the original radiograph was exposed using 80 kVp:

80 x 15% = 12	Step 1: increase by 15% of the original kVp.
80 + 12 = 92	This increase achieves the first doubling.
92 x 15% = 14	Step 2: increase by 15% of the *adjusted kEp, not the original kEp.*
92 + 14 = 106	This increase achieves the second doubling.

A fourfold increase in image density will result from 106 kVp. It would also compensate for a reduction of mAs to one fourth of the original.

Only rarely is kVp adjusted by more than 1 set of 15%, especially for reductions, which might result in an underpenetrated radiograph regardless of increases in mAs. It is to be emphasized that mAs, not kVp, is the primary density control for radiographs, and that kVp is only changed to adjust for penetration, scatter radiation levels, image contrast, or gray scale. Nonetheless, when such adjustments are made, the mAs must often be compensated to maintain density, and the 15% rule comes into play.

One practical example of a kVp adjustment using two steps of 15% is found in deriving a barium technique (upper GI or solid column barium enema) from a routine abdomen technique. If the technique for an AP projection of the abdomen were 30 mAs and 80 kVp, the following calculations would allow adequate penetration of the same abdomen when the gastrointestinal tract is filled with barium:

30 mAs @ 80 kVp	Routine AP abdomen
15 mAs @ 92 kVp	First step increase of 15% (12 kVp), accompanied by one half the mAs to maintain density
7.5 mAs @ 106 kVp	Second step increase (14 kVp) is 15% of 92, with another halving of the mAs

For a solid column barium procedure (not air contrast) approximately 7 mAs at about 110 kVp would provide good penetration through the barium while keeping overall image density at an optimum level. (For an air contrast technique, simply reduce 10 to 15 kVp with the mAs still at about 7.)

The image density on a radiograph must be changed by at least one third or about 30% for the human eye to detect any difference. In practice, efforts to ever increase overall radiographic technique by less than 50% or to decrease it by less than 30% are wasted. Changes such as these can be made using the 15% rule in portions.

Suppose you wish to reduce the density but decide that cutting it in half would be too much. You must reduce overall technique by at least one third to make any visible difference. Taking one third of 15%, we can derive a kVp change of about 5%. The kVp must be reduced by a minimum of 5% to lighten up the image. To find 5% of the original kVp, think of it as one half of 10%. For this problem, if the original kVp was 120 kVp, the solution would be as follows:

120 x 10% = 12	Figure 10% of the kVp.
12 x 1/2 = 6	Take one half of that amount.
120 – 6 = 114	Subtract this number from the original kVp.

The kVp must be reduced at least to 114 to visibly lighten up the density in this case.

Although a 2 kVp adjustment may visibly change image density in the 40 kVp range, the same adjustment will not make a visible difference in higher ranges. The change must be at least 5%.

Consider an increase in density of 50% or 1.5 times the original. You will recall the recommendation to think of technique changes in terms of doublings or halvings. In this context, such a 50% increase should be thought of as *halfway to doubling*. (Similarly, a 25% reduction in overall technique would be thought of as halfway to cutting it in half.) Since a 15% increase in kVp will double the density, one half of 15% should bring the density halfway to a doubling. In other words, to increase the density 50%, increase the kVp by one half of 15%.

For example, suppose a radiograph taken at 80 kVp comes out a bit light. Doubling the density would be too much. You decide to increase density by about one half, or 50%:

80 x 15% = 12	Find 15% of the kVp.
12 x 1/2 = 6	Find one half that amount.
80 + 6 = 86	Add this number to the original kVp.

For a radiograph 50% darker, increase kVp to 86.

Complete this exercise using the 15% rule. Some problems will require you to apply the rule in sequential steps, some in portions of one third or one half of 15%. Finish the entire exercise; then check and review your answers using the Math Tutor Answer Key.

1 What is 5% of 120?
2 What is 5% of 90?
3 What is 5% of 80?
4 What is 5% of 50?
5 What is 5% of 60?
6 What is 15% of 70?
7 What is 15% of 40?
8 What is 15% of 60?
9 What is 15% of 110?
10 What is *one half* of 15% of 40?
11 What is *one half* of 15% of 70?
12 What is *one half* of 15% of 80?
13 What is *one half* of 15% of 50?
14 What is *one half* of 15% of 90?
15 What is *one half* of 15% of 120?
16 Starting at 120 kVp, what new kVp would result in a density one half as dark as the original?
17 Starting at 40 kVp, what new kVp would result in a density twice as dark as the original?
18 Starting at 60 kVp, what new kVp would result in a density 50% darker than the original (halfway to double the original)?
19 Starting at 80 kVp, what new kVp would result in a density about 75% (halfway to one half) of the original?

EXERCISE   13

Technique Adjustments

ADJUSTING FOR DISTANCE CHANGES

....

THE INVERSE SQUARE LAW

....

THE SQUARE LAW

....

RULES OF THUMB FOR DISTANCE CHANGES

....

As described in the textbook radiologic technologists should be completely familiar with the inverse square law. It describes the relationship between radiation quantity or intensity in the x-ray beam and the distance from the x-ray tube. Because the x-ray beam "fans out" over larger areas with increasing distance, the concentration of x rays decreases at a rate inversely proportional to the square of the distance. The formula is as follows:

$$\frac{I_1}{I_2} = \frac{(D_2)^2}{(D_1)^2}$$

where I_1, is the original quantity or concentration of x rays, I_2 is the new radiation quantity after the distance change, and D_1 and D_2 are the old and new distances (SIDs), respectively.

The inverse square law can be used to predict radiation exposure to the patient, operator, or film. Because the density produced on the film is generally directly proportional or "reciprocal," to the exposure, the inverse square law can be used to predict image density changes when distance is altered. Some of the questions in this exercise apply this formula.

However, this section also focuses on two derivations from the inverse square that are extremely helpful in daily practice: the "square law" and rules of thumb for distance changes.

Whereas the inverse square law is used to predict image density, the *square law* is used to compensate technique so that density is maintained when distance changes. The formula for the square law is as follows:

$$\frac{mAs_1}{mAs_2} = \frac{(D_1)^2}{(D_2)^2}$$

where mAs_1 is the original mAs used at D_1, the original SID, and mAs_2 is the new mAs needed to maintain equal density if the SID is changed to D_2.

When the original mAs is not given or known, place a 1 in the formula for "mAs_1" and solve for mAs_2. The resulting number will be the *factor* by which mAs should be changed. A 2.0 would indicate that the original mAs, whatever it was, should be doubled. A result of 0.5 would indicate that it should be cut in half, and so forth.

As an example, suppose the distance (SID) is increased from the usual 40 inches to 60 inches. The technique chart is written for 40 inches. What change would need to be made in the overall technique taken from the chart to maintain adequate image density at 60 inches?

$\dfrac{1}{mAs_2} = \dfrac{40^2}{60^2}$	Since the actual mAs is not given, place a 1 for "mAs_1". D_1 is 40 inches, and D_2 is 60 inches.
$\dfrac{1}{mAs_2} = \dfrac{1600}{3600}$	Square the distances.
$1600(mAs_2) = 3600$	Cross multiply.
$mAs_2 = \dfrac{3600}{1600}$	Isolate mAs_2 by dividing both sides of the equation by 1600.
$mAs_2 = 2.25$	This is the *factor* by which mAs should be changed.

The 40-inch technique should be increased 2.25 times to maintain density at 60 inches SID.

The solutions to square law problems are always the inverse of those for solving inverse square law problems. For example, if a distance change would result in twice as dark a film by the inverse square law, then the tech-

TABLE MT-2 Rules of thumb for distance changes starting at 40 inches.

New distance (in)	Technique change computed by square law	Rule of thumb technique change
30	0.56	1/2
40	1.0 (standard)	1
60	2.25	2x
72	3.24	3x
80	4.0	4x
96	5.76	6x

nique that would be required to maintain the original density at the new distance would be one half the mAs. If the density change can be predicted, simply invert this change to find the technique adjustment.

Although the inverse square law is important to understand, in practice radiologic technologists rarely use a calculator or pencil to apply it accurately. Rather, when doing a mobile procedure at 60 inches SID, for example, they will likely make a mental estimate of the increase in technique required when compared to the usual 40-inch SID. This section provides some simple rules of thumb that, if committed to memory, will greatly improve your accuracy in making this kind of technique adjustment.

A handful of distances (30, 40, 60, 72, and 96 inches) applies to more than 95% of radiographic procedures. By taking the most commonly used 40 inches as a standard and comparing the others to it, rules of thumb are easily derived and learned.

It helps to think of distance changes in factors of two, that is, doublings and halvings. For example, the square law formula shows that if SID is increased from 40 inches to 80 inches (a doubling), the technique must be increased by four times to maintain density. However, by thinking of this quadrupling of the technique as *two doublings*, rules of thumb can be formulated for other distance changes:

For example, think of increasing the SID from 40 inches to 60 inches as going *halfway to doubling* the SID. That is, 60 inches is halfway from 40 to 80. Since 80 inches would require two doublings of technique, 60 inches will require one half of that increase, or one doubling. For a 60-inch projection, double the mAs used at 40 inches.

In a similar manner, 30 inches can be considered as halfway to cutting 40 inches in half. A 20-inch distance would require one fourth of the overall technique, or two halvings. Thus 30 inches requires only one halving of the 40-inch technique.

Table MT-2 summarizes these rules of thumb for the most used distances. A column listing the actual solution

based on the square law formula is provided as well so that you can see how close these rules of thumb are for accuracy. If you keep in mind that density must be changed by at least 30% to see a visible difference, the rules of thumb are clearly accurate enough for practical use.

By far the most useful of these rules of thumb will be those for 60 inches and 72 inches because these distances are frequently used both in mobile procedures and in the radiology department. For mobile procedures the rules of thumb can be taken one step further to derive a technique for 50 inches SID.

If you consider 50 as halfway to 60, the technique would be increased halfway to a doubling, or increased 50%. By the square law formula, the needed increase is 1.57 times the original. The rule of thumb rounds it to 1.5 times. *Radiologic technologists assigned to mobile units should remember that compared to the usual 40-inch technique, a 50-inch SID requires a 50% increase in overall technique (preferably using mAs), a 60-inch distance requires a doubling, and a 72-inch distance requires a tripling.*

Since chest radiography is commonly performed with the 72-inch SID, it is well to emphasize that the 72-inch distance requires three times the 40-inch technique and that a 40-inch distance requires one third of the 72-inch technique. This relationship is frequently encountered in performing upright or decubitus abdomen radiographs along with chest radiographs. *Remember that the relationship between a 40-inch SID and a 72-inch SID is a factor of 3.*

These rules of thumb can also be used to solve for density problems, if you remember to invert them (make fractions out of them). For example, if the distance is increased from 40 inches to 72 inches, and the technique is *not* compensated for this change, how dark will the radiograph be? Simply invert the factor for 72 inches from Table MT-2. The answer is that the new radiograph will have one third the density of the original. A radiograph taken at 60 inches without compensating technique would be one half as dense, and so on.

Complete this exercise as directed. The first 13 questions should be done mentally, using rules of thumb. Note that those starting at 60 inches or 30 inches can also be solved in your head if you analyze the distance changes as doubling, halving, halfway to doubling, or halfway to halving. Questions 14 to 25 employ the square law to find a new mAs that will compensate for the change in distance.

After completing the entire exercise, carefully check and review your answers using the Math Tutor Answer Key.

Use the technique rules of thumb to solve these problems:

	From:	To maintain density:
1	25 mAs	_____mAs
	40-in SID	72-in SID
2	15 mAs	_____mAs
	40-in SID	60-in SID
3	7.5 mAs	_____mAs
	40-in SID	80-in SID
4	6 mAs	_____mAs
	40-in SID	96-in SID
5	60 mAs	_____mAs
	40-in TFD	20-in TFD
6	2.5 mAs	_____mAs
	30-in TFD	60-in TFD
7	30 mAs	_____mAs
	40-in TFD	30-in TFD
8	12.5 mAs	_____mAs
	30-in TFD	45-in TFD
9	30 mAs	120 mAs
	80 kVp	_____kVp
	40-in TFD	60-in TFD

Use the density rules of thumb to solve these problems:

	From:	To:
10	40-in TFD	20-in TFD
	Density = 1	Density = _____
11	60-in TFD	45-in TFD
	Density = 1	Density = _____
12	40-in TFD	80-in TFD
	Density = 1	Density = _____
13	30-in TFD	45-in TFD
	Density = 1	Density = _____

Use the square law to solve these problems:

	From:	To maintain density:
14	10 mAs	_____mAs
	40-in TFD	100-in TFD
15	5 mAs	_____mAs
	60-in TFD	50-in TFD
16	2.5 mAs	_____mAs
	72-in TFD	40-in TFD
17	2.5 mAs	_____mAs
	60-in TFD	20-in TFD
18	2.5 mAs	2.5 mAs
	80 kVp	_____kVp
	60-in TFD	42.5-in TFD
19	180 mAs	20 mAs
	36-in TFD	_____TFD
20	45 mAs	5 mAs
	90-in TFD	_____TFD
21	30 mAs	120 mAs
	20-in TFD	_____TFD
22	5 mAs	45 mAs
	20-in TFD	_____TFD
23	12 mAs	_____mAs
	96-in TFD	30-in TFD
24	25 mAs	_____mAs
	96-in TFD	40-in TFD
25	40 mAs	_____mAs
	80-in TFD	36-in TFD

Use the inverse square law to solve these problems:

	From:	To:
26	40-in TFD	72-in TFD
	Density = 1	Density = _____
27	60-in TFD	72-in TFD
	Density = 1	Density = _____
28	50-in TFD	36-in TFD
	Density = 1	Density = _____
29	72-in TFD	96-in TFD
	Density = 1	Density = _____

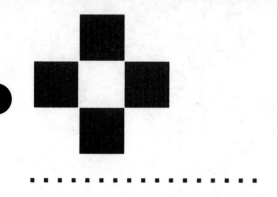

Experiment Section

EXPERIMENT   1

Inverse Square Law

OBJECT

To demonstrate the effect that distance from the x-ray source has on x-ray intensity.

DISCUSSION

X rays are emitted isotropically (i.e., with equal intensity in all directions) from the target of the x-ray tube. The anode and diagnostic housing prevent x rays from exiting in any direction other than through the window of the tube and port of the housing. The collimator or other beam-restricting devices further define the useful x-ray beam. The intensity of the x-ray beam decreases as the square of the distance from the source. If the distance from the source is doubled, the intensity will be reduced to one fourth its former value. This relationship, known as the **inverse square law**, is based solely on geometry. It has nothing to do with x-ray absorption. The x-ray intensity (I_1) passing through a unit area at some distance (r_1) from the target will be

$$I_1 = \frac{I_o}{4\pi r_1^2}$$

where I_o is the total number of x rays emitted from the target. The intensity (I_2) at any other distance (r_2) from the target will similarly be as follows:

$$I_2 = \frac{I_o}{4\pi r_2^2}$$

Combining these equations:

$$\frac{I_1}{I_2} = \frac{\frac{I_o}{4\pi r_1^2}}{\frac{I_o}{4\pi r_2^2}} \quad \text{and} \quad \frac{I_1}{I_2} = \frac{\frac{I_o}{r_1^2}}{\frac{I_o}{r_2^2}}$$

results in

$$\frac{I_1}{I_2} = \frac{r_2^2}{r_1^2} = \left(\frac{r_2^2}{r_1^2}\right)$$

MATERIALS REQUIRED

Radiographic x-ray unit
Ionization chamber
Tape measure

PROCEDURE

1. The x-ray machine may be used as it is normally filtered. Record the total filtration present if known.
2. Set the tube potential to 70 kVp. This will remain constant throughout the experiment.
3. Locate the position of the source (the target) of x rays. Many tube housings are marked at the position of the target; if not, assume the target position to be at the middle of the tube housing.
4. Position the ionization chamber on the central ray of the useful beam and as close to the source as possible.
5. Record this distance on the data sheet provided and take three readings of intensity. If possible, the mA and exposure time should remain constant throughout this experiment. However, if the response range of the ionization chamber will not accommodate such measurements, either or both may require adjustment.
6. Repeat these measurements at approximately 25 cm intervals to a distance of 200 cm from the source.
7. Express the radiation intensity as exposure rate (mR/mAs) at each distance by use of the following expression:

Exposure rate (mR/mAs) =

$$\frac{\text{Exposure (mR)}}{\text{Tube current (mA) exposure time(s)}}$$

RESULTS

Plot exposure rate (mR/mAs) as a function of distance from the source (cm) on the semilog graph paper provided.

EXERCISES

1 What was the shape of the curve obtained? Why?
2 Calculate the quantity $1\sqrt{mR/mAs}$, and plot this as a function of distance from the target on the linear graph paper provided. What is the appearance of this curve and why? Where does the curve intersect the x axis (distance axis), and where should it have intersected?
3 If the output intensity of an x-ray tube is 2.5 mR/mAs (0.65 μC/kg-mAs) at 100 cm source-to-image receptor distance (SID), what would the intensity be at 150 cm SID?
4 The output intensity is shown to be 150 mR/mAs (3.87×10^{-5} C/kg-mAs) at 100 cm SID. At what SID will the intensity be 100 mR/mAs?

DATA SHEET
Laboratory experiment 1

Constant factors
70 kVp
Filtration _____mm Al

Source to ionization chamber distance (cm)	Exposure (mR)				Tube current (mA)	Exposure time(s)	mAs	mR/mAs	$\dfrac{1}{\sqrt{mR/mAs}}$
	First measurement	Second measurement	Third measurement	Average					

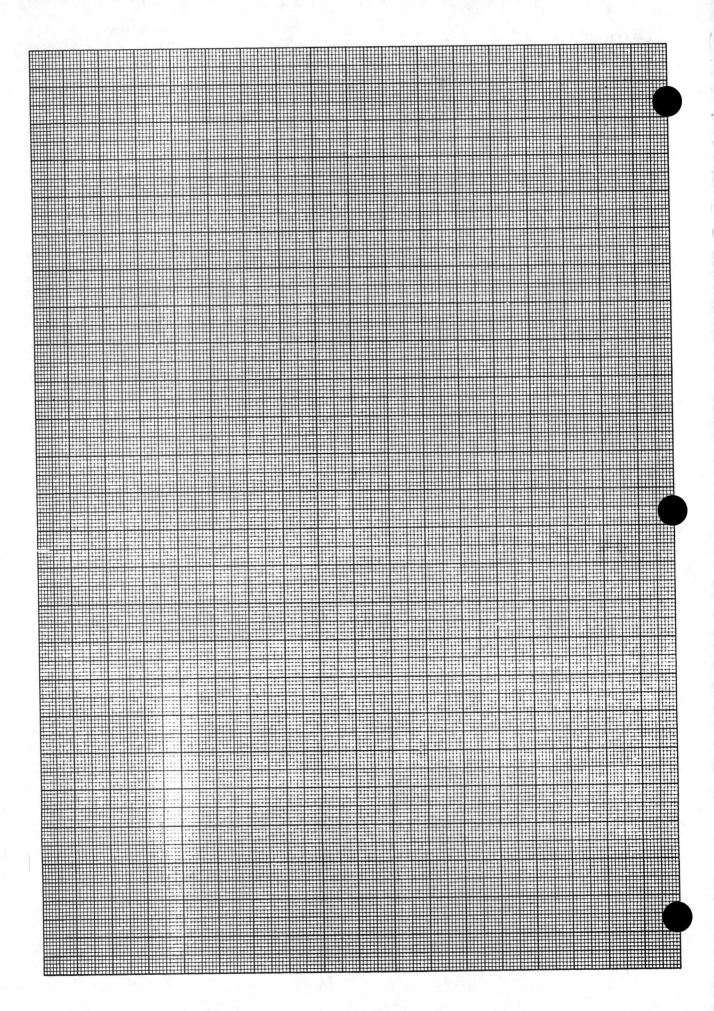

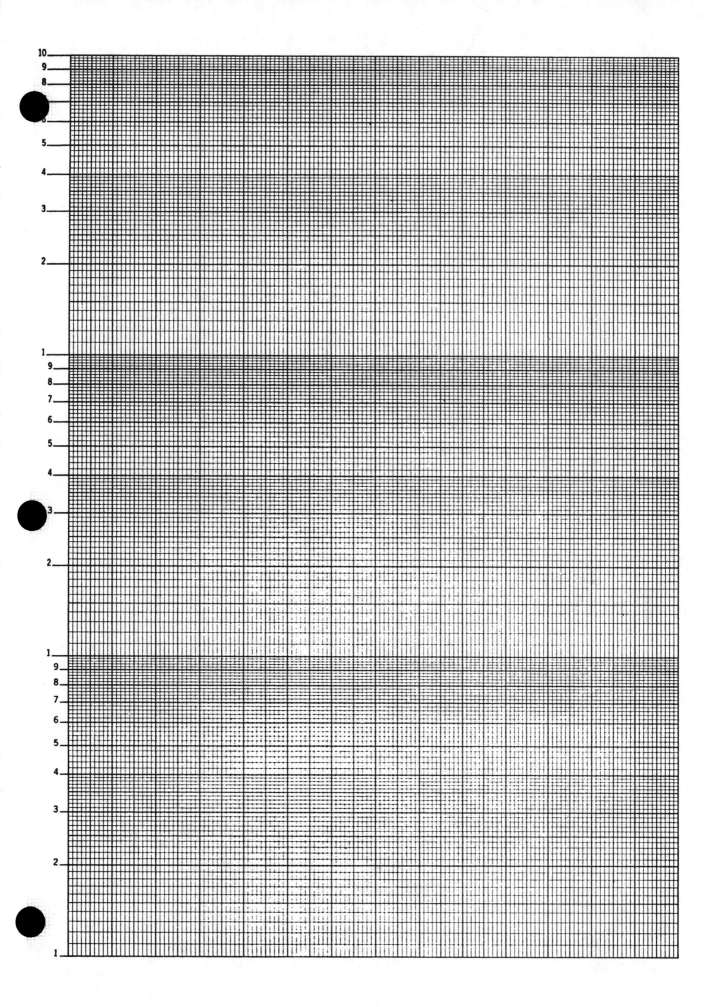

Name_____

Date_____

Effect of Source-To-Image Receptor Distance on Optical Density

OBJECT

To demonstrate the effect of changing the source-to-image receptor distance (SID) on the optical density (OD) of the image.

DISCUSSION

As demonstrated in experiment 1, an adjustment in SID changes radiation intensity is inversely proportional in proportion to the inverse square of the distance. The intensity of the x-ray beam directly controls the OD of the film; consequently film responds according to the same law. To maintain a given OD when changing SID, technique must be compensated according to a "square law." For example, if the distance were reduced to one half, the mAs should be cut to one quarter (one half squared). If this adjustment were not made to compensate for the change in distance, then the resulting radiograph would be four times darker according to the inverse square law.

MATERIALS REQUIRED

Radiographic x-ray machine
Step-wedge penetrometer
X-ray film processor
200 speed 14 in x 17 in (35 cm x 42 cm) screen film
    cassette
Leaded rubber sheets
Rectangular sponge approximately 4 inches thick
Tape measure
Lead numbers
View box
Densitometer
Calculator

PROCEDURE

1. Warm up the processor if needed, and run a couple of "scrap" films through it to stabilize temperature and circulation.
2. Load and place the cassette on the tabletop. Three exposures will be taken on one film. Collimate the light field to a 5 in x 10 in area crosswise at one end of the film. Use the leaded sheets to mask the adjacent film area.
3. Place the thick, flat sponge over the light-field area. This creates a large object-to-film distance, which must be kept constant on all exposures.
4. Place the step-wedge penetrometer crosswise on the sponge, centered to the light field.
5. Number each exposure with a lead marker on the cassette. Take three exposures using the following techniques or alternate techniques to accommodate your equipment.

Exposure 1   Carefully set the SID at 100 cm to the tabletop.
               Technique: 100 mA, 0.1 s (1/10 s; 100 ms), 50 kVp

Exposure 2   Carefully set the SID at 50 cm to the tabletop. Be sure to collimate the light field, opening it up to include the entire step wedge if possible.
               Technique: 100 mA, 0.025 s (1/40 s; 2.5 ms), 50 kVp.

Exposure 3   Place the cassette on the floor with the sponge and step wedge over the last third of the film. Carefully measure and set the SID to 180 cm from the cassette. Collimate the light field.
               Technique: 100 mA, 0.35 s (3/10 s; 350 ms), 50 kVp.

TABLE E2-1

	Total mAs	SID	OD
Exposure 1			
Exposure 2			
Exposure 3			

6. Process the film.
7. On the resulting images, select a step on the step wedge from which to take OD measurements. On exposure 1, the selected step must have a medium OD, between 1.0 and 2.0. Using the densitometer, determine the optical density at this step for each exposure.

RESULTS

In Table E2-1, record for each exposure the total mAs used at each SID and the measured OD.

EXERCISES

1 Compute the relative change in OD for exposures 2 and 3 by dividing the OD for 1 into that for 2 and by dividing the OD for 1 into 3, and record here:

2/1:_____   3/1:_____

2 Compute the average OD change by summing these two ratios and then dividing by two:

Average density change ratio:_____

3 OD change ratio of 1.0 would indicate that the ODs produced by the different techniques are exactly the same. Is your computed average change within 15% of the original; that is, does it fall between 0.85 and 1.15?

4 Visually compare exposure 2 to exposure 1. In 2 the SID was reduced to one half of the original, and, using the square law, the mAs was reduced to one fourth. Did the "square law" for the technique reasonably maintain image OD in this case?

5 On exposure 2, if the mAs had not been adjusted, how dark would the exposure have turned out compared to 1?

6 If the SID were doubled, what change in mAs would be required to maintain OD?

7 Restate your answer to 5 in terms of sets of doubling mAs. For example, would you double the original mAs once, twice, three times, or four times to compensate?

8 Now consider a change in SID from 100 cm to 150 cm. This can be thought of as going halfway to doubling the distance. In light of your answer to 6, how many doublings of mAs would be required at 150 cm to maintain a constant OD?

9 Visually compare 3 with 1. The SID for exposure 3 was 180 cm, roughly halfway between 150 cm and 200 cm. Was OD reasonably maintained? By what ratio was the mAs increased for exposure 3?

10 As a rule of thumb, by what factor must mAs be changed to compensate for adjusting the SID from 100 cm to 180 cm?

EXPERIMENT 3

Effect of Source-To-Image Receptor Distance on Image Blur

OBJECT

To demonstrate the effect of changing the source-to-image receptor distance (SID) on the degree of blurring of an image.

DISCUSSION

In addition to optical density (OD), distance affects two geometric properties of an image. The amount of focal spot blurring in an image is inversely proportional to the SID. Long SIDs result in less blur and increased sharpness. The magnification of the image is reduced with a long SID. Usually blur and magnification are undesirable; therefore as a rule the longest practical SID should be used.

MATERIALS REQUIRED

Radiographic x-ray machine
Small dry bone such as a phalanx (or other small object)
Line pairs per millimeter (lp/mm) resolution test pattern
X-ray film processor
200-speed 14 in x 17 in (35 cm x 42 cm) screen film cassette
Leaded rubber sheets
Rectangular sponge approximately 4 inches thick
Tape measure
Lead numbers
View box
Calculator

PROCEDURE

1. Warm up processor if needed, and run a couple of "scrap" films through it to stabilize temperature and circulation.
2. Load and place the cassette on the tabletop. Two exposures will be taken on one film. Collimate the light field to a 5 in x 10 in area crosswise at one end of the film. Use the leaded sheets to mask the adjacent film area.
3. Place the thick, flat sponge over the light-field area to create a large object-to-film distance, which must be kept constant on all exposures.
4. Place the resolution template crosswise on the sponge with the small bone alongside. Pay close attention to the position in which the bone is laid, since you must lay it precisely the same way on subsequent exposures.
5. Number each exposure with a lead marker on the cassette. Take two exposures using the following techniques or alternate techniques to accommodate available equipment.

Exposure 1   Carefully set the SID to 50 cm. Open the light field to include the resolution template and the bone.
Technique: 50 mA, 0.008 s (1/120 s; 8 ms), 60 kVp.

Exposure 2   Place the cassette on the floor with the sponge, resolution template and bone over the other half of the film. Carefully measure and set the SID at 180 cm.
Technique: 50 mA, 0.1 s (1/10 s; l00 ms), 60 kVp.

6. Process the film.

RESULTS

On the images of the resolution test pattern, scan across the black and white line pairs from thickest to thinnest, and determine the first position where they are so blurred that you cannot distinguish separate lines from one another. Note this value of Ip/mm. Refer to the test pattern itself or to the table provided by your instructor.

TABLE E3-1

	SID	Resolution in lp/mm	Bone image length
Exposure 1			
Exposure 2			

Actual bone length: _____

The unit "line pairs per millimeter" (lp/mm) is a direct measurement of spatial resolution or image blur. The greater the number of Ip/mm resolved, the better the resolution of the system and the less blur there is in the image. In the table below, record each SID and the Ip/mm resolved.

When you have completed this, obtain a millimeter ruler and measure the length of the bone images on both exposures. Then, taking care to hold the bone as it was placed on the cassette and lining the ruler up precisely to the same points as you did on the radiographs, measure the length of the actual dry bone. Record these measurements also in Table E3-1.

EXERCISES

1 Visually examine the marrow portion of the bone images for fine trabecular details. At which SID is more detail resolved? At which SID does the image appear to have sharper edges, less blur, and better spatial resolution?

2 Refer to Table E3-1. Which SID resolved the greater number of line pairs per millimeter? Does this agree with your visual observations in exercise 1?

3 What general rule of thumb can you make for SID to consistently produce radiographs with minimum image blur (best resolution)?

4 From Table E3-1 compute the magnification factor (MF) for the two exposures, using the formula below:

$$MF = \frac{\text{Imaged bone length}}{\text{Actual bone length}}$$

Exposure 1 magnification: _____

Exposure 2 magnification: _____

5 Convert the above MFs to percentages by subtracting 1.0 from the ratio and then multiplying the result by 100. (For example, a ratio of 1.33 – 1.0 = 0.33 x 100 = 33. This would be 33% magnification.) Record your answers below:

Exposure 1 percent magnification: _____
Exposure 2 percent magnification: _____

6 Which SID caused the greater percent magnification?

7 What general rule of thumb can you make for SID to consistently produce radiographs with minimum magnification?

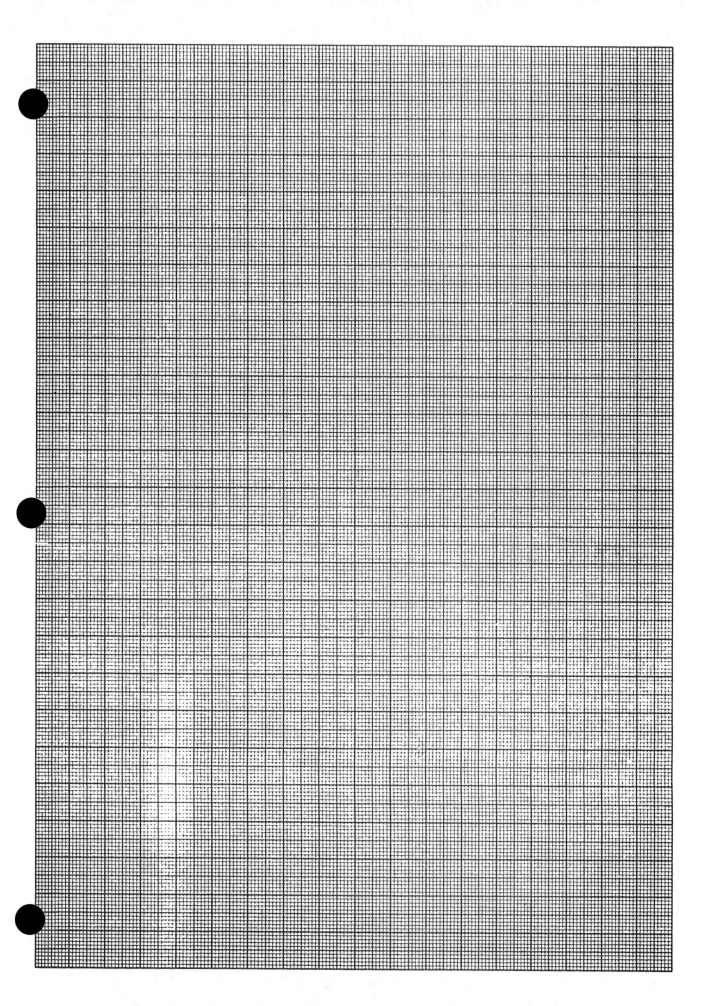

EXPERIMENT 4

Effect of mAs on X-ray Quantity

OBJECT

To measure the effect on radiation intensity of mAs.

DISCUSSION

The product of x-ray tube current (mA) and exposure time(s) controls the radiation intensity (mR) emitted by the x-ray tube directly. That is, as the mAs is increased, the radiation intensity increases proportionally. Selection of a certain mA station (e.g., 50, 100, 200 mA) causes a precise current to flow through the filament of the x-ray tube cathode. This change in filament current alters the heating of the filament and changes the tube current accordingly. The x-ray tube current is the number of electrons accelerated across the tube from cathode to anode per second. When multiplied by exposure time(s), the product (mAs) represents the total number of electrons used for that exposure. As these electrons strike the target of the anode, x rays are produced. The number of x rays produced is the x-ray output intensity or x-ray quantity.

By following this logic further, one can see that if the number of electrons is increased, the quantity of x rays is increased proportionally. Tube current is controlled by selecting an appropriate mA station. When energized for a certain exposure time, the total mAs obtained determines the x-ray quantity (mR).

MATERIALS REQUIRED

Radiographic x-ray machine
Tape measure
Ionization chamber

PROCEDURE

1. Position the ionization chamber 100 cm from the x-ray source.

2. The x-ray machine may be used as it is normally filtered. Record the amount of total filtration present if possible.
3. Adjust the tube potential to 70 kVp. If, as you change mA stations, the kVp drifts, readjust it to 70 kVp so that it will remain constant throughout the experiment.
4. Select the lowest mA station and, using the data sheet provided, record three readings of radiation intensity.
5. The exposure time selected should be held constant throughout these measurements in case there is a timer error. However, the response range of the ionization chamber may require that exposure time be reduced as mA is increased. If this occurs, note it on the data sheet.
6. Repeat these measurements for at least four additional mA stations, including the small and the large focal spots. The highest possible mA should be one of these five.
7. Determine the average intensity (mR) at each mAs.
8. Express the x-ray intensity as exposure rate in mR/mAs. The following relationship may be used:

$$\text{Exposure rate (mR/mAs)} = \frac{\text{Exposure (mR)}}{\text{mAs}}$$

RESULTS

Plot exposure rate (mR/mAs) vs. mAs on the linear graph paper provided.

EXERCISES

1 What was the shape of the curve obtained? Why?
2 What effect was observed when focal spot size was changed? In a properly designed x-ray machine, what should you expect?
3 Calculate the quantity mR/s at each mA station. If

these data were graphed, what would be the shape of the curve?

4 If 200 mA, 0.5 s results in an exposure of 50 mR $(1.29 \times 10^{-5}$ C/kg-mAs), what exposure would 100 mA, 1 s produce?

5 An x-ray machine produces an output intensity of 4.5 mR/mAs $(1.2 \times 10^{-6}$ C/kg-mAs). What radiation exposure would result from the following conditions?
a. 50 mA, 200 ms
b. 300 mA, 1.5 s
c. 800 mA, 16 ms

Constant factors
70 kVp
Total filtration _____mm Al
100 cm source-to-detector distance

DATA SHEET
Laboratory experiment 4

Tube current (mA)	Exposure time (s)	Exposure (mR)			Average exposure (mR)	Exposure rate	
		First	Second	Third		mR/mAs	mR/s
Small focal spot							
1							
2							
3							
4							
5							
6							
7							
8							
9							
10							
Large focal spot							
1							
2							
3							
4							
5							
6							
7							
8							
9							
10							

EXPERIMENT 5

Effect of mAs on Optical Density

OBJECT

To demonstrate the relationship among mA, exposure time, and total mAs and their combined effect on radiographic optical density (OD).

DISCUSSION

When the radiographic unit is properly calibrated, the radiation intensity will be directly proportional to the mA and to the exposure time selected at the console. For example, a doubling of either mA or exposure time will result in twice as much radiation intensity for a particular exposure. The radiographic film normally responds proportionally to exposure; that is, twice the radiation will result in a radiograph twice as dark.

The total mAs is the product of the selected mA station and the exposure time. OD is directly proportional to mAs. To maintain constant OD when the mA is doubled, the exposure time should be cut to one half. Conversely, if the mA is cut to one third its original value, the exposure time should be tripled to maintain constant OD. In other words, mA and exposure time are **inversely** related to each other when maintaining constant mAs and therefore constant OD.

MATERIALS REQUIRED

Radiographic x-ray machine
Step-wedge penetrometer
Leaded rubber sheets
X-ray film processor
200-speed 14 in x 17 in (35 cm x 42 cm) screen film
    cassette
Lead numbers
View box
Densitometer
Calculator

GENERAL PROCEDURE

1. Set 50 kVp. This will remain constant throughout the experiment. If the kVp drifts when changing mA stations, adjust it to remain constant at 50 kVp.
2. Warm up the processor if needed, and run a couple of "scrap" films through it to stabilize temperature and circulation.
3. Position the x-ray tube 100 cm from the tabletop.

PART II PROCEDURE

1. Load and place the cassette faceup on the tabletop. Place the step-wedge penetrometer crosswise at one end of the cassette. Four exposures will be taken on one film. It is important to use one film so that processing conditions will be constant.
2. Collimate the light field to a 4 in x 10 in area, and center over the step wedge. Use the leaded sheets to mask the adjacent film area to prevent scatter fogging.
3. Number each exposure with a lead marker on the cassette. Take four exposures using the techniques listed below or recording alternate techniques you use. Begin with a very low mA and an exposure time of 0.025 s (1/40 s; 25 ms) or less that can be exactly doubled at least twice. After the first exposure, move the step wedge to the next quarter of the film, double the time as shown in technique 2 below, and so on. For the fourth exposure, double the mA station instead of the time. Always use leaded sheets to mask the cassette adjacent to either side of the exposure area.

    Exposure 1   50 mA, 0.05 s (1/20 s; 50 ms)
    Exposure 2   50 mA, 0.1 s (1/10 s; 100 ms)
    Exposure 3   50 mA, 0.2 s (1/5 s; 200ms)
    Exposure 4   100 mA, 0.2 s (1/5 s; 200ms)

4. Process the film.
5. On the resulting images, select a step on which to make OD measurements. The step selected must have a measured OD of less than 0.3 on exposure 1, yet it should be visibly darker on exposure 2. This will be an extremely light OD on exposure 1. Using the densitometer, determine the OD for each exposure, taking care to measure the same step each time.

TABLE E5-1

	mA	Time	Total mAs	OD
Exposure 1				
Exposure 2				
Exposure 3				
Exposure 4				

RESULTS

In Table E5-1, record for each exposure the mA and exposure time used, the total resulting mAs, and the measured OD.

EXERCISES

1　Compute the relative OD change for each increase in technique by dividing the density for 2 by that for 1, 3 by that for 2, and 4 by that for 3, and record the results below. You will note that these relative changes vary somewhat because x-ray machines are not perfectly calibrated.
　2/1:_____　3/2:_____　4/3:_____
2　Compute an average OD change by summing these three numbers and then dividing by 3:
　　　　Average density change:_____
　Does this change fall within 15% of a doubling; that is, does it fall between 1.7 and 2.3?
3　If the relationship between total mAs and OD were plotted on linear paper, what would be the appearance of the graph?
4　What term best describes this relationship?
5　In terms of the resulting OD, is there any difference between doubling the mA and doubling the exposure time?

PART II PROCEDURE

1.　Load and place the cassette faceup on the tabletop. Place the step-wedge penetrometer crosswise at one end of the cassette. Three exposures will be taken on one film. It is important to use one film so that processing conditions will be constant.
2.　Collimate the light field to a 4 in x 10 in area and center over the step wedge. Use the leaded sheets to mask the adjacent film area to prevent scatter fogging.
3.　Number each exposure with a lead marker on the cassette. Take three exposures using the techniques listed below or recording alternate techniques you use. After the first exposure, move the step wedge to the next third of the film. Double the mA station, but cut the exposure time to exactly one half of the orig-

TABLE E5-2

	mA	Time	total mAs	OD
Exposure 1				
Exposure 2				
Exposure 3				

inal so that the same total mAs results. For exposure 3, double the mA and halve the exposure time again. Always use leaded sheets to mask the cassette adjacent to either side of the exposure area.

Exposure 1　　　　50 mA, 0.2 s (1/5 s; 200 ms)
Exposure 2　　　　100 mA, 0.1 s (1/10 s; 100 ms)
Exposure 3　　　　200 mA, 0.05 s (1/20 s; 50 ms)
4.　Process the film.
5.　On the resulting images, select a step on which to make OD measurements; the step selected must have a medium-gray OD between 0.5 and 1.5 as measured on the densitometer. Determine the OD for each exposure, taking care to measure the same step each time.

RESULTS

In Table E5-2, record for each exposure the mA and exposure time used, the total resulting mAs, and the measured OD.

EXERCISES

1　Compute the relative OD changes between these techniques by dividing the density for 2 by that for 1, 3 divided by 2, and 3 divided by 1, and record here:
　2/1:_____　3/2:_____　3/1:_____
2　Compute the average OD change by summing these three numbers and then dividing by 3:
　　　　Average OD change:_____
　An OD change ratio of 1.0 would indicate that the ODs produced by the different techniques are exactly the same. Is your computed average change close to 1.0?
3　Visually examine the three images. Is there a substantial difference in OD among them?
4　As long as the total mAs is the same, does the particular mA station or exposure time make any difference in terms of overall OD?
5　In maintaining a given OD, what term would describe the relationship between milliamperage and exposure time?
6　Why should you generally choose short exposure times with high mA station?
7　When would you choose a very long exposure time with a low mA station?

X-ray Beam Penetration

OBJECT

To demonstrate the relationships among kVp, x-ray beam penetration, and the resulting gray scale of the radiographic image.

DISCUSSION

To produce useful optical densities (ODs) on the radiograph, x rays must first penetrate through each tissue of interest and interact with the film. If the x-ray beam does not have enough energy to penetrate a tissue, an inadequate image will result regardless of how many x rays are used. Therefore no amount of mAs, which controls only x-ray quantity, will ever compensate for insufficient kVp.

As kVp is increased, more different types of tissue are penetrated and recorded on the film. Thus more ODs are present in the image. The image has a longer **gray scale**. Tissues that are not penetrated result in white areas on the radiograph. Such areas have no information recorded and therefore are diagnostically useless.

Adequate penetration is essential to the production of a useful radiograph. Penetration is also directly related to the number of different gray shades produced on the image. The penetrating ability of the x-ray beam, often termed **radiation quality**, is controlled by kVp.

MATERIALS REQUIRED

Radiographic x-ray machine
Pelvis phantom or other large phantom such as a skull
X-ray film processor
200-speed 10 in x 12 in (24 cm x 30 cm) screen film
    cassette
Lead numbers
View box
Densitometer

PROCEDURE

1. Warm up the processor if needed, and run a couple of "scrap" films through it to stabilize temperature and circulation.
2. Position the x-ray tube 100 cm from the tabletop.
3. Load and place a cassette lengthwise in the Bucky tray. Place the pelvis phantom on the table in supine position.
4. Collimate the light field to the film size and center.
5. Number each exposure with a lead marker on the cassette. Take four exposures on separate films using the techniques listed here or alternate techniques to accommodate your equipment.

Exposure 1	200 mA, 0.1 s (1/10 s;100 ms), 84 kVp
Exposure 2	200 mA, 0.2 s (1/5 s; 200 ms), 50 kVp
Exposure 3	200 mA, 0.5 s (1/2 s; 500 ms), 50 kVp
Exposure 4	200 mA, 1.0 s (1 s; 1000 ms), 50 kVp

6. Process the films.

RESULTS

For comparison purposes, exposure 1 must be of good average OD. If it is not, change the mA station used, but keep the mA constant throughout the experiment.

Visually examine each radiograph in comparison with exposure 1 to determine the amount of diagnostic information present and the number of different shades of gray produced.

EXERCISES

1 For each succeeding exposures 2, 3, and 4, the total mAs was approximately doubled each time, but a very low kVp was used. Note that for exposure 4 the total mAs is 10 times the mAs used for exposure 1. Has a satisfactory OD been achieved on exposure 2, 3, or 4?

2 Would a satisfactory OD be achieved at 40 kVp if the total mAs were increased to 1000 mAs?

3 Explain why this is so in terms of x-ray intensity and beam penetration.

4 Restate your answer from 3 in terms of mAs and kVp.

5 Count the number of different ODs, or shades of gray, on exposure 1 and 2, and record them here:

Exposure 1:_____   Exposure 2:_____

6 Which of these two radiographs displays the longest gray scale?

7 Explain why this is so.

EXPERIMENT   7

Effect of kVp on X-ray Quantity

OBJECT

To measure the effect of varying x-ray tube potential (kVp) on radiation intensity.

DISCUSSION

Experiment 4 demonstrated that x-ray quantity is directly related to mAs. X-ray quantity varies more rapidly with changes in kVp. The output intensity of an x-ray unit increases approximately as the square of the increase in kVp according to the relationship

$$\frac{I_1}{I_2} = \left(\frac{kVp_1}{kVp_2}\right)^2$$

where I_1 and I_2 are the x-ray intensities at kVp_1 and kVp_2, respectively. The exponent 2 is a reasonable approximation. Experimentally it has been shown to range from 1.5 to 3, depending on the x-ray tube design.

The number of electrons accelerated from cathode to anode is measured by the mAs. The number of accelerated electrons does not change with increasing tube potential (kVp). However, as kVp is increased, each electron possesses increased kinetic energy, which is transformed into more heat and x rays. As kVp is increased, each electron has a higher probability of multiple interactions with target atoms, thereby producing more x rays. Further, each x ray so produced will average a higher energy and therefore be more penetrating.

Changing kVp changes x-ray quantity and quality; changing mAs affects only x-ray quantity.

MATERIALS REQUIRED

Radiographic x-ray unit
Tape measure
Ionization chamber

PROCEDURE

1. Position the ionization chamber 100 cm from the x-ray tube target.
2. The x-ray machine may be used as it is normally filtered. Record the amount of total filtration present if known.
3. Select a low mA station (i.e., less than 100 mA) so that a number of repeat exposures will be possible at all kVp settings without overheating the tube.
4. Beginning at 40 kVp and increasing in 20 kVp increments, record the measured radiation intensity on the data sheet provided. Three measurements should be recorded at each kVp and the average value calculated. In addition to constant mA, the exposure time should remain fixed if the response range of the detector will allow; otherwise, the exposure time will have to be reduced with increasing kVp.
5. Determine the average exposure (mR or C/kg) at each kVp setting.
6. Express the x-ray output intensity as exposure rate in mR/s (C/kg-s). The following relationship may be used:

$$\text{Exposure rate (mR/s)} = \frac{\text{Exposure (mR)}}{\text{Exposure time (s)}}$$

RESULTS

Plot exposure rate (mR/s or C/kg-s) vs. tube potential (kVp) on the linear graph paper provided.

EXERCISES

1 What was the shape of the curve obtained? Why?
2 Calculate the quantity mR/mAs (C/kg-mAs) at each kVp selected. If these data were graphed, what would be the shape of the curve?

3 From the data recorded, estimate the actual value of n for this machine in the following expression:

$$\frac{I_1}{I_2} = \left(\frac{kVp_1}{kVp_2}\right)^n$$

4 From the data obtained, estimate the x-ray quantity resulting from the following factors:
   a. 55 kVp, 100 mA, 50 ms
   b. 73 kVp, 200 mA, 0.25 s
   c. 96 kVp, 50 mA, 750 ms
   d. 124 kVp, 300 mA, 16 ms
   e. 114 kVp, 300 mA, 16 ms

5 A useful rule of thumb states that a 15% increase in kVp accompanied by a 50% reducdon of mA will result in the same density on the film and reduced patient exposure. Can this be confirmed by your data? Begin with 70 kVp/50 mAs.

DATA SHEET
Laboratory experiment 7

Constant factors
100 cm source-to-detector distance
ma _____
Filtration _____mm Al

kVp	Exposure time (s)	Exposure (mR)			Average exposure (mR)	Exposure rate	
		First	Second	Third		mR/s	mR/mAs
1							
2							
3							
4							
5							
6							
7							
8							
9							
10							

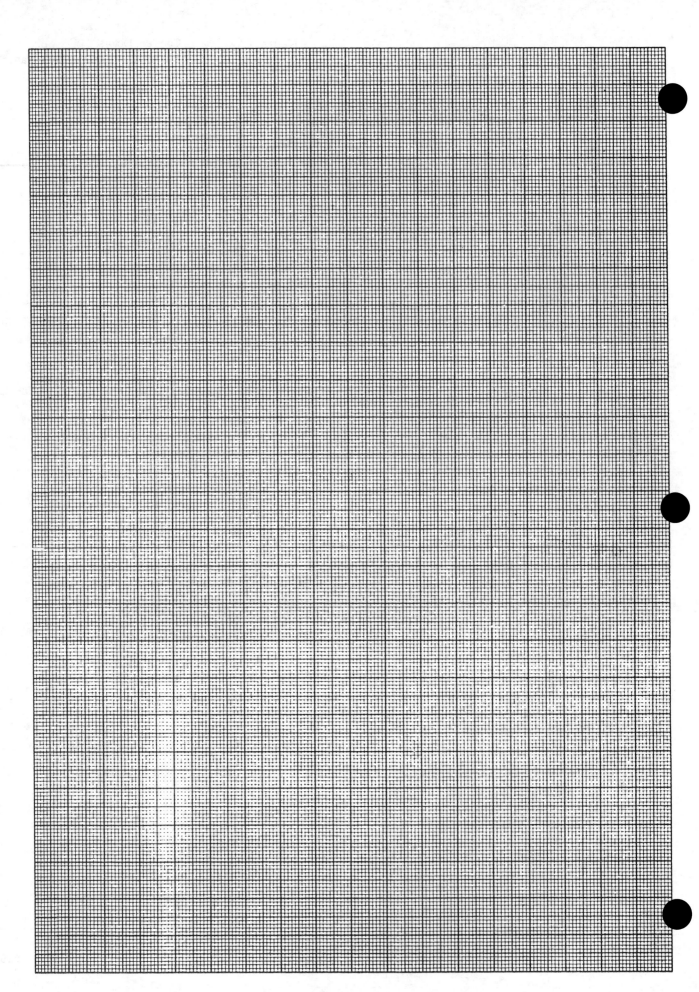

EXPERIMENT 8

Effect of kVp on Optical Density

OBJECT

To demonstrate how kVp influences optical density (OD; the 15% rule).

DISCUSSION

Peak kilovoltage controls the energy level of the x-ray beam. This property of the x-ray beam is also called **penetrability**, or x-ray beam quality. At higher energy levels, a greater percentage of the x rays penetrates through the anatomy and reaches the film, thus contributing to OD. Also, at higher kVp the x-ray tube emits more x rays. When this higher radiation intensity is added to the increased penetration, the resulting image becomes much darker. That is, a small change in kVp causes a big change in OD.

When kVp is changed, it is not easy to predict exactly how much OD will change because it depends on two different processes: changing beam intensity and changing beam penetration. However, a rule of thumb traditionally used by radiologic technologists has proved very useful. The **15% rule** states that if the kVp is changed by 15%, the resulting OD will change roughly by a factor of two. Therefore a 15% increase in kVp should be accompanied by a 50% reduction in mAs to maintain constant OD.

MATERIALS REQUIRED

Radiographic x-ray machine
Skull phantom, other large phantom, or large step wedge
X-ray film processor
200-speed 10 in x 12 in (24 cm x 30 cm) screen film cassette
Lead numbers
Positioning sponges
View box
Densitometer
Calculator

PROCEDURE

1. Warm up the processor if needed, and run a couple of "scrap" films through it to stabilize temperature and circulation.
2. Position the x-ray tube 100 cm from the tabletop.
3. Load and place a cassette crosswise on the tabletop. Place the anatomic phantom on the cassette in lateral position, using sponges as needed to balance it.
4. Collimate the light field to the film size, and center to the anatomic phantom.
5. Number each exposure with a lead marker on the cassette. Take four exposures on separate films using the techniques listed here or alternate techniques to accommodate your equipment. If possible, use the same mA station for all exposures. Kilovoltage increases are made in 15% increments. Beginning with exposure 3, these changes are compensated by cutting the exposure time in half each time.

Exposure 1   50 mA, 0.1 s (1/10 s; 100 ms), 70 kVp
Exposure 2   50 mA, 0.1 s (1/10 s; 100 ms), 80 kVp
Exposure 3   50 mA, 0.05 s (1/20 s; 50 ms), 80 kVp
Exposure 4   50 mA, 0.025 s (1/40 s; 25 ms), 92 kvp

6. Process the films.
7. On the resulting images, select an area within the bony anatomy that shows a smooth medium gray OD on exposure 1. Circle this area, and, using the densitometer, determine the OD in this same area for each exposure.

RESULTS

In Table E8-1, record for each exposure the total mAs and kVp used and the measured OD.

TABLE E8-1

	mAs	kVp	OD
Exposure 1			
Exposure 2			
Exposure 3			
Exposure 4			

EXERCISES

1 Compute the relative OD change for exposure 2 by dividing the OD for 1 into that for 2, and record here:

2/1:_____

2 Visually compare exposure 2 to exposure 1. When kVp is increased without adjusting any other factors, what happens to overall OD?

3 According to your preceding calculation, how much darker is exposure 2 compared with exposure 1?

4 Compute the relative OD changes for the adjustments in technique made in the subsequent exposures by dividing the OD for 3 by that for 1, and the OD for 4 by 3, and record here:

3/1: _____   4/3: _____

5 Compute an average OD change by summing these two numbers and then dividing by 2:

Average OD change: _____

6 An OD change ratio of 1.0 would indicate that the ODs produced by the different techniques are exactly the same. Is your computed average change within 15% of the original; that is, does it fall between 0.85 and 1.15?

7 In exposures 3 and 4, a 15% increase in kVp was accompanied by halving the mAs. Does the 15% rule of thumb work in approximately maintaining overall OD when changing kVp?

EXPERIMENT   9

Effect of kVp on Image Contrast

Name_____

Date_____

OBJECT

To demonstrate how image contrast changes when kVp is changed.

DISCUSSION

Kilovoltage also affects image contrast for two important reasons. First, at higher energies, the x rays penetrate more tissues and thus lengthen the gray scale recorded. Gray scale is the opposite of contrast. Second, at higher x-ray beam energies, very few photoelectric interactions occur in the tissues. The fogging of the image from Compton interactions then becomes more apparent. Combining the effects of a longer gray scale with more visible fog, contrast is reduced. Conversely, using low kVp's will restore higher image contrast.

MATERIALS REQUIRED

Radiographic x-ray machine
Skull phantom, other large phantom, or large step wedge
X-ray film processor
Two-speed 10 in x 12 in (24 cm x 30 cm) screen film cassette
Lead number
Positioning sponges View box
Densitometer Calculator

PROCEDURE

1. Warm up the processor if needed, and run a couple of "scrap" films through it to stabilize temperature and circulation.
2. Position the x-ray tube 100 cm from the tabletop.
3. Load and place a cassette crosswise on the tabletop. Place the anatomic phantom on the cassette in lateral position, using sponges as needed to balance it.
4. Collimate the light field to the film size, and center

to the anatomic phantom.
5. Number each exposure with a lead marker on the cassette. Take two exposures on separate films using the techniques listed below or alternate techniques to accommodate your equipment. If possible, use the same mA station for both exposures.

Exposure 1   50 mA, 0.1 s (1/10 s; 100 ms), 70 kVp
Exposure 2   50 mA, 0.025 s (1/40 s; 25 ms), 92 kVp

6. Process the films.
7. On the resulting images, select an area within the bony anatomy that shows a uniform light gray OD on exposure 1 and a uniform medium gray OD on exposure 2. Circle these areas, and using the densitometer, determine the OD in each area for each exposure.

RESULTS

In Table E9-1, record for each exposure the kVp used and the measured OD in area A and area B.

EXERCISES

1 Compute the contrast for each exposure by subtracting the area A OD by the area B OD, and record here:

Exposure 1 contrast (A-B):_____
Exposure 2 contrast (A-B):_____

TABLE E9-1

	kVp	Area A OD	Area B OD
Exposure 1			
Exposure 2			

2 Compare the computed contrast levels. Even though mAs was compensated for kVp to maintain OD, what happened to the measured contrast for exposure 2 when a much higher kVp was used?

3 Visually compare exposure 2 to exposure 1. When using a much higher kVp, is the change in contrast visible?

4 The difference between exposure 1 and exposure 2 is 22 kVp. Would a difference in contrast be visible for a much smaller change, such as an increase of 4 kVp?

5 Briefly explain why this contrast change occurs at high kVp levels.

EXPERIMENT   10

Half-value Layer

OBJECT

To determine the half-value layer (HVL) of an x-ray beam under three conditions of kVp.

DISCUSSION

HVL is defined as that thickness of an absorbing material required to reduce the intensity of the x-ray beam to one half its original value. HVL is the single most appropriate unit of measure for beam quality. Total filtration, effective energy, and kVp are also useful for describing beam quality. The absorbing material most often used to determine the HVL of diagnostic x-ray machines is aluminum.

MATERIALS REQUIRED

Radiographic x-ray machine
Ionization chamber
Aluminum absorbers
Ring stand and clamps

PROCEDURE

1. Position the ionization chamber 100 cm from the x-ray source. Place aluminum absorbers approximately midway between the ionization chamber and the x-ray tube target.
2. The x-ray machine may be used as it is normally filtered. Record the amount of total filtration if possible.
3. Using the light localizer, collimate to just cover the area of the ionization chamber.
4. Adjust the tube potential to 60 kVp.
5. Select a technique of mAs that will provide a reading that is nearly full scale on the ionization chamber.
6. Expose the ionization chamber sequentially three times, and record each measurement on the data sheet provided.
7. Insert 0.5 mm Al filtration midway between the target and detector, and record three additional measurements.
8. Repeat this process with added aluminum filtration thicknesses of 1.0, 2.0, 3.0, 4.0, 6.0, and 8.0 mm. If an increase in mA, exposure time, or both is required at greater thicknesses of aluminum filtration, record these changes.
9. Repeat steps 4 through 8 at 90 kVp and again at 120 kVp.
10. Calculate the average intensity (mR) for each level of filtration at each kVp. Express the x-ray intensity in mR/mAs as follows:

X-ray intensity (mR/mAs) =

$$\frac{\text{Average intensity (mR)}}{\text{Tube current (mA)} \times \text{Exposure time (s)}}$$

RESULTS

Plot the x-ray intensity vs. mm Al added filtration for each kVp on the linear and semilog graph paper provided. Estimate the HVL for each curve.

EXERCISES

1 Complete Table E10-1.

TABLE E10-1

kVP	HVL (mm Al)
60	
90	
120	

2 On the linear graph paper provided, plot HVLvs. kVp. From the extrapoladon of this curve, what would be the estimated HVL at 40 kVp? At 140 kVp?

3 Given the data obtained at 90 kVp, if an additional 1 mm A1 were added to the existing total filtration, what would the HVL be?

4 The homogeneity coefficient is defined as the ratio of the first HVL to the second HVL. From the data collected at 60 and 120 kVp, estimate the homogeneity coefficient for each condition.

DATA SHEET
Laboratory experiment 10

Constant factors
100 cm source-to-ionization chamber distance
Total filtration _____mm Al

kVp	Added filtration (mm Al)	Tube current (ma)	Exposure time (s)	Exposure (mR) First	Second	Third	Average exposure (mR)	mR/mAs
60	0							
60	0.5							
60	1.0							
60	2.0							
60	3.0							
60	4.0							
60	6.0							
60	8.0							
90	0							
90	0.5							
90	1.0							
90	2.0							
90	3.0							
90	4.0							
90	6.0							
90	8.0							
120	0							
120	0.5							
120	1.0							
120	2.0							
120	3.0							
120	4.0							
120	6.0							
120	8.0							

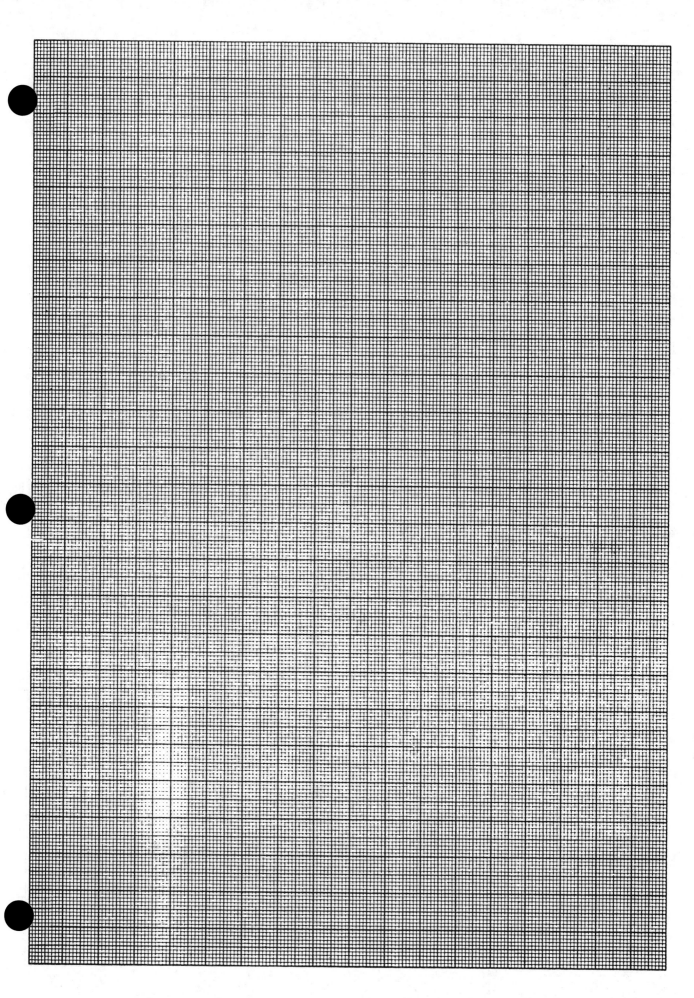

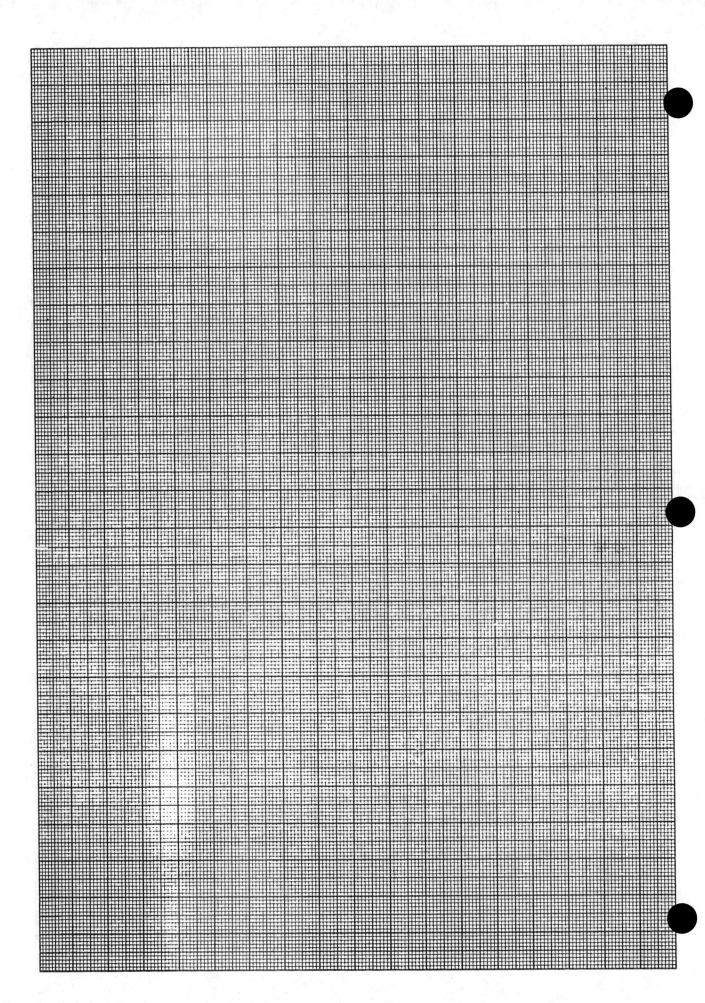

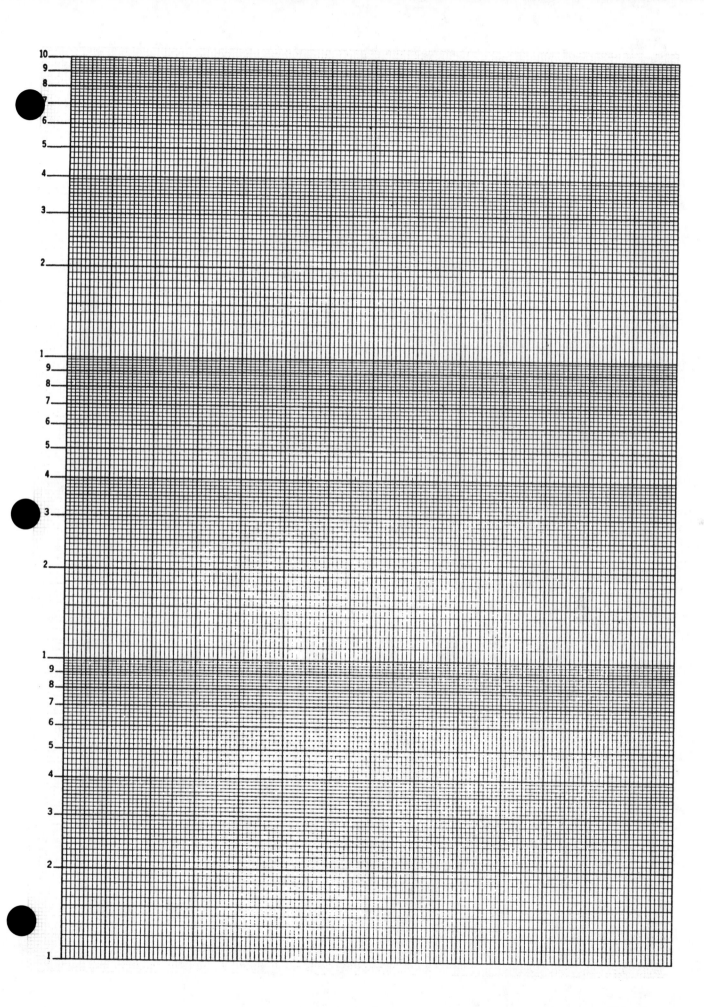

Name_____

Date_____

Field Size

OBJECT

To demonstrate the effects of field size limitation (collimation) on image optical density (OD) and contrast.

DISCUSSION

When the size of the x-ray field is reduced, a smaller volume of tissue is exposed to radiation. The volume of tissue exposed determines the amount of scatter radiation produced and thus affects the amount of fog density of the radiograph. By collimating the x-ray field to a smaller size, less fog density is produced on the final image, which will therefore demonstrate higher contrast. The total image OD is contributed to both by primary x rays penetrating to the film and by secondary scatter x rays produced within tissues. In reducing scatter radiation by collimation of the x-ray field to a smaller size one also produces an image with lower OD (lighter).

MATERIALS REQUIRED

Radiographic x-ray machine
Pelvis phantom or other phantom large enough to generate substantial scatter radiation
X-ray film processor
200-speed screen film cassettes, one 14 in x 17 in (35 cm x 42 cm) and one 10 in x 12 in (24 cm x 30 cm) or smaller
Sponges, sandbags, or positioning clamps
Lead numbers
View box
Densitometer Calculator

PROCEDURE

1. Warm up the processor if needed, and run a couple of "scrap" films through it to stabilize temperature and circulation.

2. Set 86 kVp, 100 mA, and 0.1 s (1/10 s; 100 ms) exposure time. These will remain constant throughout the experiment.
3. Position the x-ray tube 100 cm from the tabletop.
4. Have sponges and sandbags, or clamps, at hand to hold the pelvis phantom in a **lateral** position. If using another test object, position it with the thickest dimension vertical.
5. Number each film with a lead marker on the cassette. Take two exposures on separate films, using the techniques listed here or alternate techniques used to accommodate your equipment.

Exposure 1   Load and place the large cassette lengthwise on the tabletop. Place the pelvis phantom in lateral position on the film. Open the field size to 14 in x 17 in, and center over the lumbar vertebrae. Expose the film.

Exposure 2   Load and place the small cassette lengthwise on the tabletop. Place the pelvis phantom in lateral position on the film. Collimate the field size to a 5 in x 5 in square, and center over the lumbar vertebrae. Expose the film using the same technique.

6. Process the films.
7. On exposure 2, select and circle two uniform OD areas within the anatomy to take densitometer measurements as follows: area A must show a medium dark gray soft tissue density. Area B must show a light gray bony density. Now circle the same two smooth density areas on exposure 1. Using the densitometer, determine the OD in these two areas for each exposure, and record below.

TABLE E11-1

	Field size	Area A OD	Area B OD
Exposure 1			
Exposure 2			

RESULTS

In Table E11-1, record for each exposure the field size used and the measured OD in areas A and B.

EXERCISES

1 In Table E11-1, what happened to the OD in area A when the field size was reduced? Can you visually see the difference in area A between the two films?

2 Why does this effect occur when reducing field size?

3 Compute the radiographic technique change that would be required to maintain OD when field size is reduced in this case as follows: divide area A OD for exposure 2 into that for exposure 1. This is the factor by which mAs must be changed in order to maintain constant OD:

$$\frac{\text{Exposure 1, area A}}{\text{Exposure 2, area A}} = \underline{\hspace{2cm}} =$$

4 Change the above answer into a percentage as follows: from this ratio, subtract 1.0 and then multiply the remaining decimal number by 100:

$$\underline{\hspace{1.5cm}} - 1.0 = \underline{\hspace{1.5cm}} \times 100 = \underline{\hspace{1cm}}\%$$

This is the percentage by which mAs must be changed to compensate. When collimating down to the smaller 5 in square field, should mAs be increased or decreased by this percentage to maintain OD?

5 Compute the contrast for each exposure as follows: subtract the area A OD by the area B OD, and record here:

Exposure 1 contrast (A-B): _____

Exposure 2 contrast (A-B): _____

6 Compare the computed contrast levels. What happened to the measured contrast for exposure 2 when a much smaller field size was used?

7 Visually compare exposure 2 to exposure 1. When using a much higher kVp, would the change in contrast be visible?

8 Briefly explain why this contrast change occurs with smaller field sizes.

EXPERIMENT   12

Effect of Radiographic Grids on Optical Density and Contrast

OBJECT

To demonstrate the effects of radiographic grids on optical density (OD) and contrast.

DISCUSSION

When radiographing thick body parts, the quality of the image will be reduced by the scatter radiation produced. Radiographic grids should be used in such cases to improve image contrast. The narrow slits of the grid allow most of the primary x rays to pass through while absorbing much of the scattered x rays. The effectiveness of a grid can be measured by comparing the image contrast produced with the grid to that produced without the grid.

It is unfortunate that this reduction in scatter radiation, along with the absorption of some of the primaly beam, results in a loss of OD. To restore proper OD, radiographic technique must be increased. This leads to an increase in patient dose, but this increase is necessary for adequate image quality. The higher the grid ratio, the more the radiographic technique must be increased to maintain OD.

MATERIALS REQUIRED

Radiographic x-ray machine
Pelvis phantom or other phantom large enough to generate substantial scatter radiation
X-ray film processor
Wafer grids, (clamp-on or tape-on type) of different ratios as available; 10 in x 12 in size preferred
200-speed screen film cassettes of the same size as the wafer grids available
Sponges, sandbags, or positioning clamps Leaded rubber sheets
Lead numbers
View box
Densitometer
Calculator

PROCEDURE

1. Warm up the processor if needed, and run a couple of "scrap" films through it to stabilize temperature and circulation.
2. Position the x-ray tube 100 cm from the tabletop.
3. Position sponges, sandbags, or clamps to hold the pelvis phantom in a lateral position. If using another phantom, position it with the thickest dimension vertical.
4. Set 86 kVp. This will remain constant throughout the experiment.
5. Number each film with a lead marker on the cassette. Take exposures on separate films using the techniques listed here or record the alternate techniques you use.

Exposure 1   No grid: Place the cassette on the tabletop. Collimate to a 14 in x 17 in lengthwise field, regardless of the film size used. Technique: 200 mA, 0.05 s (1/20 s; 50 ms), 10 mAs
NOTE: Process and check this film. It should be of medium overall density yet appear quite gray with low contrast. If it is very light or very dark, adjust the mAs and repeat Record this alternate technique:
Alternate technique: _____

Additional exposures   Wafer grid: Place the film on the tabletop with the grid centered on the top of the film. Precisely center the light field to the grid. Then arrange the phantom in lateral position on top of the grid. Do not change collimation.
Technique: Find the grid ratio labelled or embossed on one side of the grid. Refer to Table E12-1, and multiply the mAs used in the first exposure by the factor listed. (NOTE: The new mAs only needs to be

TABLE E12-1

Grid ratio	Multiply nongrid mAs by:
5:1 or 6:1	2
8:1	3
10:1 or 12:1	4
15:1 or 16:1	5

TABLE E12-2

	Grid ratio	Area A OD	Area B OD
Exposure 1			
Exposure 2			
Exposure 3			
Exposure 4			

approximate. Do *not* change the mA station unless there is no other way to approximate the needed mAs.) Record each ratio and the mAs used:

	Grid ratio	mAs
Exposure 2:	_____	_____
Exposure 3:	_____	_____
Exposure 4:	_____	_____

1. Process the films.
2. On the first exposure, select and circle two uniform OD areas within the anatomy to take densitometer measurements. Area A must show a dark gray soft tissue density but must not be black. Area B must show a medium gray bony density. Now circle the same two uniform optical density areas on all other exposures. Using the densitometer, determine the OD in these two areas for each exposure, and record in Table E12-2.

RESULTS

In Table E12-2, record for each exposure the grid ratio used and the measured OD in areas A and B.

EXERCISES

1 Consider only the ODs for area A. Compute the relative OD change for exposures 2, 3, and 4 by dividing the area A OD for 1 into each of them, and record here:

2/1:_____ 3/1:_____ 4/1:_____

2 An OD change of 1.0 would indicate that the ODs produced by the different techniques are exactly the same. Consider the value above the exposure 2: Is your computed average change within 20% of the original; that is, does it fall between 0.8 and 1.2? Did the value for the other grids also fall within this range? If not, list below the factors you would use in place of those from the table.

3 Visually compare exposures 2, 3, and 4 to exposure 1. Did the technique factors from the table reasonably maintain OD when changing from nongrid to grid exposures?

4 If these technique adjustments were not made, how would these radiographs have appeared? Why?

5 Compute the contrast for each exposure as follows: subtract the area A optical density by the area B optical density, and record here:

	Grid ratio	Contrast (A-B)
Exposure 1	_____	_____
Exposure 2	_____	_____
Exposure 3	_____	_____
Exposure 4	_____	_____

6 Compare the computed contrast levels for exposures 2, 3, and 4 to the contrast when a grid is used.

7 How do grids accomplish this change in contrast?

EXPERIMENT 13

Effect of Radiographic Grids and Grid Cutoff

OBJECT

To demonstrate grid cutoff.

DISCUSSION

Grid cutoff, a massive loss of optical density (OD), can be caused by laterally off-centering the grid in relation to the central ray, by laterally angling the grid to the central ray so that they are not perpendicular to each other, by placing the grid at an improper distance from the x-ray tube (outside of the grid radius), or by placing the grid upside down. The pattern of grid cutoff can often be used to determine which of these errors caused it.

MATERIALS REQUIRED

Radiographic x-ray machine

Pelvis phantom or other phantom large enough to generate substantial scatter radiation

X-ray film processor

Wafer grids (clamp-on or tape-on type) of different ratios as available; 10 in x 12 in size preferred (Bucky may be used if you can determine the ratio of the grid in it.)

200-speed screen film cassettes of the same size as the wafer grids available

Sponges, sandbags, or positioning clamps

Leaded rubber sheets

Lead numbers

View box

Densitometer

Calculator

PROCEDURE

1. Warm up the processor if needed, and run a couple of "scrap" films through it to stabilize temperature and circulation.
2. Position the x-ray tube 100 cm from the tabletop.
3. Set 50 mA and 0.05 s (1/20 s; 50 ms). This will remain constant throughout the experiment except on the last exposure.
4. No phantom or test object is used for this experiment. Use the highest ratio 10 in x 12 in wafer grid available to you, placing it over each film and exposing it directly to the x-ray beam.
5. Open the light field in 10 in x 12 in, and leave it at this position throughout the experiment.
6. Number each film with a lead marker on the cassette. Take exposures on separate films, following the directions below. Different angles and kVp levels are required at different grid ratios for the experiment. Instructions are listed for an 8:1 grid and for a 12:1 grid. Use those closest to the grid you have.

		If using 8:1 GRID	If using 12:1 GRID
Exposure 1:	Angle beam parallel to grid strips and center	30-degree angle, 70 kVp	25-degree angle, 80 kVp
Exposure 2:	Angle beam perpendicular to grid strips and center	30-degree angle, 70 kVp	25-degree angle, 80 kVp
Exposure 3:	Off-center a perpendicular beam across grid strips by 3 inches	65 kVp	75 kVp

	If using 8:1 GRID	If using 12:1 GRID
Exposure 4: Turn grid over and expose up side down using a perpendicular, centered beam	62 kVp	70 kVp
Exposure 5: Use a perpendicular, centered beam, but change source-to-image receptor distance (SID) to 72 inches by placing the film and grid on the floor. NOTE: Change exposure time to 0.1 (1/10) s.	62 kVp	70 kVp

RESULTS

Visually observe the radiographs on a view box.

EXERCISES

1 Which of the preceding situations did not result in grid cutoff? Why?
2 Which of the preceding situations resulted in grid cutoff more severe toward one side of the film than the other?
3 Which of the preceding situations resulted in grid cutoff that is equal toward both sides of the film?
4 Which of the preceding situations caused the most severe grid cutoff overall?
5 If a higher ratio grid were used for this experiment, what change would you expect in all of the results? Why?

EXPERIMENT 14

Intensifying Screens Effect on Optical Density and Image Contrast

OBJECT

To demonstrate how intensifying screens work and their effect on optical density (OD) and contrast.

DISCUSSION

Intensifying screens convert x rays into light, which in turn exposes the radiographic film. The principal result is a reduction in patient dose. They convert both the energy and the intensity of the x-ray beam into visible light that interacts with radiographic film more readily than x rays. Either an increase in kVp or an increase in mAs will result in the screen glowing brighter, resulting in a darker radiograph.

Intensifying screens can be made "faster" in several ways. Their absorption efficiency for x rays can be increased by using thicker emulsions. Their emission efficiency for light can be increased by improvements in phosphor composition. Their x ray to light conversion efficiency can be enhanced by using more effective phosphors, such as rare earth elements. To maintain OD, techniques must be reduced by specified amounts when employing faster screens.

Generally, intensifying screens increase contrast. This is not always measurable but is particularly pronounced when comparing screen exposures to nonscreen direct exposures.

RECOMMENDED DEMONSTRATION

Open the different types of screens available, and lay them side by side on the tabletop. Open the light field to include portions of as many of the screens as possible. Turn off all lights in the examination room. Observe the different colors of light emitted by each screen when exposed using the following techniques:

1. 50 mA, 3 s, 50 kVp
2. 50 mA, 3 s, 90 kVp
3. 100 mA, 3 s, 50 kVp

At the same time compare the brightness of light emitted by each screen. Discuss the reasons for the different brightness levels with different types of screens and with different radiographic techniques.

MATERIALS REQUIRED

Radiographic x-ray machine
Hand phantom or similar thin phantom
Knee phantom or phantom of similar thickness
X-ray film processor
Direct exposure holder
100 speed screen cassette, preferably the same size as the direct exposure holder
400 screen cassette, preferably the same size as the direct exposure holder
Small, dry bone such as a phalanx
Rectangular sponge about 6 inches thick
Lead numbers
View box
Densitometer
Calculator

PROCEDURE

1. Warm up the processor if needed, and run a couple of "scrap" films through it to stabilize temperature and circulation.
2. Position the x-ray tube 100 cm from the tabletop.
3. Number each film with a lead marker on the cassette. Take exposures on separate films using the techniques listed here or recording alternate techniques you use.

Exposure 1 Load and place the high speed or rare earth screen cassette on the tabletop. Place the knee phantom on the cassette, using sponges as needed to balance it. Collimate to the film size. Technique: 200 mA, 0.025 s (1/40 s; 25 ms), 5 mAs, 65 kVp.

NOTE: Process and check this film. It should be of medium OD. If it is very light or very dark, adjust the mAs and start over. Write your alternate technique here:

Alternate technique:_____

Exposure 2 Load and place the slow speed ("extremity" or "fine") or par speed screen cassette on the tabletop. Place the knee phantom on the cassette, in precisely the same position as you did for exposure 1. Do not change collimation from exposure 1.

Technique: Refer to Table E14-1, which gives technique factors for intensifying screens, and determine the mAs to be used as follows: Divide the factor listed for the new screen to be used by the factor listed for the screen used in exposure 1. Multiply the original mAs by your answer. (For example, if you used a rare earth medium, 200-speed screen on exposure 1 and are using a slow (50-speed) screen now, divide 2 by 1/2 = 4. Use four times as much mAs as in exposure 1.) Record the technique you use here:

Technique used:_____

Total mAs used:_____

Exposure 3 Again, use the slow speed ("extremity" or "fine") or par speed screen cassette on the tabletop. Collimate to the film size and center. Then place thick rectangular sponges on the film to create an OID of about 6 inches. Place the hand phantom on the sponges, with the resolution test pattern alongside it. Technique: 50 mA, 0.025 s (1/40 s; 25 ms), 1.25 mAs, 54 kVp.

NOTE: Process and check this film. It should be of medium overall OD. If it is very light or very dark, adjust the mAs and start over. Write your alternate technique here:

Alternate technique:_____

Exposure 4 Load the direct exposure holder with the same type of film used in the cassettes, and place it on the tabletop. Center the light field first (do not change collimation from exposure 3). Place the 6 inches of sponge on the film, with the hand phantom and resolution template alongside it as before.

TABLE E14-1 Technique factors for intensifying screens

Type of screen	Technique factor
Direct exposure holder	
With screen film	80
With direct exposure film	30
50 speed	2
100 speed	1
400 speed	1/4

Technique: 250 to 300 mAs, 54 kVp. (This technique approximates the application of the factor for a direct exposure holder with screen film as listed in Table E14-1.)

4. Process the films.
5. On exposure 1, select and circle two smooth OD areas within the anatomy to take densitometer measurements as follows: area A must show a medium dark gray soft tissue density. Area B must show a light gray bony density. Now circle the same two smooth OD areas on exposure 2. Repeat this procedure with exposures 3 and 4, circling a dark soft tissue area for area A and a light bony area for area B. Using the densitometer, determine the OD in these two areas for each exposure, and record in Table E14-2.

RESULTS

In Table E14-2, record each type of screen used, the total mAs used, and the measured OD in areas A and B.

EXERCISES

1 On a view box, visually compare the overall ODs for exposures 1 and 2. Refer to Table E14-2. By what ratio was the mAs increased when changing from the higher speed screen to the slower screen?

2 Did this technique change reasonably maintain OD when changing screens? If not, what factor would you use in place of the one from Table E14-2?

3 If this change in screens were made without adjusting technique, what would happen to the resulting OD?

4 Compute the contrast for each exposure as follows: subtract the area A OD by the area B OD, and record here:

Exposure 1 contrast (A-B): _____
Exposure 2 contrast (A-B): _____
Exposure 3 contrast (A-B): _____
Exposure 4 contrast (A-B): _____

TABLE E14-2

	Type of screen	Total mAs used	Area A OD	Area B OD
Exposure 1				
Exposure 2				
Exposure 3				
Exposure 4				

5 Compare the computed contrast level for exposure 2 to the contrast on exposure 1. Is there any difference? If so, which of these two screen speeds produces the highest image contrast?

6 Now compare the computed contrast level for exposure 3 to the contrast on exposure 4. Which of these two methods of exposure produces the highest image contrast?

EXPERIMENT   15

Intensifying Screens Effect on Image Blur

OBJECT

To demonstrate how intensifying screens work and their effect on image blur.

DISCUSSION

Intensifying screens convert x rays into light, which in turn exposes the radiographic film. The principal result is a reduction in patient dose. They convert both the energy and the intensity of the x-ray beam into visible light that interacts with radiographic film much easier than x rays. Either an increase in kVp or an increase in mAs will result in the screen glowing brighter, resulting in a darker radiograph.

The use of screens increases image blur when compared to direct exposure techniques. As the light passes from the screen to the film, it spreads, reducing the sharpness of the image. This property is called **screen blur**. This problem is not present with direct exposures, so they are much sharper.

MATERIALS REQUIRED

Radiographic x-ray machine
Hand phantom or similar thin phantom
Knee phantom or phantom of similar thickness
X-ray film processor
Direct exposure holder
100 speed screen cassette, preferably the same size as the direct exposure holder
400 screen cassette, preferably the same size as the direct exposure holder
Resolution test pattern (line pairs per millimeter [Ip/ mm])
Rectangular sponge about 6 inches thick
Lead numbers
View box
Densitometer
Calculator

PROCEDURE

1. Warm up the processor if needed, and run a couple of "scrap" films through it to stabilize temperature and circulation.
2. Position the x-ray tube 100 cm from the tabletop.
3. Number each film with a lead marker on the cassette. Take exposures on separate films using the techniques listed here or recording alternate techniques you use.

Exposure 1   Load and place the high speed or rare earth screen cassette on the tabletop. Place the resolution test pattern on the cassette, using sponges as needed to balance it. Collimate to the film size.
Technique: 200 mA, 0.025 s (1/40 s; 25 ms), 5 mAs, 65 kVp.
NOTE: Process and check this film. It should be of medium overall optical density. If it is very light or very dark, adjust the mAs and start over. Write your alternate technique here:
Alternate technique:_____

Exposure 2   Load and place the slow speed ("extremity" or "fine") or par speed screen cassette on the tabletop. Place the the resolution test pattern on the cassette. Do not change collimation from exposure 1.
Technique: Refer to Table E14-2 to determine the mAs to be used as described for that experiment.
Technique used:_____
Total mAs used:_____

Exposure 3   Again, use the slow speed ("extremity" or "fine") or par speed screen cassette on the tabletop. Collimate to the film size and center. Then place a thick rectangular sponge on the film to create an OID of about 6 inches. Place the resolution test pattern on the sponge. Technique: 50 mA, 0.025 s (1/40 s; 25 ms), 1.25 mAs, 54 kVp. NOTE: Process and check this film. It should be of gray optical density. If it is very light or very dark, adjust the mAs and start over. Write your alternate technique here:

Alternate technique:_____

Exposure 4   Load the direct exposure holder with the same type of film used in the cassettes, and place it on the tabletop. Center the light field first (do not change collimation from exposure 3). Place the 6-in sponge on the film, with the resolution test pattern on it as before.

Technique: 250 to 300 mAs, 54 kVp.

4. Process the films.

RESULTS

On the images of the resolution test pattern, scan downward across the black and white line pairs, from thickest to thinnest, and determine where they are blurred so that you cannot distinguish separate lines with clear edges. Note which line pair number this is. Refer to the resolution test pattern itself or to the table provided by your instructor to read off how many line pairs per millimeter correspond to this line pair number.

In Table E15-1, record each type of screen and the resolution in line pairs per millimeter.

TABLE E15-1

	Type of screen	Resolution (lp/mm)
Exposure 1		
Exposure 2		
Exposure 3		
Exposure 4		

EXERCISES

1 On a view box, visually compare only exposures 3 and 4. Wlth which type of image receptor are more lines resolved? Wlth which receptor do these lines appear to have sharper edges?

2 Refer to Table E15-1. Which receptor resolved the greatest number of line pairs per millimeter, the screen or the direct exposure holder? Does this agree with your visual observations in exercise 1?

3 Why does this effect occur when changing from screen to direct exposures?

4 Refer to Table E15-1. Which of the two screen speeds, the higher or the lower speed, resolved the greatest number of line pairs per millimeter?

EXPERIMENT   16

Processor Quality Assurance

OBJECT

To demonstrate a quality assurance program for automatic film processors.

DISCUSSION

When a film is "too light" or "too dark," the most frequent cause is improper radiographic technique. However, the radiographic unit or automatic processor is occasionally at fault. By establishing a processor quality assurance program, problems with processors can be documented and sometimes corrected even before processing of patient films.

A processor control program is begun by reserving a box of film to be used exclusively for processor monitoring. The standard or control film is exposed with a sensitometer. The sensitometer is a device that has an accurately reproducible light intensity combined with optical filters to produce a step-wedge image. Each day before patient film processing a test film is made with the sensitometer. With a busy processor this test may be repeated several times each day. The test film is then compared with the standard film. No change should be observed, since the same lot of film, an identical exposure of film, and same processing are used. A variation between the standard film and the test film represents a change in the automatic film processor.

Since daily monitoring of a processor is not practical for a student laboratory exercise, perform the suggested monitoring weekly at the beginning of each laboratory period. You will maintain a record of each week's results and graph the data weekly during the course of the experiment. This data will be used to evaluate the stability of performance of one processor. During the final laboratory period, you will evaluate the uniformity of all of the processors within your department.

MATERIALS REQUIRED

Empty film box that can be resealed without light leaks
Sensitometer that produces steps discernible to the eye (i.e., approximately 15% exposure increase from one step to the next)
Film illuminator
25 sheets of 8 in x 10 in (20 cm x 25 cm) film from the same manufacturer's lot

PROCEDURE
First Week

1. Set aside 25 sheets of film from the same manufacturer's lot exclusively for this experiment in an empty box that can be restored to its light-tight condition.
2. Allow the sensitometer to warm up for 5 minutes to ensure stability of the light source.
3. Expose a film with the sensitometer.
4. Process the film in the automatic processor under investigation. Be careful to note the orientation of the transfer of the film from the sensitometer into the processor so that the procedure can be identical each week.
5. Record all the data registered on the data sheet.
6. Save the film, and label it as standard or control.

Each Successive Week

1. Repeat steps 2 to 5 of the instructions from the first week.
2. Label the film as Test Film Week No. _____, and date it.
3. Using the same area of the illuminator each week, visually match the images of the step wedges of the test film with the standard film. Each step represents a change of 15% in exposure. A variance of two steps or greater indicates that the processor requires attention.

4. Record the contrast comparison difference, developer temperature, and water temperature on the data sheet, and plot the data on the graph sheet provided.

Final Week

1. Expose the test film, and record the data as usual.
2. During this laboratory period, compare the response of this processor with four other processors in your department. This can be done by using the sensitometer to expose films from the reserved package and processing them in the other processors in the same manner as all previous test films.
3. Identify the processor on each test film.

4. Compare the step-wedge images of these four processors with the test film from the processor monitored weekly, and record the results on the data sheet.

EXERCISES

1 Discuss the stability of the processor that was monitored.
2 If the contrast difference varies by more than two steps, what can the technologist check before requesting a service call?
3 How do the processors within your department compare in uniformity?

DATA SHEET
Laboratory experiment 16

Processor identification_____

Week no.	Contrast comparison	Developer temperature (˚F or ˚C)	Water temperature (˚F or ˚C)
1			
2			
3			
4			
5			
6			
7			
8			
9			
10			
11			
12			
13			
14			
15			
16			

	Processor				
	1*	2	3	4	5
Contrast comparison difference					

* Processor that has been monitored weekly

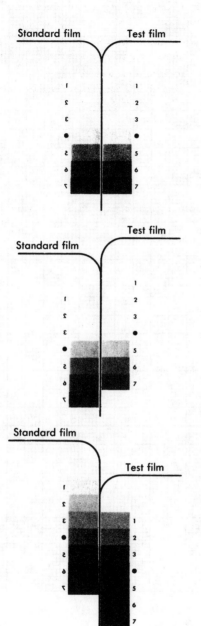

The test film is one step lighter or "slower" than the standard. This should be recorded as "−1".

The test film is 2 steps darker or "faster" than the standard. This should be recorded as "+2".

The test film matches the standard film. This should be recorded as a difference of "0".

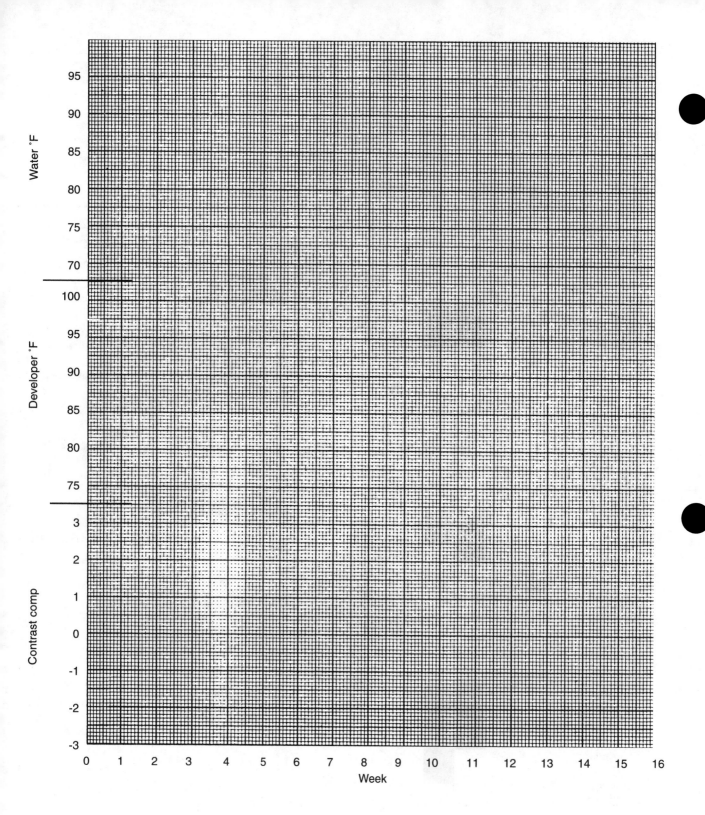

Water °F

95
90
85
80
75
70

Developer °F

100
95
90
85
80
75

Contrast comp

3
2
1
0
-1
-2
-3

0 1 2 3 4 5 6 7 8 9 10 11 12 13 14 15 16

Week

EXPERIMENT 17

Effect of Focal Spot Size on Image Blur

OBJECT

To demonstrate the effect that changing the focal spot size has on image blur.

DISCUSSION

The size of the focal spot is the only variable in radiography that affects image blur exclusively, without affecting any other image quality. It thus becomes the most important factor controlling the spatial resolution of the imaging system. The smaller the focal spot used, the less focal spot blur is transferred to the image.

Generally, small focal spots should be used for any anatomy that is small enough to be radiographed tabletop (without a Bucky) in order to maximize diagnostic image quality. Small focal spots are also used for cerebral angiography (small vessels), mammography (microcalcifications), and other examinations of small, high contrast structures.

MATERIALS REQUIRED

Radiographic x-ray machine
Small dry bone such as a phalanx (or other small object)
Resolution test pattern to measure line pairs per millimeter
X-ray film processor
200 speed screen film cassettes, 10 in x 12 in (24 cm x 30 cm)
Leaded rubber sheets
Rectangular sponge approximately 4 inches thick
Spherical object or head of a dry femur bone
Lead numbers
View box
Densitometer
Calculator
Magnifying glass

PROCEDURE

1. Warm up the processor if needed, and run a couple of "scrap" films through it to stabilize temperature and circulation.
2. Set 50 kVp. This will remain constant throughout the experiment.
3. Set the SID to 100 cm from the tabletop. This will remain constant.
4. Load and place the 10 in x 12 in cassette on the table. Two exposures will be taken on one film.
5. Collimate the light field to a 4 in x 8 in area crosswise at one end of the film. Use the leaded sheets to mask the other half of the film.
6. Place the thick (4-in) flat sponge on the film to create a large object-film distance, which must be kept constant on both exposures.
7. Place the resolution test pattern crosswise on one end of the sponge and the bone alongside it. Pay close attention to the position in which the bone is laid, because you must lay it precisely the same way on the second exposure. Both test objects must be within the light field.
8. Number each exposure with a lead marker on the cassette. Take two exposures, using the following techniques or any necessary alternate techniques.

Exposure 1	50 mA, small focal spot, 0.035 s (1/30 s; 35 ms)
Exposure 2	200 mA, large focal spot, 0.008 s (1/120 s; 8 ms)

9. Process the film.

RESULTS

On the images of the resolution test pattern, scan the black and white line pairs, from thickest to thinnest, and determine where they are blurred first so that you cannot distinguish separate lines with clear edges. Use the magnifying glass. Note which line pair number this is. Refer to the resolution test pattern itself or to the table provided by your instructor to read off how many line pairs per millimeter correspond to this line pair number.

The unit "line pairs per millimeter" is a direct measurement of spatial resolution. The greater the number of line pairs per millimeter resolved, the less the blur of the image. In Table E17-1, record each SID and the resolution in line pairs per millimeter.

When you have completed this, obtain a millimeter ruler and measure the length of the bone images for exposures 1 and 2. Then, taking care to hold the bone as it was placed on the cassette and lining the ruler up precisely to the same points as you did on the radiographs, measure the length of the actual dry bone. Record these measurements also in Table E17-1.

EXERCISES

1 Visually examine the marrow portion of the bone images for fine trabecular detail. With which focal spot size is more detail resolved? With which focal spot does this detail appear to have sharper edges?

2 Refer to Table E17-1. Which focal spot resolved the greater number of line pairs per millimeter? Does this agree with your visual observations in exercise 1?

3 What general rule of thumb can you make for focal spot size to consistently produce radiographs with maximum resolution?

TABLE E17-1

	Focal spot	Resolution (lp/mm)	Bone image size
Exposure 1	Small		
Exposure 2	Large		

Actual bone size:_____

4 From Table E17-1 compute the magnification factors for the two exposures using the formula below, and record:

$$\text{Magnification} = \frac{\text{Measured image length}}{\text{Actual bone length}}$$

Exposure 1 magnification: _____

Exposure 2 magnification: _____

5 Did one focal spot cause more magnification than the other? Does focal spot affect the gross size of the image?

EXPERIMENT 18

Name_____

Date_____

Effect of Object-to-Image Receptor Distance on Image Blur and Magnification

OBJECT

To demonstrate the effects of changing object-to-image receptor distance (OID) on image blur and magnification, the opposing relationship of OID and SID.

DISCUSSION

OID affects both image blur and magnification in the image. Ideally, the anatomic part being examined should be placed in direct contact with the image receptor so that the OID is minimized, but a substantial OID is often unavoidable. This increases focal spot blur and loss of image detail. It also results in image magnification. The only way to compensate for both of these problems is by increasing the SID as well.

MATERIALS REQUIRED

Radiographic x-ray machine
Small dry bone such as a phalanx (or other small object)
Resolution test pattern to measure line pairs per millimeter
X-ray film processor
200-speed screen film cassettes, 14 in x 17 in (35 cm x 42 cm)
Leaded rubber sheets
Rectangular sponge approximately 4 inches thick
Additional rectangular sponge approximately 2 inches thick (must be one half the thickness of the other sponge)
Spherical object or head of a dry femur bone
Lead numbers
View box
Densitometer
Calculator

PROCEDURE

1. Warm up the processor if needed, and run a couple of "scrap" films through it to stabilize temperatures and circulation.
2. Set 50 kVp. This will remain constant throughout the experiment.
3. Load and place the 14 in x 17 in cassette on the table. Three exposures will be taken on one film.
4. Collimate the light field to a 5 in x 8 in area crosswise at one end of the film. Use the leaded sheets to mask the adjacent film area. Both test objects must be within the light field.
5. Number each exposure with a lead marker on the cassette. Take three exposures, using the following techniques or necessary alternate techniques.

Exposure 1   Place the 2-in sponge on one end of the film. Place the resolution test pattern crosswise and the bone alongside it, resting on the sponge. Pay close attention to the position in which the bone is laid, because you must lay it precisely the same way on the second exposure. Set the SID precisely to 50 cm from the tabletop. Be sure to visually check the light field and open it up to include the test objects.
Technique: 50 mA, 0.0083 s (1/120 s; 8 ms).

Exposure 2   Place the 4-in sponge in the middle of the film. Place the resolution test pattern crosswise on the sponge and the bone alongside it exactly as you did for exposure 1. Keep the same SID. Check the light field to be sure the test objects are within it.
Technique: 50 mA, 0.0083 s (1/120 s; 8 ms).

Exposure 3 Place the 4-in sponge at the remaining end of the film. Place the resolution template crosswise on the sponge and the bone alongside it exactly as you did for exposure 1. Keep the same SID. Collimate the light field down to the remaining cassette area.

Technique: 50 mA, 0.035 s (1/130 s; 35 ms).

6. Process the film.

RESULTS

On the images of the resolution test pattern, scan the black and white line pairs from thickest to thinnest, and determine where they are blurred first so that you cannot distinguish separate lines with clear edges. Note which line pair number this is. Refer to the resolution test pattern itself or to the table provided by your instructor to read off how many line pairs per millimeter correspond to this line pair number. In Table E18-1, record each SID, OID, and the resolution in line pairs per millimeter.

With a millimeter ruler, measure the length of the bone images for each exposure. Then, taking care to hold the bone as it was placed on the cassette and lining the ruler up precisely to the same points as you did on the radiographs, measure the length of the actual dry bone. Record these measurements also in Table E18-1.

EXERCISES

1 Visually examine the marrow portion of the bone images for fine trabecular detail. With which SID/OID combination is the detail most blurred?
2 Refer to Table E18-1, and compare exposures 1 and 2. At which OID were the greater number of line pairs per millimeter resolved?
3 What general rule of thumb can you make for OID to consistently produce radiographs with maximum resolution?

TABLE E18-1

	SID	OID	Resolution (lp/mm)	Bone image size
Exposure 1				
Exposure 2				
Exposure 3				

Actual bone size_____

4 Now compare from the table the line pairs resolved for exposure 3 and exposure 1. For exposure 3, both the SID and OID were doubled. Is the resolution different? Why or why not?
5 From Table E18-1 compute the magnification factor for the three exposures, using the following formula:

$$\text{Magnification} = \frac{\text{Measured image length}}{\text{Actual bone length}}$$

Exposure 1 magnification:_____
Exposure 2 magnification:_____
Exposure 3 magnification:_____

6 Compare the magnification for exposures 1 and 2. At which OID was magnification the greatest?
7 What general rule of thumb can you make for OID to consistently produce radiographs with minimum magnification?
8 Now compare the magnification for exposure 2 and exposure 3. For exposure 3, both the SID and the OID were doubled. Is the magnification different? Why or why not?
9 Based on your answers to exercises 4 and 8, in controlling magnification and resolution, what is the relationship between SID and OID?

Effect of Object Alignment on Image Distortion

OBJECT

To demonstrate the distorting effects of misalignment of the x-ray beam, object, and image receptor.

DISCUSSION

Misalignment problems include off-centering of the central ray from the anatomic part, angling the film or anatomic part so that one is not parallel to the other, and angling the central ray so that it is not perpendicular to either the anatomic part or the film. Generally, these conditions cause **distortion** of shape on the image of the anatomic part being radiographed. When the anatomic part and image receptor cannot be placed parallel to each other, shape distortion will be minimized by angling the central ray one half of the angle formed between the part and the film.

There are two types of shape distortion: **elongation** and **foreshortening** of the image. Distortion is always undesirable and should be minimized.

MATERIALS REQUIRED

Radiographic x-ray machine
X-ray film processor
200-speed screen film cassettes, 14 in x 17 in (35 cm x 42 cm)
Leaded rubber sheets
Rectangular sponge approximately 2 inches thick
45-degree angle sponge
Coin
Spherical object or head of a dry femur bone
Lead numbers
View box

PROCEDURE

1. Warm up the processor if needed, and run a couple of "scrap" films through it to stabilize temperatures and circulation.
2. Set 50 kVp. This will remain constant throughout the experiment.
3. Load and place the 14 in x 17 in cassette on the table. Six exposures will be taken on one film, dividing it into two rows of three exposures each.
4. Collimate the light field to a 5-in square area in one corner of the film. Use the leaded sheets to mask the adjacent film areas.
5. Place the 2-in flat sponge on the film to create an object-to-image receptor distance (OID). All views must be taken at the same OID.
6. Number each exposure with a lead marker on the cassette. Take six exposures using the following techniques.
7. Set 50 mA, 0.05 s (1/20 s; 50 ms), and 50 kVp.

Exposure 1	Place the spherical object or head of a femur on the sponge in the corner of the film. Pay close attention to how you place this object, because it must be placed exactly the same way on the next exposure. Center a 100 cm perpendicular beam to the sphere.
Exposure 2	Place the spherical object on the sponge in the same position as you did for exposure 1. Angle the x-ray beam 35 degrees, and maintain source-to-image receptor distance (SID) by reducing the tabletop-tube distance to 84 cm. Center to the sphere.
Exposure 3	Place the coin on the sponge lying parallel to the film. Center a 100 cm, perpendicular beam to the coin.

Exposure 4   Tape the coin to a 45-degree angle sponge at a spot that maintains exactly the same OID as the flat sponge in exposure 3. Angle the x-ray beam 45 degrees so that the central ray is perpendicular to the coin, and maintain SID by reducing the tabletop-tube distance to 79 cm. Center to the coin.

Exposure 5   Keep the coin taped to the same spot on the 45-degree angle sponge as in exposure 4. Center a vertical beam perpendicular to the film. The SID should be 100 cm.

Exposure 6   Keep the coin taped to the same spot on the 45-degree angle sponge as in exposure 4. Angle the x-ray beam isometrically to 22.5 degrees (one half of the angle formed between the coin and the film). Maintain SID by reducing the tabletop-tube distance to 90 cm, and center to the coin.

RESULTS

Visually observe the images on a view box. If distortion effects are not obvious, use a ruler to measure the objects and images along the axis at which the beam or coin was angled.

EXERCISES

1   Visually compare exposures 1 and 2. Does angling the x-ray beam distort the true shape of a spherical object?

2   Note the width of the spherical image, the axis crosswise to the direction the beam was angled. Compare exposure 2 to exposure 1. You can superimpose the images with a bright light for visual comparison or use a ruler and measure the width. For magnification to occur, both the length and the width of the image should be increased from exposure 1. Did angulation of the beam cause magnification of the image when distances were maintained?

3   Compare the coin image on exposure 4 to that on exposure 3. Is distortion caused when the object is angled in relation to the film and the beam is kept perpendicular to the object? If so, what specific type of distortion occurs?

4   Compare the coin image on exposure 5 to that on exposure 3. Is distortion caused when the object is angled in relation to the film and the beam is kept perpendicular to the film? If so, what specific type of distortion occurs?

5   Compare the coin image on exposure 6 to that on exposure 3. Is distortion caused when the object is angled in relation to the film and the beam is angled isometrically between the object and the film?

EXPERIMENT   20

Anode Heel Effect

OBJECT

To demonstrate the variation of x-ray intensity in a plane perpendicular to the central axis of the useful beam.

DISCUSSION

The radiation intensity across the useful x-ray beam is higher on the cathode side than on the anode side. Along a line perpendicular to the anode-cathode axis, the radiation intensity is constant. The x rays produced from a depth in the tube target must traverse a greater thickness of target material on the anode side than on the cathode side. Because of this self-absorption of photons within the "heel" of the anode, the resulting distribution of the x-ray intensity is known as the **heel effect**.

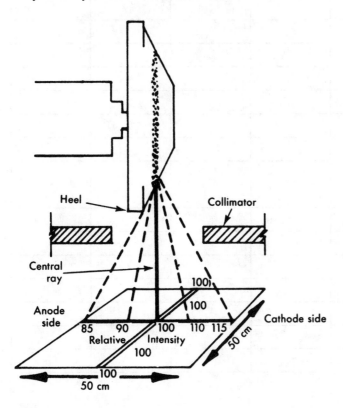

MATERIALS REQUIRED

Radiographic x-ray unit
Ionization chamber
50 cm x 50 cm grid marked in 5 cm intervals

PROCEDURE

1. Tape the 50 cm x 50 cm grid to the tabletop so that the central axis of the useful x-ray beam intersects the center of the grid.
2. Position the x-ray tube target 80 cm above the tabletop.
3. The x-ray machine may be used as it is normally filtered. Record the amount of total filtration if known. Adjust the tube potential to 70 kVp, and select an appropriate mAs that will produce a response of the ionization chamber that is at least half scale. The kVp, mA, and exposure time will remain constant throughout the experiment.
4. Position the detector on the central ray, and, using the data sheet provided, record the response. Three measurements are necessary.
5. Reposition the detector at 5 cm intervals along the four major radii from the central axis (two along the anode-cathode axis and two perpendicular to that axis).
6. Calculate the average intensity (mR) at each location.
7. Calculate the percentage of the central ray intensity at each location as follows:

Central ray intensity (%) =

$$\frac{\text{Intensity at grid location (mR)}}{\text{Intensity at central ray (mR)}} \times 100$$

RESULTS

On the linear graph paper provided, plot the percentage of the central ray intensity vs. the position of the x-ray beam along the anode-cathode axis and vs. the position of the x-ray beam along the axis perpendicular to the anode-cathode axis.

EXERCISES

1 If a 10 in x 12 in film were centered on a grid with the 12-in (30 cm) dimension along the anode-cathode axis, what percentage of the central ray exposure would exist along the four sides of the film?

2 Discuss the effect, if any, that changing from the small focal spot station to the large focal spot station would have on the magnitude of the heel effect.

3 Discuss the effect, if any, that changing the target angle would have on the magnitude of the heel effect.

4 In each of the following examinations, how should the anode-cathode axis of the x-ray tube be oriented with respect to the patient—or does it not matter?
a. extremity _____
b. chest _____
c. skull _____
d. pelvis _____
e. mammogram _____

Constant factors
70 kVp mA _____
Exposure time(s) _____
75 cm source-to-detector distance
Filtration _____ mm Al

DATA SHEET
Laboratory experiment 20

Grid position	Exposure (mR)			Average exposure (mR)	Percent of central ray
	First	Second	Third		
Central ray					100
2					
3					
4					
5					
6					
7					
8					
9					
10					
11					
12					
13					
14					
15					
16					
17					
18					
19					
20					
21					
22					
23					
24					
25					

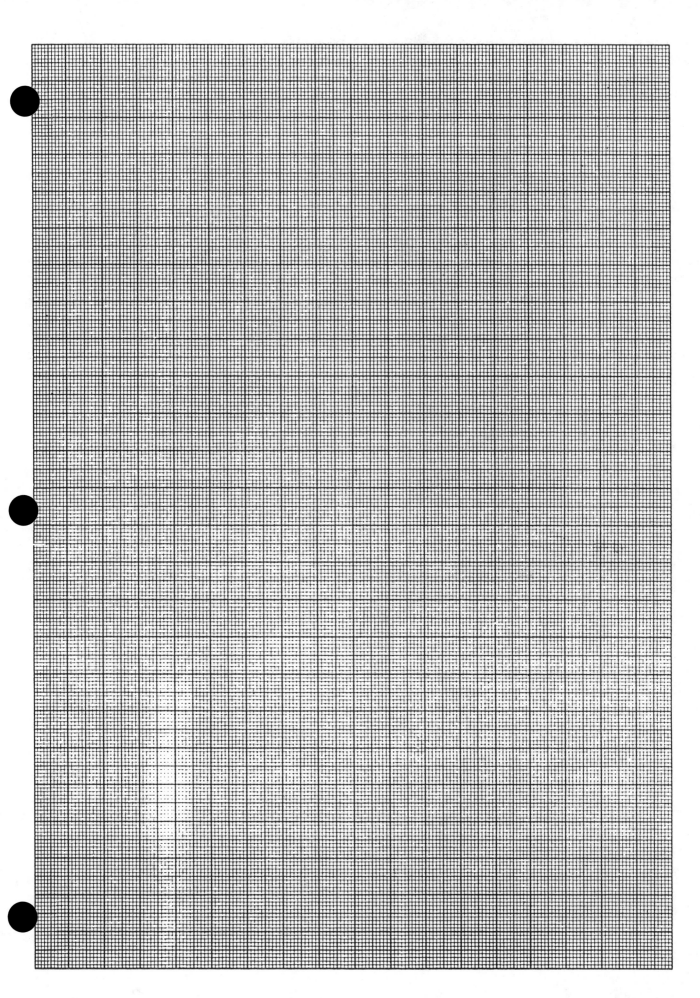

Name_____

Date_____

Effective Focal Spot Size

OBJECT

To measure the effective focal spot size under differ-
ing conditions of x-ray tube current.

DISCUSSION

There are currently three methods for measuring
effective focal spot size while the tube is energized. The
use of the **pinhole camera** is simplest in concept but
somewhat difficult to use. When x rays from the focal
spot are incident on an aperture, or pinhole, which is
much smaller than the focal spot and positioned midway
between the target and the image receptor, the resulting
image will have the same size and shape as the effective
focal spot. If the pinhole is located at any other position

between target and film, magnification or minification
will occur. Positioning of the pinhole is critical. It must
lie on the central ray of the x-ray beam, midway between
the target and image receptor and in a plane parallel with
the image receptor yet perpendicular to the central axis.

$$EFS = AFS \times \sin \theta$$

where

$$EFS = \text{Effective focal spot size}$$
$$AFS = \text{Actual focal spot size}$$
$$\theta = \text{Target angle}$$

The use of a **star test pattern** is much easier, but the
theoretic basis for its use is more complicated and
unnecessary to the success of this experiment. The star

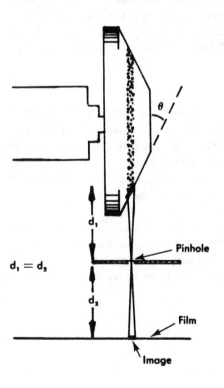

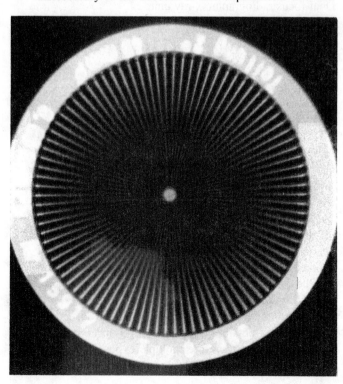

test pattern must be centered on the central ray of the x-ray beam and perpendicular to it. With this device, however, precise positioning is less necessary. The effective focal spot size (**EFS**) is calculated from measurements made from the star test pattern image as follows:

$$\text{EFS} = \frac{N}{57.3} \times \frac{D}{(m-1)}$$

where

EFS = Effective focal spot size in millimeters
N = Star pattern angle in degrees (usually 1 or 2 degrees and indicated on the pattern)
D = Blur diameter measured in millimeters from the image
$m = \dfrac{\text{Image size}}{\text{Object size}}$ (magnification factor)

The blur diameter should be measured across the image along the anode-cathode axis and its perpendicular axis. The results may demonstrate that the EFS is not square.

The third method employs a **slit camera**. The slit camera is used in much the same way as the pinhole camera, and when used correctly it is the most accurate of the three. The slit camera is used by manufacturers in their laboratories and by medical physicists in the clinic. Because of the time and precision required for its use, it is not included as a part of this experiment.

MATERIALS REQUIRED

Dual-focus radiographic x-ray unit
Pinhole camera with approximate 0.03 mm opening
Tape measure
360-degree star test pattern
Magnifying glass
0.1 mm increment rule

PROCEDURE
Pinhole Camera

1. Select 50 kVp and an mA station for which both large and small focal spot sizes are available. Usually the 100 mA station is suitable. Begin with the small focal spot station.
2. Position the pinhole camera midway between the target and image receptor, and cone down the useful beam to about 5 cm x 5 cm on the film, centered on the pinhole. The source-to-image receptor distance (SID) should be about 75 cm.
3. Adjust the pinhole alignment until an acceptable image is obtained. At least 1000 mAs may be required, and therefore multiple exposures may be necessary.

TABLE E21-1

	mm x mm		
	Small spot, low mA	Large spot, low mA	Large spot, high mA
Pinhole camera			
Star test pattern			

4. Change to the large focal spot station and repeat step 3.
5. Using the large focal spot, increase the mA to the highest possible value while maintaining a constant mAs and repeat step 3.

Star Test Pattern

1. Replace the pinhole camera with the star test pattern. It is acceptable to tape the test pattern to the light-localizing collimator.
2. Repeat steps 3, 4, and 5 of the pinhole camera procedure. A much lower mAs will be required. Try 50 mAs as a starter.

RESULTS

With the magnifying glass and scale ruled to the nearest 0.1 mm, measure the length and width of each of the three focal spot images obtained with the pinhole camera. Measure the perpendicular blur diameters from the three star test pattern exposures. Use the attached data sheet as a guide and calculate the effective focal spot size. Complete Table E21-1, which shows results.

EXERCISES

1 When mA is increased, the EFS will often increase in size. This effect is called *blooming*. Using the pinhole data and the star data, calculate the percentage increase in EFS with an increase in mA.
2 Describe the shape and optical density distribution of each of the images obtained with the pinhole camera.
3 If the actual focal spot of a 13-degree target angle tube is 4.8 mm x 1.0 mm, what will be the EFS?
4 If the EFS is 0.6 mm x 0.6 mm and the target angle is 10.5 degrees, what is the actual focal spot size?

DATA SHEET
Laboratory experiment 21

PINHOLE CAMERA

d = _____ cm. The distance on the pinhole plate separating the large localizing holes, which is usually 1.27 cm.

d' = _____ cm. The distance on the image separating the localizing holes.

Small focal spot (low mA)
    Focal spot image length _____ mm
    Focal spot image width _____ mm
Large focal spot (low mA)
    Focal spot image length _____ mm
    Focal spot image width _____ mm
Large focal spot (high mA)
    Focal spot image length _____ mm
    Focal spot image width _____ mm

Effective focal point size (mm) =

$$\text{Image size} \left(\frac{d}{d' - d} \right)$$

STAR TEST PATTERN

N = _____ degrees, the star test pattern angle.
Object size = _____, the diameter of the star test pattern.
Image size = _____, the diameter of the image of the star test pattern.
m = _____.

Small focal spot (low mA)
    Blur diameter _____ mm x _____ mm
Large focal spot (low mA)
    Blur diameter _____ mm x _____ mm
Large focal spot (high mA)
    Blur diameter _____ mm x _____ mm

Effective focal spot size (mm) =

$$\frac{N}{57.3} \times \frac{\text{Blur diameter}}{(m - 1)}$$

EXPERIMENT 22

Repeat Analysis

OBJECT

To demonstrate how to conduct a repeat analysis.

DISCUSSION

Repeat analysis can be conducted either for an individual radiographer or for an entire radiology department. Studies have shown that when an imaging department initiates a quality control program, including repeat analysis, sensitometric processor monitoring, and the use of technique charts, the exposures repeated because of improper optical density (OD) can be cut by one third to one half. This saves money for the department, reduces unnecessary patient dose, and should be taken seriously by every radiographer.

By analyzing and categorizing repeated exposures, the department can identify specific areas of need for continuing education. The individual radiologic technologist can recognize areas for improvement as well as personal strong points. The more detailed the analysis, the more useful it will be.

MATERIALS NEEDED

A box, drawer, or file in which to store throwaway films for each individual or group under study

PROCEDURE

1. For a period of 2 to 4 weeks, as directed by your instructor, place all of your throwaway films in a separate box, drawer, or file with your name on it so no one will inadvertently misplace it.
2. During this time you must also keep fairly accurate records of the total number of views taken. For accuracy, it is best to use the following record A, which you must mark after every procedure, summing the number of views taken (not films used). However, if you do not have time to do this, a fair estimate can

be made by using record B, which must be filled out at the end of each working day to the best of your memory. The totals would be estimated at the end of the study period by multiplying the number of views taken for that procedure. Choose record A or record B, and fill in the required information.
3. At the end of the study period, fill in the data under the following section and complete the exercises.

Record A for Repeat Analysis

After each procedure performed, fill in the number of views (*not* films) taken in the appropriate category below. NOTE: "Torso" includes chest film, abdomen films, and intravenous pyelograms (IVPs). "Extremity" includes pelvic and shoulder girdle films. "Fluoroscopic" includes upper gastrointestinal films, barium enemas, and air contrast barium enemas.

Record B for Repeat Analysis

At the end of each working day, fill in the number of each type of procedure performed that day. At the end of the study period, fill in the routine number of views taken for each type of procedure. Multiply the number of views by the number of each procedure done to obtain a total.

RESULTS

Refer to the record, and record here the total number of views taken: _____

Record the number of views taken in each of the following:

Torso   _____
Head   _____
Spines   _____
Extremities (and girdles)   _____
Fluoroscopic procedures   _____
Other   _____

Record the total number of repeat exposures made

Type of procedure					
Torso	Head	Spine	Extremity	Fluoroscopic	Other

Totals for period: Grand total

No. of views for period (add all columns): _____

Now carefully examine each film in the throwaway file, and determine the primary cause for its being repeated. Sort the films into the following groups. When this is done, count and record the number of films in each group:

Reason for repeat	Number of repeats
Density too dark	_____
Density too light	_____
Not flashed or not properly marked	_____
Artifacts on patient, film, or table	_____
Motion	_____
Blank film or processing artifacts	_____
Positioning, alignment, and collimation	_____

From the positioning category only, sort and total the following:

Torso   _____
Head   _____
Spines   _____
Extremities   _____
Fluoroscopic procedures _____
Other   _____

EXERCISES

1 Refer to the "Results" section, and determine the overall repeat rate as follows. Divide the total number of repeats taken for the entire period by the total number of views taken. Multiply the result by 100. Record here:

Overall repeat rate:_____%

2 Compute the percent of all repeats caused by each of the following problems, as follows. Divide the number of repeats taken for this reason by the total number of repeats taken for the entire period. Multiply this result by 100. Record here for each category:

Density too dark	_____%
Density too light	_____%
Not flashed or not properly marked	_____%
Artifacts on patient, film, or table	_____%
Motion	_____%
Blank film or processing artifacts	_____%
Positioning, alignment, and collimation	_____%

3 What type of problem caused the most repeat exposures? What type of problem caused the second-most repeats?

4 What type of problem caused the least repeats?

5 Refer to the "Results" section, and compute the repeat rate for each of the following types of procedures, as follows. Divide the number of repeats taken for each procedure by the total number of views taken for each procedure. Multiply this result by 100. Record here:

Torso	_____%
Head	_____%
Spines	_____%
Extremities (and girdles)	_____%
Fluoroscopic procedures	_____%
Other	_____%

6 Which general type of procedures has the highest repeat rate? What could be done to improve this area?

Day of month or of study period

Procedure	Routine number of views	1	2	3	4	5	6	7	8	9	10	11	12	13	14	15	16	17	18	19	20	21	22	23	24	25	26	27	28	29	30	31	Total procedures	Total views taken
Torso																																		
Chest																																		
Abdomen																																		
IVP																																		
Head																																		
Skull																																		
Sinus/facies																																		
Mandible																																		
Orbits																																		
Other																																		
Spines																																		
Cervical																																		
Thoracic																																		
Lumbar																																		
Sacrum/C																																		
Extremities																																		
Hand/finger																																		
Wrist																																		
Forearm																																		
Elbow																																		
Humerus																																		
Shoulder																																		
Clavicle/scapula																																		
Foot/toe																																		

Cont'd

Procedure	Routine number of views	Day of month or of study period																														Total procedures	Total views taken
		1	2	3	4	5	6	7	8	9	10	11	12	13	14	15	16	17	18	19	20	21	22	23	24	25	26	27	28	29	30	31		
Ankle																																		
Leg																																		
Knee																																		
Femur																																		
Hip																																		
Pelvis																																		
Fluoroscopic																																		
Upper gastrointestinal																																		
Air contrast barium enema																																		
Barium enema																																		
Other																																		

Grand total no. of views for period: _____

EXPERIMENT   23

Tomography

OBJECT

To demonstrate the effect of different motions and angles on the tomographic image.

DISCUSSION

Frequently obtaining an acceptable radiograph is difficult because of the superimposition of overlying anatomic structures. For example, examination of the bronchi is difficult with a conventional radiograph because of the adjacent sternal and vertebral bony structures. A tomographic motion will blur the image of the overlying sternum and underlying spine while maintaining detail of structures in the plane of focus— the plane containing the pivot or fulorum.

During tomography, the x-ray tube and image receptor are separated by a fixed distance and move in synchrony about the pivot or focal point. A variety of motions are available: linear, circular, elliptic, hypocycloidal, and trispiral. For most motions a range of tomographic angles is permitted. Complex motions produce more blurring of objects outside the plane of focus than simple motions. This has the effect of increasing the contrast of objects in the plane of focus.

Similarly, an increase in tomographic angle will increase the blurring of objects outside the plane of focus. Additionally, an increase in tomographic angle will reduce the thickness of the in-focus layer.

MATERIALS REQUIRED

Tomographic phantom
Multidirectional tomograph
Film marking pencil
Lead diaphragm with pinhole
200-speed cassette, 10 in x 12 in (25 cm x 30 cm)
View box

NOTE: This experiment has been designed for use with the 3M Tomographic Phantom. Other phantoms are available, but they may not be compatible with all parts of this laboratory experiment.

PROCEDURE
Part I: Pinhole Tracing

Place a lead diaphragm containing the pinhole on the examination table and position it 17 cm above the plane of focus. Shield a large area around the pinhole with lead masks or apron. With the collimators fully open, make a separate exposure on 10 in x 12 in (25 cm x 30 cm) film, using each of the possible movements of the tomograph (try 65 kVp, 120 mAs). The pinhole tracings that you obtain can be used to evaluate the following tomographic characteristics.

1. **Geometric form of the motion.** Any gross deviations from the intended motion will be observed.
2. **Mechanical stability.** Unwanted motion in the x-ray tube housing or the image receptor assembly will result in a wavy tracing, or "wobble."
3. **Completeness of exposure.** Open sections in the image tracing indicate incomplete exposure, whereas overlapped sections indicate unnecessary double exposure.
4. **Uniformity of intensity.** Undesirable changes in radiation intensity during exposure will appear on the tracing as variations in optical density (OD).

Observations on each of these characteristics are to be made on the data sheet.

Part II: Thickness of Cut

The section thickness can be measured and compared with that stated by the manufacturer.

Center the tomographic phantom on the table, set the focal plane at the level of the scale (~ 4.0 cm above the table), and make an exposure (try 120 mAs at 50 kVp). Do this procedure for each motion, using a constant tomographic angle. The phantom should be positioned perpendicular to the direction of the tube movement for the linear motion. Examine the image of the inclined wires next to the scale. One wire measures in millimeter increments, whereas the other measures in centimeter increments.

Place the film on a view box, and use a film marking pencil to mark lightly where each end of the wire comes into focus. Lay a piece of paper next to the wire image and mark the in-focus length of wire. Use the paper as a guide and lay it next to the image of the scale. Read the thickness of cut, using the appropriate scale, and record these values on the data sheet.

Compute the percent error as follows:

$$\% \text{ Error} = \frac{\text{Difference between indicated and measured thickness}}{\text{Indicated thickness}}$$

Observe the quality of the image of the bone lesion.

Part III: Effect of Tomographic Angle

Center the tomographic phantom on the table and adjust the focal plane to the level of the scale. Make an exposure of the tomographic phantom (try 120 mAs at 50 kVp), using tomographic angles of 10, 20, and 30 degrees in the linear or any of the multidirectional modes. Remember to place the tomographic phantom perpendicular to the tube movement when the linear motion is used. Compare the blur images of the circle and star patterns. The patterns nearest the scale are in the plane of focus, and their image should be sharp. The patterns farthest from the scale are 5 mm above the plane of focus. Their image should demonstrate the effect of blurring of objects out of the plane of focus.

Using the technique in Part II, measure the thickness of cut. Observe the quality of the image of the bone lesion. Record your observations and values on the data sheet.

RESULTS

Complete the data sheet below.

EXERCISES

1 Briefly discuss the clinical application of each motion you studied and the reason it was selected for that examination.

DATA SHEET
Laboratory experiment 23

PART I: PINHOLE TRACING

Type of motion	Integrity of motion	Mechanical stability	Completeness of exposure	Intensity uniformity
Linear				
Circular				
Elliptic				
Trispiral				
Hypocycloidal				

PART II: THICKNESS OF CUT   Tomographic angle _____

Type of motion	Indicated section thickness	Measured section thickness	% error	Quality of image of bone lesion
Linear				
Circular				
Elliptic				
Trispiral				
Hypocycloidal				

PART III: EFFECT OF TOMOGRAPHIC ANGLE   Type of motion _____

Tomographic angle	Angle thickness	Width of blur	Quality of image of bone lesion
10 degrees			
20 degrees			
30 degrees			

EXPERIMENT   24

Radiographic Quality Control Survey

OBJECT

To evaluate the operation of a radiographic unit for deficiencies in image quality and radiation safety.

DISCUSSION

In the United States, two organizations are directly concerned with the safe design and operation of medical x-ray apparatus: the National Council on Radiation Protection and Measurement (NCRP) and the Center for Devices and Radiological Health (CDRH), an arm of the U.S. Food and Drug Administration (FDA). The NCRP is an advisory group and has no authority to enforce compliance with its recommendations. The CDRH does have the authority to set standards and enforce them. In addition to the CDRH, many state governments in general subscribe to NCRP recommendations.

The tests included in this experiment are adopted from CDRH and NCRP documents and are designed as relatively simple evaluations that the radiologic technologist can perform to maintain good image quality and to control the radiation exposure of patients and radiology personnel.

MATERIALS REQUIRED

Single-phase radiographic unit with variable-aperture light-localizing collimator
Tape measure
Paper clips
Spinning top
Portable ionization chamber survey meter
Aluminum filters
Aluminum step wedge
200 speed cassette

PROCEDURE

The format of this experiment is slightly different from previous experiments. A statement will be made regarding proper operation of a specific component of the radiographic equipment. This is followed by instructions on how to determine whether the given operation is consistent with acceptable radiation control characteristics.

1. Coincidence of the x-ray beam and light field.
   The error of coincidence must not exceed 2% of the source-to-image receptor distance (SID) on any side of the field.
   Place a cassette at 100 cm SID, outline the light field with paper clips, and make an exposure. Measure the deviation in both directions, and determine if the degree of coincidence is acceptable.

2. Accuracy of the distance indicator.
   The SID indicator should be correct to within 2% of the indicated distance.
   Locate the position of the target of the x-ray tube. It is marked on many tube housings. If it is not, the target position may be estimated by the procedure demonstrated in experiment 1. With a tape measure, determine the actual distance from the target to the image receptor when the indicator shows 100 cm. Repeat this measurement at the maximum and minimum travel of the tube.

3. Exposure switch location.
   The exposure switch should be so located that it cannot be conveniently operated outside a shielded area.
   Examine the exposure switch to see if the cord is too long or if the console-mounted button is in such a position that it allows a technologist to make an exposure while part of her or his body is outside the shielded area. If the cord is too long, it should be shortened or permanently affixed to the console. If the console is too close to the edge of the protective barrier, warning tape should be placed on the floor.

4. Exposure timer accuracy.
   Single-phase exposure timers should be accurate to the time indicated.
   The timer on single-phase equipment can be checked

with a conventional spinning top. Place the spinning top on a cassette at any convenient SID, and expose it while it is spinning. It should be exposed for 1/60, 1/30, 1/20, and 1/10 second. Compare the number of dashes observed with the number expected.

5. Indication of "beam-on."

The control panel should include a device (usually a milliammeter) to give positive indication of the production of x rays whenever the x-ray tube is energized.

Check for a positive indication of beam-on by deflection of the needle of the mA meter during an exposure. Newer equipment provides a separate lamp and an audible signal as well.

6. Exposure linearity.

The radiation exposure obtained by operation of adjacent mA stations at constant exposure time should not vary more than 10% when expressed as mR/mAs.

If a direct-reading ionization chamber is used, the results are directly obtainable; exposure time should remain constant while mA is increased. Otherwise, the simultaneous exposure of a spinning top and penetrometer will suffice. There should be no readily detectable difference in the penetrometer image when exposed to adjacent mA stations at constant mAs. Try 80 kVp at 100 ms as follows:

$$100 \text{ mA} = 10 \text{ mAs}$$
$$200 \text{ mA} = 20 \text{ mAs}$$
$$400 \text{ mA} = 40 \text{ mAs}$$
$$800 \text{ mA} = 60 \text{ mAs}$$

7. Reproducibility.

The radiation intensity obtained during sequential exposures at a fixed technique should exhibit a coeffcient of variation (c) of not more than 0.05 where

$$c = \frac{\sqrt{\dfrac{\Sigma(X_i - \overline{X})^2}{n-1}}}{\overline{X}} \leq 0.05$$

This requirement essentially states that the variation in output intensity of a constant technique shall not exceed 5%. To test this, 10 successive exposures are made and the radiation intensity recorded for each. From these measurements the coefficient of variation is calculated.

8. X-ray quality.

The following total filtration is required:

Operating kVp	Minimum total filtration (inherent plus added)	Minimum acceptable HVL
Below 50 kVp	0.05 mm Al	0.6 mm Al at 50 kVp
50 to 70 kVp	1.5 mm Al	1.3 mm Al at 60 kVp
Above 70 kVp	2.5 mm Al	2.2 mm Al at 70 kVp

If the added filtration is not directly measurable, determine the half-value layer at 70 kVp as demonstrated in experiment 10. If the unit is ever operated above 70 kVp, 2.5 mm Al or an HVL of 2.2 mm Al must exist.

RESULTS

1. Coincidence of the x-ray beam and light field.
   SID = _____
   2% SID = _____
   Misalignment
   Width: _____ + _____ = _____
       ≤ 2% SID? ❏Yes ❏No
   Length: _____ + _____ = _____
       ≤ 2% SID? ❏Yes ❏No
       Is this acceptable? ❏Yes ❏No

2. SID indication.
   Selected SID = _____
   2% Selected SID = _____
   Measured SID = _____
   Difference = _____
       ≤ 2% Selected SID? ❏Yes ❏No

3. Is the exposure switch adequately located?
   ❏Yes ❏No

4. Exposure timer accuracy.

Time(s)	Expected dashes	Observed dashes	Acceptable?
1/10			
1/20			
1/30			
1/60			

5. Positive indication of beam-on.
   Visible: ❏Yes ❏No
   Audible: ❏Yes ❏No

6. Exposure linearity. 70 kVp

No.	mA	Time (s)	mAs	Exposure (mR) 1st	2nd	3rd	Average exposure (mR)	mR/mAs
1								
2								
3								

Is $(mR/mAs_1 - mR/mAs_1) < 0.1 (mR/mAs_1 + mR/mAs_2)$? ❏Yes ❏No
_____ – _____ < 0.1 (_____ + _____)

288

Is $(mR/mAs_2 - mR/mAs_3) < 0.1 (mR/mAs_2 + mR/mAs_3)$? ❏Yes ❏No

_____ – _____ < 0.1 (_____ + _____)

Is this acceptable?   ❏Yes ❏No

7.

Exposure number (n)	Xi (mR)	Xi–$\overline{X}$	(Xi–$\overline{X}$)^2
1			
2			
3			
4			
5			
6			
7			
8			
9			
10			

Total Xi = _____

$$\overline{X} = \frac{\text{Total Xi}}{10} = \text{_____}$$

Total $(Xi - \overline{X})^2$ = _____

$$\frac{\text{Total } (Xi - \overline{X})^2}{9} = \text{_____}$$

$$\sqrt{\frac{\text{Total } (Xi - \overline{X})^2}{9}} = \text{_____}$$

$$\frac{\sqrt{\dfrac{\text{Total } (Xi - \overline{X})^2}{9}}}{X} = \text{_____}$$

c ≤ 0.05 ❏Yes ❏No

8. Beam quality.

70 kVp _____mA
40 in (100 cm) SID _____s
Normal filtration _____mm Al

Added filtration (mm Al)	Exposure (mR)			Average exposure (mR)	mR/mAs
	1st	2nd	3rd		
0					
0.5					
1.0					
2.0					
3.0					
4.0					
5.0					

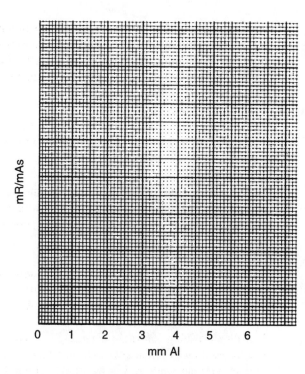

Plot the resulting mR/mAs as a function of mm Al on the graph above and estimate the half-value layer.
HVL = _____ mm Al
HVL ≥ 2.2 mm Al? ❏Yes ❏No

EXERCISES

1 A 25 cm x 40 cm (10 in x 16 in) light field is set at an SID of 100 cm (40 in). The x-ray beam has exactly the same dimensions, but it misses superimposition by 1 cm on all sides. Is this acceptable? What is the limit of acceptability in this instance?

2 The SID indicator shows 91 cm, but actual measurement shows 89 cm. Is this acceptable? What is the range of accpetability for this situation?

3 A portable unit (single-phase, half-wave rectified) is operated with the exposure timer at 1/30 second. How many dashes from the image of the spinning top would be expected?

4 The following exposure data are obtained from a conventional radiographic unit operated at 70 kVp:

50 mA, 0.5 s, 210 mR (5.4×10^{-5} C/kg)
100 mA, 0.5 s, 390 mR (1.0×10^{-4} C/kg)
200 mA, 0.5 s, 704 mR (1.8×10^{-4} C/kg)

Are these acceptable?

EXPERIMENT   25

Fluoroscopic Quality Control Survey

OBJECT

To evaluate the design and operation of a fluoroscope for deficiencies in image quality and radiation safety.

DISCUSSION

As with the previous experiment, this experiment consists of a series of measurements and observations, each designed to test compliance with a specific radiation control recommendation of the NCRP or the CDRH. The procedure section contains statements of requirements followed by directions for measuring compliance with those requirements.

MATERIALS REQUIRED

Image-intensified fluoroscope
Aluminum block patient phantom
Lead attenuation block
Ionization chamber
Portable ionization chamber survey meter
Tape measure
Aluminum filters

PROCEDURE

Caution must be exercised during this experiment to ensure that the image intensifier is not damaged because of exposure to an unattenuated primary beam. Always position the aluminum block patient phantom, the lead attenuator, or both in the useful beam during exposure.

1. Protective curtain and Bucky slot cover.
    Shielding devices of at least 0.25 mm Pb equivalent must be available to intercept scatter radiation that would otherwise reach the technologist and radiologist standing to the side of the table.
    This is a visual inspection. See that a protective curtain of adequate design is affixed to the intensifier

tower and that it drapes all the way to the tabletop regardless of source-to-image receptor distance (SID). When the Bucky is moved to the end of the table, a cover for the space between the tabletop and the side panel, the Bucky slot cover, should automatically move into place.

2. Exposure switch and timer.
    A dead-man type of switch is required for energizing the fluoroscopic x-ray tube. A 5-min preset timer is also required, and an audible alarm should sound at the end of 5 min. The sound should continue untl the timer has been reset.
    Check all exposure switches to be sure that a continuous pressure by the operator is required during the entire exposure. Set approximately 15 s on the timer, and observe whether the audible alarm functions properly when the time expires.

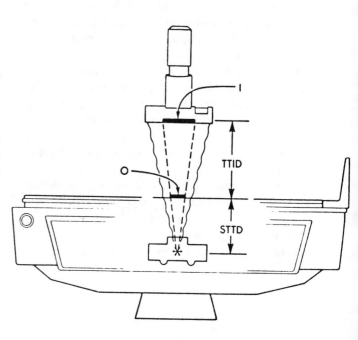

3. X-ray tube target position.

The source-to-tabletop distance should be at least 15 inches (38 cm).

Place a flat, regularly shaped metal object on the tabletop, and take a spot film of it. Measure the tabletop-to-image receptor distance, and calculate the distance of the x-ray tube target to the tabletop as follows:

$$SOD = (SID) \frac{O}{I}$$

where

SOD = Source-to-tabletop distance
SID = Source-image receptor distance
O = Object size
I = Image size

4. Beam quality.

The total filtration, including the tabletop, should be at least 2.5 mm Al equivalent.

Position the ionization chamber approximately 8 inches (20 cm) above the tabletop, and sequentially insert graduated thicknesses of aluminum filtration between the ionization chamber and the tabletop. When the fluoroscope is operated at 80 kVp, if the estimated half-value layer (HVL) is 2.4 mm Al or greater, total filtration is sufficient. If it is only possible to operate in the automatic exposure mode, the total thickness of aluminum filtration must remain constant. Begin with the total thickness of aluminum filtration positioned in the x-ray beam above the ionization chamber. Each aluminum filter positioned between the ionization chamber and the tabletop should come from the stack above.

5. Beam quantity.

When operated at 80 kVp, the tabletop exposure rate should not exceed 3.2 R/mA-min (0.83 mC/kg-mA min), and under no conditions of operation should the output intensity exceed 10 R/min (2.6 mC/kg-min).

Adjust the fluoroscopic tube potential and, with the ionization chamber on the tabletop, record the tube mA and the output intensity in R/m (C/kg-m). It is helpful if the mA is first adjusted to an integer value, that is, 1, 2, or 3. Next adjust the kVp and mA to their maximum values and record the R/m (C/kg-m).

6. Primary protective barrier.

The entire cross section of the useful beam should be intercepted by a primary protective barrier at all SIDs.

When the image intensifier tower is in the parked position, it should not be possible to energize the undertable x-ray tube. On equipment that fails this test, a simple microswitch interlocked with the x-ray exposure switch will satisfy the requirement. With the tower at maximum SID and in position to intercept the wide open beam, the exposure rate above the tower must not exceed 2 mR/hr (0.52 μC/kg-hr) for every R/m (0.26 μC/kg-m) at the tabletop. This is measured with the portable survey meter.

7. Primary beam limitation.

When the adjustable collimators are fully open, the primary beam should be restricted to the diameter of the input phosphor.

Open the collimators wide and elevate the tower so that the input phosphor is 15 inches (38 cm) from the tabletop. With the x-ray tube energized, an unexposed border should be visible on four sides of the image field. In newer equipment, as the elevation of the tower is changed, the collimators should automatically compensate to continue the unexposed borders on the viewing system.

RESULTS

1. Protective curtain and Bucky slot cover.
   Is an adequate protective tower curtain present?
   ❑Yes ❑No
   Is there a tightly fitting Bucky slot cover?
   ❑Yes ❑No
2. Exposure switch and timer.
   Is a dead-man type of exposure switch in use?
   ❑Yes ❑No
   Is there a properly functioning 5-min reset timer?
   ❑Yes ❑No
   Is the signal Audible?   ❑Yes ❑No
               Visual?   ❑Yes ❑No
   Does the timer terminate the exposure?
   ❑Yes ❑No
   For how long? _____
3. X-ray tube target position.
   Object size (O) _____ Image size (I) _____
   Tabletop-to-image receptor distance
         (TTID) _____

$$STTD = \frac{(TTID)\ O/I}{(1 - O/I)}$$

   Source-to-tabletop distance (STTD) _____
   ≤ 38 cm?   ❑Yes ❑No

4. Beam quality.

80 kVp

Normal filtration _____ mA

Added filtration (mm Al)	Exposure rate (R/min)
0	
0.5	
1.0	
2.0	
3.0	
4.0	
5.0	

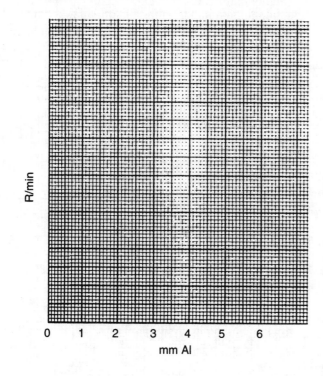

Plot the resulting R/min as a function of mmAl on the graph and estimate the half-value layer.

HVL = _____ mm Al

HVL ≥ 2.4 mm Al?　　❑Yes ❑No

5. Beam quantity.

Tube current _____ mA

Tabletop exposure rate _____ R/min

Output intensity _____ R/mA-min ≤ 3.2 R/mA

Maximum output intensity _____ R/m

　　Obtained at _____ kVp and _____ mA

<10 R/min?　❑Yes ❑No

6. Primary protective barrier.

Is the intensifier tower assembly properly connected and interlocked with the x-ray tube?　　❑Yes ❑No

Table output intensity_____ R/min

Exposure rate above and around the intensifier tower _____ mR/hr

_____ (mR/r) ÷ _____ (R/min) =_____

$$\frac{\text{mR/hr}}{\text{R/min}} \leq \frac{2\text{mR/hr}}{\text{R/min}} ?$$

❑Yes ❑No

7. Primary beam limitation.

Do the primary beam collimators function properly?

❑Yes ❑No

EXERCISES

1 Calculate the quantity of R/mA-min for each of the following conditions of operation:

　a. 70 kVp, l.5 mA, 3.2 R for 2 min

　b. 95 kVp, 4.2 mA, 4.1 R for 30 s

　c. 115 kVp, 2.7 mA, 6.8 R for 5 min

2 A silver dollar measures 3.8 cm in diameter. Its image on a spot film measures 9.1 cm, and the object and image planes are separated by 30 cm. What is the x-ray tube target-to-tabletop distance, and is it sufficient?

3 The following beam quality data were obtained at 80 kVp and 5 mA, and the detector was positioned 20 cm above the tabletop. The x-ray target-to-tabletop distance was 40 cm (16 inches).

Added filtration (mm Al)	0	0.5	1	2	3	4	5
R/min		5.3	4.5	3.9	3.1	2.5	1.9	1.5

Is the total filtration adequate? Is the tabletop exposure rate acceptable? Use the graph paper provided to assist in the solution.

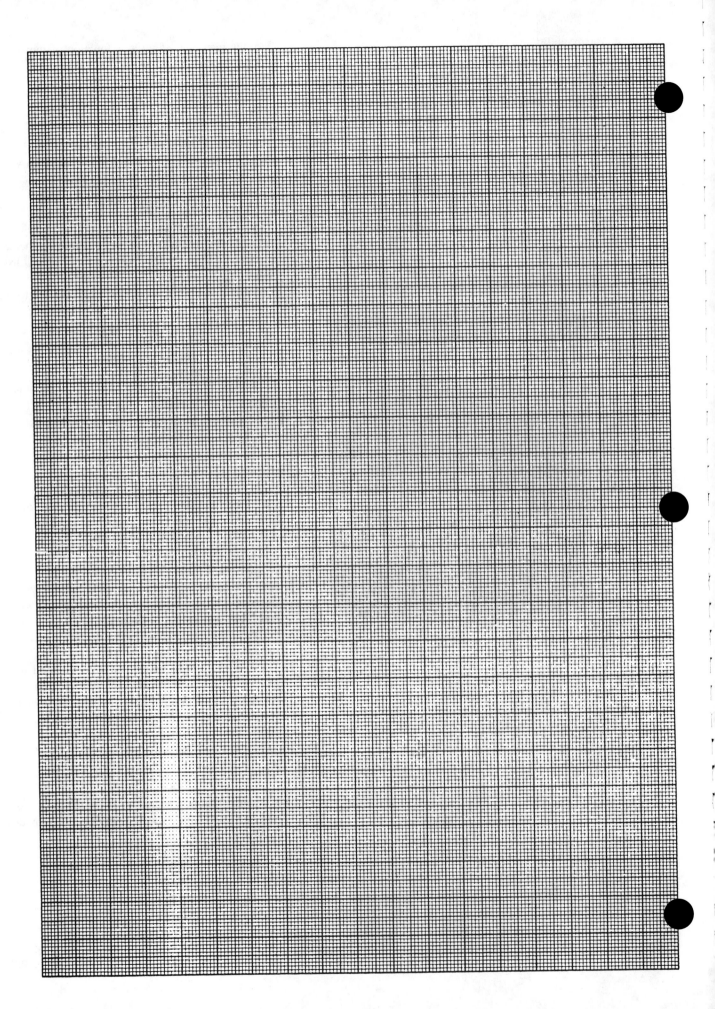

Worksheet Answers

Chapter 1

1. a (p. 6)
2. d (p. 5)
3. b (p. 9)
4. c (p. 9)
5. c (p. 4)
6. d (p. 4)
7. c (p. 4)
8. c (p. 4)
9. b (p. 5)
10. b (p. 4)
11. c (pp. 4-5)
12. b (p. 5)
13. b (p. 5)
14. b (p. 5)
15. b (p. 5)
16. c (p. 5)
17. a (p. 5)
18. b (p. 6)
19. b (p. 6)
20. a (p. 6)
21. b (p. 6)
22. c (p. 6)
23. a (p. 7)
24. a (p. 8)
25. c (p. 8)
26. d (p. 8)
27. a (p. 9)
28. b (p. 9)
29. d (p. 9)
30. b (p. 9)
31. d (p. 9)
32. d (p. 9)
33. b (p. 10)
34. b (p. 10)

Challenge Questions

1. In general, x-ray examinations should be limited to symptomatic patients, eliminating screening exams, except for mammograms. (p. 8)
2. Column 1 on page 9 will provide you with a variety of valuable tips in reducing unneces-sary patient exposure.
3. The electrical energy in the x-ray machine produces electromagnetic energy in the form of an x-ray beam, which is then converted into light and chemical energy, resulting in an image on the x-ray film. (p. 5)
4. Roentgen discovered x-rays on Nov. 8, 1895. He also made the first x-ray, which was of Bertha R.'s hand. (pp. 6-7)
5. Answers are found on pp. 7, 8, and 11.
6. Somewhat lengthy answers are found on page 8.
7. The most common were alopecia, anemia, and erythema. These are fully described on page 6.
8. Michael Pupin first used fluorescent screens in conjuction with glass photographic plates in 1896. (p. 9)

Chapter 2

Guidance in solving questions 1–9 can be found on page 13.

1. c, vi
2. f, viii
3. a, ix
4. g, ii
5. h, i
6. e, iv
7. j, iii
8. d, vii
9. b, v
10. d (p. 13)
11. a (p. 13, illustration 2-1)
12. e (pp. 13-14)
13. c (p. 14)
14. d (p. 14)
15. d (p. 14)

Guidance in solving questions 16–20 can be found in Tables 2-1, 2-2, and 2-3.

16. 10,000 meters
17. 0.01 mA
18. 0.07 Mg

19. 10^{-9} m
20. 1800 mm

Guidance in solving questions 21–33 can be found on pages 15–16.
21. 8/12 = 2/3
22. 3/16
23. 1/8
24. 18 61/128
25. 1 1/2
26. 1:4
27. 5.58
28. 2.35
29. a = 9.7
30. b = −126
31. 6 mR
32. 224 mAs
33. 7

Guidance in solving questions 34–38 can be found on page 15 and in Table 2-3.
34. 3.7617 x 10^4
35. 1.6 x 10^{-3}
36. 10^{20}
37. 10^9
38. 20:1

Guidance in solving questions 39–45 can be found on page 16.
39. 0.13 (0.125)
40. 0.017 (0.0167)
41. 1/20
42. 1/3
43. x = 3.5
44. x = .24
45. 7
46. 2
47. 75

Answers for questions 46–50 are based on information on p. 17 in the text.

48.
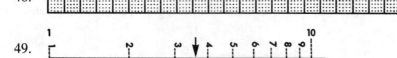

49.
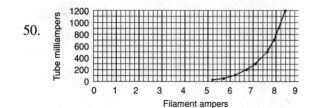

50.
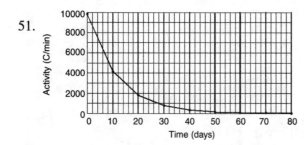
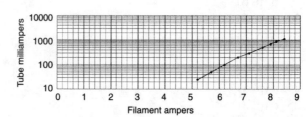

51.
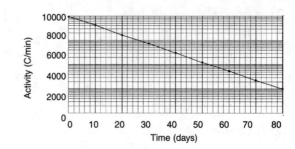

Challenge Questions

1. 9 (p. 16)
2. 100 ms (Table 2-1)
3. 2 x 10^4 μR (Table 2-1)
4. 444 mR (p. 16)
5. 14.3 mR (p. 16)

Chapter 3

1. Answers are shown in Fig. 3-1 on p. 20.
2. (p. 21)

Unit	British	MKS	CGS	SI Units
length	foot (ft)	meter (m)	centimeter	meter (m)
mass	pound (lb)	kilogram (kg)	gram (g)	kilogram (kg)
time	second (s)	second (s)	second (s)	second (s)

3. d (p. 20)
4. c (p. 21)
5. d (p. 21)
6. c (p. 21)
7. b (p. 21)
8. b (p. 21)
9. c (p. 21)
10. d (p. 22)
11. c (p. 22)
12. d (p. 23)
13. b (p. 23)
14. c (p. 23)
15. b (p. 23)
16. c (pp. 23-24)
17. a (p. 24)
18. b (p. 24)
19. a (p. 24)
20. c (p. 24)
21. d (p. 25)
22. b (p. 25)
23. e (p. 24)
24. 6 ft/s
25. 7.9×10^2 m/s^2
26. 80 km/hr
27. 19.6 m/s; 58.8 m/s
28. 158 N
29. 2800 J (p. 24)
30. 28 W (p. 24)
31. a (p. 24)
32. c (p. 22)
33. e (pp. 23-24)
34. d (p. 24)
35. c (p. 25)

Challenge Questions

1. a.   Harriet knows not just distance (magnitude) but also direction; in other words, she has a specific vector.
   b.   Jack is working with only a scalar. (p. 21)
2. a (p. 21)
3. b (p. 22)
4. d (p. 21)
5. a (p. 22)
6. Jack's acceleration has been both positive and negative. From 2:15 to 3:15, his acceleration is negative. From 3:15 to 3:30, his acceleration is positive.
7. Between 2:00 and 3:00, Jack's acceleration is a –20 mph. Between 3:00 and 4:00, it is 20 mph.

Chapter 4

1. A. medieval
   B. Dalton's
   C. Thomson's
   D. Bohr's
2. c (p. 29)
3. c (pp. 29-30)
4. a (p. 30)
5. a (p. 30)
6. a (p. 30)
7. b (p. 31)
8. d (p. 31)
9. b (p. 32)
10. d (p. 32)
11. d (p. 32)
12. e (p. 33)
13. d (p. 34)
14. b (p. 34)
15. a (p. 35)
16. d (p. 35)

Answers to questions 17–22 are found on page 33.

17. Ag stands for silver. Its atomic mass is 107.
18. Cu stands for copper. Its atomic mass is 63.
19. Au stands for gold. Its atomic mass is 197.
20. C stands for carbon. Its atomic mass is 12.
21. Fe stands for iron. Its atomic mass is 56.
22. Pb stands for lead. Its atomic mass is 208.
23. Al stands for aluminum. Its atomic mass is 27.
24. Mo stands for molybdenum. Its atomic mass is 98.
25. W stands for tungstun. Its atomic mass is 184.
26. The number of electrons that occupy the outermost shell of any atom is exactly the same as its group number. Simply identify its chemical abbreviation, find it on the periodic table, and identify the group (column) number. (p. 36)
    a.   2
    b.   2
    c.   7
    d.   2 (pp. 31 and 33)
27. a (p. 36)
28. Those atoms in the fourth period of the periodic table are called transitional elements. These interrupt the orderly scheme of atomic progression from smallest to largest. Instead of simply adding electrons to the next outer shell, electrons are added to an inner shell. (p. 36)
29. Electrons revolving around the nucleus in fixed orbits or shells produce centripetal force through their electrostatic attraction. This is a center-seeking force that just matches the force of motion or velocity. Centrifugal force is a flying-out-from-the-center force; it is balanced by the normal atom's centripetal force. (p. 36)
30. E_b stands for the electron binding energy, the strength of attachment of an electron to the nucleus. (p. 36)
31. This process is possible; it is referred to as radioactive disintegration or radioactive decay. (p. 37)
32. Any nuclear arrangement is called a nuclide, but only nuclei that undergo radioactive decay are radionuclides. (p. 37)

33. During beta emission, a neutron undergoes conversion into a proton. Simultaneously, an electron-like particle is ejected from the nucleus, escaping from the atom with considerable kinetic energy. (p. 37)
34. This is determined through the radioactive decay law, which states that the half-life of a radioisotope is the period of time required for a quantity of radioactivity to be reduced to one half of its original value. (p. 38)
35. The half-value layer is the thickness of a material used to reduce x-ray beam intensity to one-half its original intensity. (p. 39)
36. e (p. 39)
37. b (p. 40)
38. e (p. 40)
39. d (p. 41)
40. c (p. 41)
41. a (p. 41)

Challenge Questions

1. The n stands for the shell number or principal quantum number. (p. 35)
2. a. The L shell is #2, so $2n^2 = 2(2^2) = 2(4) = 8$ maximum electrons.
   b. The N shell is #4, so $2n^2 = 2(4^2) = 2(16) = 32$ maximum electrons.
   c. The Q shell is #7, so $2n^2 = 2(7^2) = 2(49) = 98$ maximum electrons. (p. 35)
3. The principal quantum number of the K shell is 1; M shell, 3; O shell, 5. Physicists call the shell number the principal quantum number. (p. 36)
4. The number of the outermost occupied electron shell of an atom is equal to its period (row) in the periodic table. Examples will depend on the elements chosen. (p. 36)
5. The number of electrons in the outermost shell is called the valence of the element. It determines chemical reactivity; it is numerically equal to the number of its group. Finally, this differs from the period number in that the period number is the number of the outermost occupied shell itself; the valence is the number of electrons in the outermost shell. (p. 36)

6. The half-life of a radioisotope is the period of time required for a quantity of radioactivity to be reduced to one-half its original value. (p. 38)
7. Answers should reflect discussion on pages 39-41.
8. Tables and labels should reflect discussion on page 30, as well as Figure 4-4.

Chapter 5

1. The three lines in the illustration represent three sine waves. Their most important difference lies in their varying amplitudes. The amplitude is obtained by determining one-half the range from crest to valley over which each sine wave varies. (p. 44)
2. (a) The important properties of this model are velocity, frequency, and wavelength. (b) Frequency is the rate of rise and fall of a sine wave. The wavelength is the distance from one crest to another, from one valley to another, or from any point on the sine wave to the next corresponding point. Velocity is the speed with which a wave moves. (pp. 45-46)
3. The illustration shows sine waves of three different wavelengths and frequencies. (p. 46)
4. As *frequency* is increased, the *wavelength* is decreased. (p. 45)
5. The relationships are best expressed in the wave equation, which is as follows: Velocity = Frequency x Wavelength (p. 46)
6. The wave equation becomes simpler whenever one deals with electromagnetic radiation because all such radiation travels with the same velocity (186,400 miles/second). (p. 47)
7. e (p. 44)
8. e (p. 44)
9. d (p. 44)
10. c (p. 45)
11. a (p. 45)
12. d (p. 46)
13. d (pp. 46-47)
14. e (p. 47)
15. a (p. 47)

16. decreases; inversely; square; inverse square (p. 47)
17. intensity (p. 47)
18. wave; particle; particles; waves; wave-partical duality (p. 50)

Challenge Questions

1. If the product of frequency and wavelength always equals the velocity of light for electromagnetic radiation, frequency and wavelength are inversely proportional. Because their product always equals the velocity, then as frequency increases, the wavelength decreases and vice versa. (p. 47)
2. Stated simply, this law is saying that whenever electromagnetic radiation is emitted from a source such as the sun or a light bulb, the intensity decreases rapidly with the distance from the source. That's why you can read better in a dark room if you sit near the only lamp in the room rather than in a dark corner farthest from the only light source available! This is called the inverse square law. The reason for the rapid decrease in intensity with increasing distance is that the total energy emitted is spread out over an increasingly larger area. (p. 47)
3. The frequency range of electromagnetic radiation extends from approximately 10 to 10^{24} Hz, and the photon wavelengths associated with these ranges of wavelengths are approximately 10^7 to 10^{-16} meters respectively. (p. 48)
4. The known electromagnetic spectrum has three regions of importance to radiologic technology: visible light, x-radiation, and radio frequency. Photons of each of these radiations are essentially the same. Each can be represented as a bundle of energy consisting of varying electric and magnetic fields traveling at the speed of light. The only difference among photons of these various portions of the electromagnetic spectrum is in frequency and wavelength. (p. 48)
5. The units of measure in question are (a) the meter; (b) the hertz; (c) the electron volt. (d) These three scales are directly related mathematically, meaning that if the value of radiation of even one scale is known, a value on the other two can easily be computed.

(e) The reason there is no generally accepted, single standard for measuring radiation is that scientific investigation of the electro-magnetic spectrum has been conducted for over 100 years, and scientists working with radiation in one portion of the spectrum were often unaware of the investigation of the others. (p. 48)

6. The only true statement out of those given is this: "The shorter the wavelength of light, the greater the photon of energy." Expanded discussion might include the comparison of light wave behaviors to that of water waves. (p. 51)

7. I_1 = $I_2 (d_2/d_1)^2$
    = $(400 \text{ mR}) (36 \text{ in} / 18 \text{ in})^2$
    = $(400 \text{ mR}) (2)^2$
    = $(400 \text{ mR}) (4)$
    = 1600 mR will be the intensity of the x-ray beam at 18 in. (pp. 47-48)

8. E = hf
    = $(4.15 \times 10^{-15} \text{ eV-s}) (12.6 \times 10^5/\text{s})$
    = 5.23×10^{-9} eV is the energy of one photon from the broadcast frequency of 1260 kHz. (p. 54)

9. Answers are in Table 5-1.
10. Answers are in Figure 5-16.

All answers to the crossword puzzle are found on pages 48–50.

Across

1. m band
2. refraction
3. radio
4. energy
5. ultraviolet
6. gamma
7. smallest

Down

1. microwave
2. long
3. wavelength
4. violet
5. duality

Chapter 6

1. c (p. 57)
2. b (p. 57)
3. a (p. 57)
4. c (p. 57)
5. a (p. 58)
6. c (p. 58)
7. e (p. 58)
8. e (p. 58)
9. b (p. 58)
10. a (p. 58)
11. Running the comb vigorously through one's hair removes electrons and deposits them on the comb. This is the production of electrifi-cation by friction; another name for this is static electricity. The hair is electrified because it has an abnormally low number of electrons. The reason it stands on end is because of mutual repulsion. (p. 58)
12. The charge of one electron is much too small to be useful; consequently, the fundamental unit of electric charge is the coulomb (C). One coulomb equals 6.3×10^{18} electron charges. (p. 58)
13. Coulomb's law says that electrostatic force is directly proportioanl to the product of the charges and inversely proportional to the square of the distance between them:

$$F = k \frac{O_A O_B}{d^2}$$

F = electrostatic force (newtons)
O_A and O_B = quantities of electrostatic charge (coulombs)
d = distance between the charges
k = constant of proportionality (p. 60)
14. These laws are discussed on pages 60-61.
15. This law is on page 63.
16. d (p. 60)
17. d (p. 60)
18. e (p. 60)

Help with 19–28 can be found on pages 61 and 62.

19. f
20. d
21. c
22. g
23. e
24. h
25. a
26. j
27. i
28. b

29. In a series circuit, all circuit elements are connected in a line along the same conductor. A parallel circuit contains elements that bridge conductors rather than lie in a line along a conductor. Applicable "rules" for each are found on p. 64. One possible analogy is the example of Christmas lights, discussed on p. 65.
30. Answers will vary but should reflect the discussion on pp. 65 and 66.
31. F (p. 62)
32. F (p. 63)
33. F (p. 64)
34. F (p. 65)
35. T (p. 66)

Challenge Questions

1. During a thunderstorm, wind and cloud movements remove electrons from one cloud and deposit them on another. Both clouds become electrified, one negatively and one positively. If electrification is great enough, a discharge between the clouds can occur. Electrons move rapidly back and forth to whichever cloud is deficient. This is lightning. Lightning occurs between clouds, but it can also occur between an electrified cloud and the earth. (p. 58)
2. $V = IR$
   $= (0.75 A) (8 W)$
   $= 6 V$ of potential across the conductor (p. 66)
3. $I = P/V$
   $I = 50,000 W / 220 V$
   $I = 227 A$
   (p. 66)
4. See Table 6-2. (p. 64)

Chapter 7

1. b (p. 69)
2. c (p. 69)
3. b (p. 69)
4. d (pp. 69-70)
5. a (p. 71)
6. c (p. 71)
7. a (p. 71)
8. d (p. 71)
9. They are classified as (1) naturally occurring magnets; (2) artificially induced permanent magnets; and (3) electromagnets. (p. 70)
10. the magnetic moments of hydrogen atoms in the body are the basis of MRI. (p. 69)
11. Fe_3O_4 (p. 69)
12. *Magnetism* comes from the ancient village name, Magnesia. Ancient people knew lodestone or magnetite attracted iron. They considered magnetism and electrostatics to be the same. (p. 69)
13. Electromagnets are wire around an iron core. When electric current is conducted through the wire, a magnetic field is created. (p. 71)
14. Godolinium is paramagnetic. (p. 71)
15. This is the degree to which a material can be magnetized. (p. 71)
16. Maxwell's field theory is that magnetic force is proportional to the product of the magnetic pole strengths divided by the square of the distance between them. This magnetic force is inversely proportional to the squre of the distance between the poles. For instance, if the distance between two magnets is halved, the magnetic force will be increased by four times. (p. 73)
17. Both magnetism and electrostatics obey the inverse square law. (p. 73)
18. The earth's magnetic field is strongest at the poles. (p. 73)
19. The tesla (T) = 10,000 gauss (G). (p. 73)
20. b (p. 69)
21. a (p. 69)
22. b (p. 69)
23. c (p. 70)
24. b (p. 70)
25. d (p. 71)
26. c (p. 73)

Challenge Questions

1. See Table 7-1.
2. See pages 71-73.
3. We know that a moving charged particle induces a magnetic field in a plane perpendicular to its motion; for purposes of analysis and visualization, we create imaginary lines of this magnetic field. These are established so that we have a unified basis for discussion and visualization. In the same way, the phrase "by convention" suggests that we

establish a unified direction for these imaginary lines, so we say that "by convention" the imaginary lines of the magnetic field leave the north pole of a magnet and return to the south pole. (p. 72)

4. Running a CD over a magnet demagnetizes the sensor tag after a CD has been purchased. Thus, when Harriet leaves the store with her CDs, no alarms will go off, pinpointing her as a shoplifter! Since credit cards have magnetic strips of information, it can be risky to put them too close to the desensor magnet. The clerk has merely been trying to protect Harriet's credit cards.

5. A permanent magnet is created when a ferromagnetic material is actually charged in the field of an electromagnet. If Mariel does this to her piece of iron, it will become a permanent magnet until it is heated or hit hard enough by an object to jar the individual magnetic domains from their alignment, causing them to become randomly aligned again, destroying their magnetism.

Marianne's iron, however, will merely be placed in the vicinity of an intense magnetic field. The lines of induction will be altered by attraction to the soft iron, and thus the iron will be made temporarily magnetic. When removed from the magnetic field, however, it will probably not retain its strong magnetic property. It is a magnet only while its magnetism is being induced. In many MRI units, an iron magnetic shield is used to reduce the level of nonuseable fringe magnetic field. Ferromagnetic material acts as a magnetic sink by drawing the fringe lines of the magnetic field to it. (pp. 71 and 73)

Across
1. undisturbed (p. 70)
2. suscepti- (p. 71)
3. electrostatics (p. 69)
4. magnetite (p. 69)
5. ferromagnet- (p. 70)
6. moment (p. 69)
7. aligned (p. 69)

Down
1. dipole (p. 69)
2. di- (p. 71)
3. axis (p. 70)

4. lodestone (p. 69)
5. charge (p. 69)
6. acted on (p. 69)
7. slightly (p. 71)
8. field (p. 71)
9. origin (p. 70)

Chapter 8

1. c (p. 76)
2. c (p. 76)
3. b (p. 76)
4. a (p. 76)
5. c (p. 76)
6. d (p. 76)
7. b (p. 76)
8. d (p. 77)
9. b (pp. 76, 78–79)
10 c (p. 78)
11. a (p. 78)
12. c (p. 78)
13. d (p. 78)
14. c (p. 78)
15. a (p. 78)
16. c (p. 79)
17. c (p. 80)
18. a (p. 80)
19. c (p. 80)
20. b (p. 80)
21. d (p. 80)
22. c (p. 81)
23. b (p. 82)
24. Answers should show that the electric motor is most closely associated with Oersted's experiments. (pp. 76 and 80)
25. Answers will vary but should describe Faraday's experiment, particularly as it affects today's electormachanical dives. (p. 80)
26. Answers should include a description of how a coil of wire is rotated in a magnetic field. (p. 80)
27. See pages 78 and 81 for descriptions of the various components of a DC electric motor.
28. Answers should show that the electic generator is most closely associated with Faraday's experiments. (p. 80)
29. The true statement is a: "Generators and motors convert energy from one form into another." Paragraphs should expand on this. (p. 81)

30. Answer should include a description of how electric current is supplied to a coil of wire, among other factors responsible for the function of an electric motor. (p. 80)
31. Answers should discuss how and why generators and motors are classified as electro-mechanical devices. (p. 82)
32. b (p. 80)
33. a (p. 81)
34. b (p. 81; Fig. 8-14, b)
35. d (p. 81)
36. b (p. 81)
37. c (p. 81)
38. d (p. 81)
39. a (p. 82)
40. a (p. 82)
41. b (p. 82)
42. c (p. 82)
43. See page 76.
44. See Figure 8-4
45. See page 78.
46. See pages 78-79.
47. See page 79.
48. The secondary voltage will be greater than the primary voltage. (p. 83)
49. The change in current across a transformer is not in the same direction as the voltage change, but it is not exactly proportional to either voltage change or the turns ratio. The truth is that it is inversely proportional to the turns ratio. (p. 83)
50. See page 83.
51. The main difference can be seen by converting the AC (alternating current) to DC (direct current) by replacing the slip rings on an AC current with a simple device called the communtator ring, which acts like a switch, thus changing the polarity of the contact on the brush wire at precisely those points at which the electrical charge on one side changes. The resulting reversed current, flowing out of the commutator ring assembly, is humped in one direction. (p. 81)
52. a (p. 82)
53. a (pp. 82-83)
54. d (p. 83)
55. a (p. 83)
56. c (p. 83)
57. d (p. 83)
58. c (pp. 83–84)
59. c (p. 84)

60. d (p. 84)
61. c (p. 84)
62. a (p. 84)
63. d (p. 85)
64. b (p. 85)
65. d (p. 85)
66. c (p. 85)
67. b (p. 86)

Challenge Questions

1. See page 77.
2. See Figure 8-21.
3. See Figures 8-19 and 8-22.
4. See Figure 8-18.
5. Answers will vary but should accurately reflect information given on pp. 80–81. Perhaps most important is to point out that the net effect of an electric generator is to convert mechanical energy into electric energy. This conversion process is not 100% efficient because of frictional losses in the mechanical moving parts and heat losses caused by resistances in the electrical components. (p. 81)
6. (a) The turns ratio is 67:1. (b) The secondary voltage is 14.7 kV. (c) The secondary current is 75 mA. (p. 83)
7. The output waveform will contain 60 negative pulses per second. (p. 84)

Chapter 9

1. a (p. 92)
2. c (p. 92)
3. a (p. 92)
4. b (p. 94)
5. e (p. 94)
6. e (p. 96)
7. b (p. 96)
8. d (p. 97)
9. a (p. 98)
10. e (p. 98)
11. See Figure 9-10.
12 a (p. 99)
13. F (p. 92)
14. T (p. 94)
15. F (p. 94)
16. F (p. 99)
17. F (p. 105)
18. F (p. 105)

19. (350 mA) (0.085 seconds) = 29.75 mAs (p. 97)
20. (450 mA) (0.12 seconds) = 54 mAs (p. 97)
21. (8.3 amperes)(1/15) = (8.3/15) = 0.553 amperes (p. 97)
22. (7.6 amperes)(1/20) = 0.38 amperes (p. 97)
23. 90 mAs/220 mA = .409 seconds or 409 ms (p. 97)
24. 85 mAs/350 mA = .243 seconds or 243 ms (p. 97)
25. (230 Vp) (850:1) = 195,500 Vp = 195.5 kVp is the secondary voltage. (p. 100)
26. (180 Vp) (770:1) = 138,600 Vp = 138.6 kVp is the secondary voltage. (p. 100)
27. 900 mA x 110 kVp = 99,000 mA x kVp = 99,000 watts = 99 kW (p. 105)
28. 950 mA x 120 kVp = 114,000 x kVp = 114,000 watts = 114 kW (p. 105)
29. (0.7) x (mA x kVp)/1000 = (0.7) (600 mA x 240 kVp)/1000 = 0.7 x (144,000/1000) = (0.7)(144) = 100.8 kW is the power rating. (p. 105)
30. (0.7) x (mA x kVp)/1000 = (0.7) (550 mA x 200 kVp)/1000 = 0.7 x (110,000/1000) = (0.7)(110) = 77 kW is the power rating. (p. 105)
31. The autotransformer is designed to supply a precise voltage to the filament circuit and to the high-voltage circuit of the x-ray machine. As the line compensator measures the voltage provided to the x-ray machine, its adjustment is usually provided automatically through the autotransformer, to which it is wired. The autotransformer works on the principle of electromagnetic induction, but with one winding and one core. The single winding has a number of connections along its length. Two of these, the primary connections, conduct input power to the autotransformer. Some of the secondary connections allow the autotransformer to increase and decrease voltage. Because the autotransformer operates as an induction device, the voltage it receives and the voltage it provides are in direct relation to the number of turns of the transformer enclosed by the connections. (p. 94)
32. The prereading voltmeter allows the voltage to be monitored before an exposure. On most operating consoles, such a kVp meter registers even though no exposure is being made

and no current is flowing in the circuit. (p. 96)
33. Voltage for the filament circuit, which controls x-ray tube current, is provided from connections on the autotransformer. This voltage is reduced via precision resistors to a valve corresponding to the mA station provided. In some units, mAs can be varied continuously during an exposure to the minimum exposure time. This is referred to as a falling-load mA. The voltage from the mA-selector switch is then delivered to the filament transformer, which supplies voltage to the filaments that is lower than the voltage supplied to the filament transformer itself. Thus it is called a step-down transformer—because the voltage supplied to the filaments is lower than that supplied to the transformer. (p. 97)
34. These detectors operate with a very accurate internal clock based on a quartz-crystal oscillator. They can measure exposure times as short as 1 millisecond and can also display the radiation waveform when used with an osciloscope. They are usually used by medical physicists and service engineers to test x-ray equipment. (p. 99)
35. There are two possibilities. A spinning top test can be used to check x-ray exposure times. A 100-ms image of a spinning top test should result in 12 dashes for a full-wave–rectified unit. A second option is the use of a solid-state radiation detector, if one is available. These devices are capable of measuring exposure times as short as 1 millisecond. (p. 99)
36. X-rays cannot be produced by electrons flowing in reverse direction from anode to cathode because the construction of the cathode assembly could not withstand the heat generated by such a process; besides, the anode cannot emit electrons thermionically. It would be disastrous to the x-ray tube for electron flow to be reversed. (p. 100)
37. The voltage across an x-ray tube during the negative half cycle is called inverse voltage. It can be removed from the supply to the x-ray tube by rectification, a process that converts alternating current into direct current and thus does not allow the voltage to swing negatively. (p. 101)
38. Half-wave rectification does not allow volt-

age to swing negatively during the negative half of its cycle. It is called half-wave rectification because only one-half of the AC waveform appears in the output; the negative portion has been removed. Half-wave–rectified circuits contain either zero, one, or two diodes, and the x-ray output is pulsating, with 60 x-ray pulses produced each second. Full-wave–rectified x-ray machines contain at least four diodes in a high-voltage circuit. In a full-wave–rectified circuit, the negative half cycle corresponding to the inverse voltage is reversed so that a positive voltage is always directed across the x-ray tube. The output voltage across the x-ray tube is positive, and there are no gaps in the output waveform. All of the input waveform is rectified into usable output. (p. 101)

39. One shortcoming of half-wave rectification is that it wastes half the supply power. Full-wave rectification is preferred because it does not waste any of the input source. Its main advantage is that the exposure time for any given technique is cut in half. (pp. 101 and 102)

40. Illustrations will vary but should be as thorough as Figure 9-20 (p. 102)

Challenge Questions

1. See page 92.
2. See Figure 9-9.
3. See Figure 9-24.
4. See Figure 9-25.
5. See Figure 9-26.

Across

1. diodes (p. 100)
2. ioniz- (p. 98)
3. size (p. 103)
4. square (p. 103)
5. time (p. 97)
6. half-value (p. 92)
7. timing (p. 92)
8. step (p. 97)
9. quantity (p. 92)
10. autotransformer (p. 94)
11. reverse (p. 101)
12. falling (p. 97)
13. supply (p. 94)
14. therm- (p. 96)

Down

1. sinus- (p. 100)
2. single (p. 94)
3. image (p. 98)
4. half (p. 101)
5. electromagnetic (p. 94)
6. quality (p. 92)
7. inverter (p. 103)
8. low (p. 94)
9. negatively (p. 101)
10. temperature (p. 96)
11. current (p. 97)
12. turn (p. 94)
13. filament (p. 97)
14. ripple (p. 104)
15. serial (p. 98)

Chapter 10

1. a, p. 108
2. d, p. 108
3. d, p. 108
4. e, p. 108
5. a, p. 108
6. b, p. 108
7. b, p. 108
8. d, p. 108
9. c, p. 108
10. b, p. 108
11. a, p. 110
12. c, p. 110
13. a, pp. 110–11
14. d, p. 116
15. c, p. 116
16. d, p. 117
17. d, p. 121
18. F, p. 110
19. T, p. 111
20. T, pp. 115 and 120
21. T, p. 116
22. T, pp. 116–17
23. F, p. 120
24. T, p. 122
25. (1) Because the accelerating electrons coming from the cathode to the anode in an x-ray tube are electrically negative, the electron beam tends to spread out. The principle demonstrated by such a phenomenon is referred to as electrostatic repulsion. Some electrons can even miss the anode com-

pletely. (2) A focusing cup is negatively charged so that it condenses the electron beam to a small area of the anode. (p. 111)

26. The anode is (1) an electrical conductor, receiving electrons from the cathode and conducting them through the tube to the connecting cables and back to the high-voltage generator. It also (2) provides mechanical support for the target and is (3) a good thermal conductor, conducting the intense heat from electrons' kinetic energy away from the anode. (p. 113)

27. It is important, when using a two-position exposure switch, to push the switch to its final position in one motion. This minimizes the time that the filament is heated, which prevents excessive space charge and thus prolongs tube life. (p. 115)

28. Manufacturers of mammography equipment take advantage of this property by angling the x-ray tube so that the smaller focal spot coincides with the thick tissue of the chest wall. (p. 118)

29. See page 112.
30. See page 112.
31. Copper, molybdenum, and graphite are the most common. (p. 113)
32. See yellow box on page 113.
33. See page 113.
34. See Figure 10-16.
35. See pages 117-118.
36. See page 118.
37. See pages 120-121.

Challenge Questions

1. (p. 122)
   a. unsafe
   b. safe
   c. safe
   d. unsafe
   e. unsafe

2. First locate the proper rating chart (lower left in Figure 10-26). Then locate the 100 kVp line. Beginning from the left (shorter exposure time), calculate the mAs for the intersection of each mA curve with the 100 kVp level. The first intersection is approximately 300 mA at 1 second, which equals 300 mAs. This is not enough. The next intersection is approximately 250 mA at 6 second(s), which equals 1500 mAs. This is enough. Consequently, 6 seconds is the minimum possible exposure time. (pp. 121–22)

3. Number of heat units = 75 kVp x 400 mAs = 30,000 HU is generated in this exam. (p. 122)

4. 100 kVp x 2.5 mA x 2 minutes x 60 seconds/minute = 30,000 HU are generated during the exam. (p. 123)

5. The 200,000 HU level intersects the anode cooling curve at approximately 2 minutes. From that point on the curve to complete cooling requires an additional 13 minutes. Therefore 13 minutes are required for complete cooling. (p. 123)

6. 50 kVp x 400 mAs = 20,000 joule = 20 kJ of heat is produced. (p. 123)

7. See page 123.

Chapter 11

1. d (p. 127)
2. c (p. 127)
3. b (p. 127)
4. b (p. 128)
5. b (p. 128)
6. a (p. 129)
7. a (p. 129)
8. b (p. 129)
9. a (p. 129)
10. c (p. 130)
11. a (p. 130)
12. e (p. 132)
13. F (p. 127)
14. T (p. 128)
15. T (p. 128)
16. T (p. 128)
17. F (p. 128)
18. T (p. 132)
19. The resultant x-ray is called a (a) K x-ray because (b) it results from ionization of a K-shell electron. (c) The energy of the characteristic x-ray is 69.4 keV. (p. 129)
20. The resultant x-ray is called an (a) O x-ray because (b) it results from ionization of an O-shell electron. (c) The energy of the characteristic x-ray is 0.08 keV. (p. 129)
21 a. 57.4 keV (p. 130)
    b. 68.9 keV (p. 130)
    c. 69.4 keV (p. 130)

22. The answer is yes, there is enough information to determine the machine's kVp: the maximum energy that an x-ray can have is numerically equal to the kVp of operation; thus, it was operated at approximately 90 kVp. (p. 132)

23. (a) The projectile electrons can have kinetic energies up to 82 keV. (b) A bremsstrahlung x-ray produced can have any energy in the range of 0 to 82 keV. (p. 132)

24. Graphs will have a vertical axis labeled "relative emission" or similar term, while the horizontal axis is labeled "x-ray energy (keV)." The curve should intersect the energy axis at 0 and 87.6 keV and have the same general bell shape, but a bremsstrahlung spectrum is much lower. A line should extend above the curve at 17 keV to represent the characteristic x-rays. (p. 133)

25. 0.0124 nm is the minimum wavelength associated with 100 kVp. (p. 133)

26. 0.0248 nm would be the minimum wavelength. (p. 133)

27. See Figure 11-8. (p. 131)

28. Characteristic x-rays have precisely fixed or discrete energies that are characteristic of the differences between electron-binding energies of a particular element. A plot of the frequency with which characteristic x-rays are emitted as a function of their energy is called the characteristic x-ray emission spectrum, which has disccrete vertical lines represent K x-rays, L-x-rays and other lower-energy emissions from the outer electron shells. If it were possible to measure the energy contained in each bremsstrahlung photon emitted from an x-ray tube, one would find that these energies range from the peak electron energy all the way down to zero. For this reason, a typical bremsstrahlung x-ray emission spectrum is plotted as a continuous spectrum, rather than a bar graph. (p. 132)

29. Depending on the type of rectification and high-voltage generator, many of these electrons may have very low energies when they strike the target. (p. 132)

30. The added filtration selectively removes low-energy x-rays from the beam. (p. 132)

31. See page 133.

32. (a) The farther to the right a spectrum is, the higher the effective energy or quality of the beam. The greater the area under the curve, the higher the x-ray intensity or quantity of photons in the beam. (b) A change in mA results in a directly proportional change in the amplitude of the x-ray emission spectrum at all energies. For instance, a rise in mA while all other conditions remain constant results in a proportionate rise in the number of electrons flowing from cathode to anode, as well as a proportionate rise in the number of x-rays of every energy. Graphically, this will mean that the spectrum will be changed in amplitude but not in shape. (p. 133)

33. (a) A change in kVp affects both the amplitude and the position of the x-ray emission spectrum. More specifically, when kVp is increased, the relative distribution of emitted x-rays shifts to the right to higher x-ray energies. The area under the curve increases to an area approximating the square of the factor by which kVp was increased. Accordingly, the x-ray quantity increases with the square of this factor as well. (b) This partially explains the 15% kVp rule, which states that a 15% increase in kVp is equivalent to doubling the mAs. (c) This rule of thumb is used by radiographers to calculate the kVp and mAs changes necessary to produce a constant optical density on a radiograph. (p. 134)

34. Hardening the x-ray beam (a) does not affect the characteristic spectrum, but it does (b) reduce the bremsstrahlung x-ray emission spectrum more on the left than on the right. It has (c) no effect on the maximum energy of x-ray emission, while still (d) absorbing low-energy x-rays and allowing higher energy x-rays to pass through. (p. 135)

35. (a) As the atomic number of the target material increases, the efficiency of the production of bremsstrahlung radiation increases. (b) The characteristic spectrum is shifted to the right, representing the higher-energy characteristic radiation--a much more pronounced change than that of the bremsstrahlung x-ray spectrum. (p. 135)

Challenge Questions

1. (a) The first machine will increase to 58 kvP, while the second will now operate at about 127 kVp. (b) A 15% in crease in kVp does

not double the output intensity from an x-ray machine, but it is equivalent to doubling the mAs to obtain a given optical density on the radiograph. To double the output intensity, the first machine would have to raise the kVp by as much as 40%. (c) Only a 15% increase in kVp is necessary because with increased kVp, the penetrability of the beam is increased and less radiation is absorbed by the patient, leaving proportionately more to expose the film. (pp. 136–37)

2. See Figures 11-3 and 11-5.
3. See page 132.
4. See pages 133-136.
5. a. 63.25 kVp
   b. 69 kVp
   c. 82.8 kVp
   d. 92 kVp
   e. 103.5 kVp
   f. 138 kVp
6. See Tables 11-2 and 11-3.

Chapter 12

1. a (p. 140)
2. a (p. 140)
3. c (p. 142)
4. c (p. 141)
5. b (p. 142)
6. a (p. 142)
7. b (p. 142)
8. e (p. 143)
9. a (p. 143)
10. b (p. 143)
11. c (p. 143)
12. T (p. 141)
13. F (p. 143)
14. T (p. 144)
15. F (p. 145)
16. 80 mR is the increased x-ray intensity. (p. 140)
17. 111 mR is the increased x-ray intensity. (p. 140)
18. $x/200$ mR = 30 mAs/60 mAs
    $x = (200)(30)/(60) = 100$ mR is the reduced x-ray intensity. (pp. 140–141)
19. $x/220$ mR = 40 mAs/50 mAs
    $x = 220(4)/5 = 880/5 = 176$ mR is the reduced x-ray intensity. (pp. 140–141)

20. $I/36$ mR = $(150/100 \text{ kVp})^2$
    $I = 36 (150/100 \text{ kVp})^2 =$
    $36(1.5)^2 = 36(2.25) = 81$ mR is the increased intensity. (p. 141)
21. 129.6 mR is the increased intensity. (p. 141)
22. $I/40$ mR = $(85 \text{ kVp}/100 \text{ kVp})^2$
    $I = 40(85/100)^2 = 40(0.85)^2 =$
    $40(0.72) = 28.8$ mR is the reduced x-ray intensity. (p. 141)
23. A constant exposure of the film can be maintained by reducing the mAs by one-half whenever the kVp is increased by 15%. Thus, the expected intensity can be calculated as follows:
    $I/150$ mR = (25 mAs/50 mAs) (92 kVp/80 kVp)^2
    $I = 150(25/50) (92/80)^2 = 150(0.5)(1.32) = 75(1.32) = 99$ mR is the intensity resulting from the change in mAs and kVp. (p. 141)
24. $I/15$ mR = $(100 \text{ cm}/80 \text{ cm})^2$
    $I = 15(1.25)^2 = 15 (1.56) = 23.4$ mR is the increased intensity at the reduced distance. (p. 142)
25. $I/14$ mR = $(200 \text{ cm}/100 \text{ cm})^2$
    $I = 14$ mR $(200 \text{ cm}/100 \text{ cm})^2 = 14(4) = 56$ mR is the increased intensity at the decreased distance. (p. 142)
26. $I/17$ mR = $(240 \text{ cm}/80 \text{ cm})^2$
    $I = 17$ mR $(240 \text{ cm}/80 \text{ cm})^2 = 17(3)2 = 17(9) = 153$ mR is the increased intensity at the decreased distance. (p. 142)
27. Because the addition of filtration attenuates the x-ray beam, it affects x-ray quantity. This value can be predicted if one knows the half-value layer of the beam. The addition of filtration equal to the beam half-value layer reduces the beam quantity to half its pre-filtered value. Since there is an addition of one half-value layer, the x-ray quantity will be 1.5 mR/mAs. (p. 145)
28. The steps involved are described in detail on pp. 142–43.
29. These are described in detail on p. 145.
30. The addition of a filter to an x-ray beam attenuates x-rays of all energies emitted by the tube, but it attenuates more low-energy x-rays than high-energy x-rays. This shifts the x-ray emission spectrum to the high-energy side, resulting in an x-ray beam with higher

energy and greater penetrability. Because this addition of filtration attenuates the x-ray beam, it affects x-ray quantity. This value can be predicted if one knows the half-value layer of the beam. The addition of filtration equal to the beam half-value layer reduces the beam quantity to half its prefiltered value and results in a harder x-ray beam. (p. 145)

31. See Table 12-1.
32. directly proportional (p. 140)
33. $1R = 2.58 \times 10^{-4}$ C/kg. (p. 140)
    $1C = 6.25 \times 10^{18}$ electrons. (p. 141)
34. See page 142.
35. See page 142.
36. See page 144 and Table 12-4.
37. See page 145.

Challenge Questions

1. A compensating filter can make up for the differences in subject radiopacity. Its use here suggests that there is a difference in radiopacity between Mr. Henson's lungs—one lung probably has significantly more fluid than the other. For instance, if his right lung has more fluid and his left lung is more clear, the thinner part of the filter is positioned over the fluid-filled lung. (p. 145)

2. The radiographer is no doubt using a trough filter. This is sometimes used in chest radiography, even on healthy subjects with clear lungs. The thin central region is positioned over the mediastinum, which houses the heart and great vessels, while the lateral thick portion is placed over the air-filled lung fields. This results in a more uniform optical density. (p. 145)

3. An AP projection of the foot would most likely call for a wedge filter, since the foot varies considerably in thickness from the toes to the heel. You would be wise to position the wedge with its thick portion over the toes and the thin portion toward the heel. (p. 145)

4. See Figure 12-9 and its discussion on pages 145-146.

5. a. ≈ 7 mR/mAs at 100 cm
   b. 10 mR/mAs at 100 cm
   c. ≈ 4 mR/mAs at 100 cm
   d. .5 mR/mAs at 100 cm
   e. .5 mR/mAs at 100 cm

Chapter 13

1. l (p. 150)
2. j (p. 150)
3. i (p. 150)
4. f (p. 151)
5. a (p. 151)
6. c (p. 151)
7. h (p. 153)
8. m (p. 155)
9. k (p. 155)
10. b (p. 156)
11. o (p. 156)
12. g (p. 156)
13. d (p. 159)
14. n (p. 160)
15. e (p. 160)
16. d (p. 150)
17. c (p. 150)
18. a (p. 151)
19. b (p. 151)
20. d (p. 151)
21. d (p. 151)
22. d (p. 151)
23. a (p. 152)
24. b (pp. 153 and 154)
25. c (p. 155)
26. e (p. 155)
27. e (p. 156)
28. e (p. 157)
29. e (p. 158)
30. $40 \text{ keV} = E_s + (0.04 \text{ keV} + 16 \text{ keV})$
    $E_s = 40 \text{ keV} - (0.04 \text{ keV} + 16 \text{ keV})$
    $= 40 \text{ keV} - (16.04 \text{ keV})$
    $= 23.96 \text{ keV}$ is the energy of the scattered x-ray (p. 151)
31. $36 \text{ keV} = E_s + (0.04 \text{ keV} + 14 \text{ keV})$
    $E_s = 36 \text{ keV} - (0.04 \text{ keV} + 14 \text{ keV})$
    $= 36 \text{ keV} - (14.04 \text{ keV})$
    $= 21.96 \text{ keV}$ is the energy of the scattered x-ray (p. 151)
32. a. We know that the carbon atom's binding energies are as follows: K shell = 0.284 keV; L shell = 0.01 keV.
    $E_{KE} = E_i - E_b = 60 \text{ keV} - 0.284 \text{ keV}$
    $= 59.716 \text{ keV}$ is the kinetic energy of the photoelectron displaced in a carbon atom.
    $E_x = 0.284 \text{ keV} - 0.01 \text{ keV}$
    $= 0.274 \text{ keV}$ is the energy of the characteristic x-ray emitted from

the carbon atom.

b. We know that the barium atom's binding energies are as follows:

K shell = 37.4 keV; L shell = 5.989 keV

$$E_{KE} = E_i - E_b = 60 \text{ keV} - 37.4 \text{ keV}$$
$$= 22.6 \text{ keV is the kinetic energy of the photoelectron displaced in a barium atom.}$$

$$E_x = 37.4 \text{ keV} - 5.989 \text{ keV}$$
$$= 31.411 \text{ keV is the energy of the characteristic x-ray emitted from the carbon atom. (p. 153)}$$

33. a. $(30 \text{ keV} / 60 \text{ keV})^3 = (1/2)^3 = 0.125$ or 12.5% is the probability of 60 keV interaction compared with 20 keV interaction.

b. The atomic number of air = 7.6
The atomic number of lung tissue = 7.4
$(7.6 / 7.4)^3 = (1.027)^3 = 1.08$ or 108% is the probability of interaction with air compared with lung tissue. (p. 155)

34. Bone has an atomic number of 13.8; fat has an atomic number of 6.3; muscle, 7.4.
$13.8^3 / 7.4^3 = 2628 / 405 = 6.5$ times more likely to interact with bone than muscle.
$13.8^3 / 6.3^3 = 2628 / 250 = 10.51$ times more likely to interact with bone than fat. (p. 157)

35. Differential absorption due to atomic number: $7.4^3 / 6.3^3 = 405 / 250 = 1.62$
Differential absorption due to mass density:
$320 / 910 = .35$
Total differential absorption:
$(1.62)(.35) = .5670 = .57$ (p. 159)

36. They are equal at 20 keV and 40 keV. (p. 158)

37. Yes. When x-rays penetrate any type of tissue, they interact with the atoms of that tissue in one way or another. The relative frequency of interaction depends primarily on the atomic number of the tissue atoms and the x-ray energy. The photoelectric effect is called absorption because the x-ray disappears. (p. 159)

38. Attenuation is the total reduction in the number of x-rays remaining in an x-ray beam after penetration through a given thickness of tissue. When a broad beam of x-rays penetrates any tissue, some of the x-rays are absorbed and some are scattered. The result is a reduction in the number of x-rays, so attenuation equals absorption plus scattering. (p. 159)

39. See Table 13-6. (p. 159)

40. See Figures 13-1, 13-2, 13-5, 13-8, and 13-9.

Challenge Questions

1. Radiologic contrast agents, such as iodine and barium, use the principles of differential absorption and attenuation to image soft tissue organs within the body. Iodine is used in vascular, renal, and biliary imaging. Air, too, has been used, with air replacing the normal body fluids in internal cavities being examined. Although this is less common since the advent of computed tomography and magnetic imaging, air is still used as a contrast agent in one type of GI exam called a double-contrast exam. (p. 160)

2. Compton-scattered x-rays produce a uniform optical density of the radiograph—in other words, fog—which results in reduced image contrast. Radiographs appear duller and flatter because of Compton-scattered x-rays. In addition, these scattered x-rays can create a serious radiation exposure hazard in radiography, particularly in fluorsocopy. Such radiaton is the source of most of the occupational radiation exposure that radiographers receive. These levels are high enough to have federal requirements for protective shielding in the x-ray examining room. (p. 151)

3. All answers are listed in Table 13-1 on p. 152.

4. The ejection of a K-shell photoelectron by the incident x-ray results in a vacancy in the K shell. This is immediately corrected when an outer-shell electron, usually from the L shell, drops into the vacancy. The electron transition is accompanied by the emission of an x-ray with energy that equals the difference in the binding energies of the shells involved. This transition does not occur often. The characteristic x-rays are secondary radiation and behave in the same manner as scattered radiation. (p. 153)

5. This means that a small variation in atomic number of the tissue atom or a small variation in x-ray energy results in a large change in the chance of photoelectric interaction. (p. 154)

6. If an incident x-ray has enough energy to come close enough to the nucleus of the atom, it can be influenced by the strong elec-

trostatic field of the nucleus. This interaction causes the x-ray to disappear. In its place appear two electrons, one positively charged positron and one negatively charged electron. This process is called pair production. Because we know that the energy equivalence of the mass of one electron equals 0.51 MeV, for two electrons to form in pair production, we must have at least 1.02 MeV of energy in the incident photon (2 x 0.51 = 1.02). An x-ray with less than 1.02 MeV cannot undergo pair production. Any energy in excess of 1.02 MeV is distributed equally between the two electrons as kinetic energy. Finally, because pair production involves only x-rays with energies greater than 1.02 MeV, it rarely occurs in the diagnostic x-ray range. (p. 155)

7. Usually, less than 5% of the incident x-rays passing through a patient reach the film, and less than half of those that reach the film interact to form an image. The radiographic image results from only 1% of the x-rays emitted by the x-ray unit. Consequestly, careful control and selection of the x-ray beam is necessary to produce high-quality radiographs. Producing a high-quality radiograph requires the proper selection of kVp so that the effective x-ray energy results in maximum differential absorption. (p. 156)

Chapter 14

1. c (p. 166)
2. a (p. 166)
3. b (p. 167)
4. c (p. 167)
5. d (p. 167)
6. d (p. 167)
7. c (p. 166)
8. b (pp. 169-170)
9. d (p. 170)
10. a (p. 170)
11. b (pp. 167-169 and 175)
12. in order: i, iii, v, iv, ii (p. 168, Figure 14-5)
13. base, emulsion (p. 166)
14. base (p. 166, Figure 14-1)
15. silver bromide (p. 167)
16. atoms of the silver halide crystal (p. 168)
17. secondary electrons (p. 168)

18. $AgNO_3$, KBr (p. 167)
19. photographic effect (p. 168)
20. spectral matching: the color of light to which the radiographic film is sensitive is properly matched to the color of light emitted by the intensifying screen; speed: film's sensitivity to light photons; contrast: range of shades of gray that appear on a radiograph; latitude: range of exposure techniques that produce an acceptable image (pp. 169-170)
21. Figures 14-8 and 14-9 (pp. 170-171)
22. The Gurney-Mott theory attempts to explain latent-image formation. It is by no means complete, but it is the accepted explanation. Production of the latent image and its conversion into a manifest image follows several simultaneous steps: Light or radiation interaction releases electrons, which migrate—bringing more migrating electrons with them—to the sensitivity speck where loss of ionic charge as negative ions are converted to neutral atoms causing the formation of atomic silver. The resultant group of silver atoms is called a latent-image center, where visible quantities of silver form during processing to create portions of the radiographic image. This process is repeated many times, causing the negative surface electrification to disappear and the silver atoms to build up. The remaining silver halide crystal is converted with processing to silver grains. (pp. 168–169)
23. A 15-watt bulb should be no closer than 5 feet from the work surface. Charts should include the following information (p. 171):
    1. Blue-sensitive film with calcium tungstate screen: Amber filter
    2. Green-sensitive film with rare-earth screen: Red filter
24. Patient dose with direct-exposure film is high, since it is made for use without intensifying screens. Today, it is used only when the benefits outweigh the risks of exposure; the emulsion of a direct-exposure film is thicker than that of screen-film and contains a higher concentration of silver-halide crystals to enhance direct x-ray interaction. It is not sensitive to light and therefore should not be used with screens. Most extremity exams now use fine-grain, high-detail screens and double-emulsion film as the image receptor instead of direct-exposure film, and most mammogra-

phy exams now use fine-grain, single-emulsion films designed to be exposed with a single intensifying screen. (pp. 171–172)

25. The effect is called halation. A special light-absorbing dye, called an antihalation coating, is used on all single-emulsion screen films, not just mammography film. The antihalation coating is removed during processing. (p. 172)

26. In video imaging, or CRT imaging, the image is formed by computer-assisted analysis of detected radiation and is displayed on a video monitor. To provide the radiologist with a permanent image, a negative photograph of the video image is made. (p. 172)

27. (a) Patient dose is not a consideration in video imaging because it is totally independent of the manner in which the video image is obtained. (b) However, the video film must be sensitive so that images can be obtained in a short time and the film can be properly matched to the spectral emission of the cathode-ray tube. Images are obtained with blue-dot or green-dot CRT phosphor with single-emulsion video-imaging film that is exposed in a multiformat camera. Films must be orthochromatic, not panchromatic, so that they can be used with any type of CRT and so that the film does not become fogged. CRT phosphor images must be recorded with blue- or green-sensitive film. (p. 172)

28. Descriptions are found on pages 172-174.

29. Discussion on handling and storage of films is found on pages 174-175.

Challenge Questions

1. The sequence of events—to the best of our knowledge, of course—are discussed on pages 168–169.

2. The information needed to check each other's work on this exercise is found on page 168, covering the silver-halide crystal's structure.

Chapter 15

1. f (p. 178)
2. e (p. 180)
3. k (p. 179, Table 15-1)
4. d (p. 178)
5. j (p. 181)
6. h (p. 180)
7. b (p. 179)
8. g (p. 180)
9. c (p. 178)
10. a (p. 179)
11. i (p. 181)
12. c (p. 180, Figure 15-3)
13. e (p. 178)
14. b (p. 182)
15. b (p. 181)
16. a (p. 180)
17. d (p. 182)
18. b (p. 180)
19. b (p. 179)
20. d (p. 178)
21. T (p. 182)
22. F (p. 185)
23. T (p. 180)
24. F (p. 185)
25. F (p. 182)
26. a (pp. 181-182)
27. d (p. 181)
28. f (pp. 180–181)
29. d (p. 182)
30. latent image, development, and fixing (p. 183, Figure 15-5)
31. The microswitch at entrance rollers controls the replenishment rate of processing chemicals. The short side of the film is placed against the guide rail of the feed tray to maintain the proper replenishment rate. (pp. 183-184, Figure 15-7)
32. A master roller with planetary rollers and guide shoes is used to reverse the direction of a film in the processor. (p. 184, Figure 15-9)
33. 95°F or 35°C (p. 185)
34. 12 liters/minute (p. 185)
35. 60-70 ml of developer, 100-110 ml of fixer (p. 186)
36. Rapid processing—as quickly as 30 seconds is now available. The processing chemicals are more concentrated and the developer and fixer temperatures are higher; Extended processing—up to 3 minutes processing time creates greater image contrast and lower patient dose when used with single-emulsion film; Daylight processing—allows cassette load, reload, and processing time to be reduced to 2 minutes. Because the film is automatically extracted and sent to the

processor, the radiographer does not have to leave the patient unassisted. (pp. 186-187)

37. Developer and fixer can quickly lose their chemical balance as they are absorbed during processing. Thus, they are replenished regularly to keep the level of solution in each tank from dropping and to avoid short contact times with the chemistry. The replenishment system puts into each tank the proper amount of chemistry for both developer and fixer. (pp. 185–186)

38. When an electron is given up (by a chemical such as a developing agent) to neutralize a positive ion, the process is called reduction. The silver ion is said to be reduced to metallic silver, and the chemical responsible for this is called a reducing agent. Oxidation is just the opposite—it produces an electron. The two can occur simultaneously. (p. 180)

39. Illustrations might include depiction of a slow buildup of metallic silver at the site of the sensitivity speck. After complete development, illustrations might show that exposed crystals have been destroyed and a grain of black metallic silver is all that remains. Unexposed crystals would look the same, since they are unaffected. The reduction of a silver ion is accompanied by the release of a bromine ion. The bromine ion migrates through the remnant of the crystal into the gelatin portion of the emulsion. From there, it is dissolved into the developer and removed from the film. (pp. 180–181)

Challenge Questions

1. Answers are found throughout the chapter.
2. Case studies and answers will depend entirely on journal articles applied to this project.
3. Information on components of the automatic processor are found on pages 183–186.
4. Rapid processing, extended processing, and daylight processing are discussed on page 186.

Chapter 16

1. a (p. 190)
2. d (p. 190)
3. e (p. 191)
4. c (p. 192)

5. b (p. 198)
6. b (pp. 198-199)
7. a (p. 199, Table 16-3)
8. in order: b, a, d, c (pp. 191-192)
9. Refer to Figure 16-1. (p. 190)
10. calcium tunstate, $CaWO_4$

    zinc sulfide, ZnS

    barium lead sulfate, $BaPbSO_4$

    gadolinium, Gd
    lanthanum, La
    yttrium, Y (p. 190 and elemental table in the dictionary)
11. sturdy; moisture resistant; discolor; chemically inert; flexible; impurities (p. 191, Box)
12. X-ray absorption—the percent absorption of x-rays in the phosphor layer of intensifying screens. (Figure 16-4, A); Screen conversion efficiency—efficiency of converting x-ray energy to light energy; Image noise—deterioration of the radiographic image caused by (1) the number of x-rays used to expose the patient or MAs, (2) the limited absorption efficiency of x-rays in the intensifying screen, and (3) the randomness of the x-ray to light conversion process; Spatial resolution or image blur—the ability of the screen to produce an accurate and clear image. (pp. 192-194)
13. (1) phosphor composition
    (2) phosphor thickness
    (3) reflective layer
    (4) dye
    (5) crystal size
    (6) concentration of phosphor crystals
    (p. 193)
14. See discussion on page 196 and Figure 16-8.
15 Refer to Figure 16-10. (p. 197)
16. DQE is the term commonly used by manufacturers of imaging receptors to define the noise efficiency of an imaging system. DQE calculations include noise from all aspects of the imaging chain, a few of which are as follows: some types of processing nonuniformities, the random placement size of the phosphor grains in the phosphor layer, and random placement and size of the silver-halide crystals in the film emulsion. (p. 194)
17. IF $= 7600 / 240 = 31.6$
    32 is the intensification factor (p. 193)
18. IF $= 7200 / 180 = 40$ (p. 193)

19. IF = 6400 /200 = 32 (p. 193)
20. See Table 16-2 on page 197.
21. Only a narrow range of excited energy states for an outer-shell electron is possible, and these states depend on the structure of the luminescent material. The wavelength of the emitted light is determined by the level of excitation to which the electron was raised and is characteristic of a given luminscent material. Thus, luminescent materials emit light of a characteristic color. (p. 192)
22. See page 200.
23. See Table 16-4.
24. A discussion of the use of carbon fiber in radiographic devices is found in column 2 of page 196.
25. (a) Screen-film contact can be checked by radiographing a wire-mesh device. This should be done when new screens are installed in a cassette to obtain a baseline evaluation. Additional wire-mesh radiographs of screen-film contact should be made once a year and compared with the baseline film. (b) The process is described on page 202.
26. The most common causes of poor screen-film contact are described on page 202.
27. (a) Below the K-shell absorption edge for the rare-earth elements, x-ray absorption is higher in tungsten. At x-ray energies above the K-shell absorption edge for tungsten, the rare-earth elements again exhibit lower absorption than that for tungsten. At an x-ray energy equal to the K-shell electron binding energy of the rare-earth elements, the probability of photo-electric absorption is considerably higher than that for tungsten. (b) Each of the rare-earth screens has an absorption cuve characteristic of the phosphor that determines the speed of the screen and how it changes with kVp. (c) Rare-earth screens exhibit better absorption properties than calcium-tungstate screens only in the energy range between the respective K-shell absorption edges. This energy range extends from about 35 to 70 keV and corresponds to most of the useful x-rays emitted during routine x-ray examinations. (p. 199)
28. Instructions for cleaning screens are given on page 201.

Challenge Questions

1. Design characteristics of intensifying screens that will affect x-ray absorption and x-ray-to-light conversion efficiency are listed in the box on p. 193.
2. Dose reduction from nonscreen radiography to intensifying screen radiography is calculated using the intensification factor (IF). This factor is defined as the ratio of the exposures required to produce the same optical density with and without the use of screens as follows (p. 193):

$$IF = \frac{\text{Exposure required without screens}}{\text{Exposure required with screens}}$$

3. IF = 6300/700 = 9 is the intensification factor. (p. 193)
4. The line-pair test pattern is used to measure degrees of spatial resolution—the ability of a system to image an object exactly. If an image is in focus, it shows good spatial resolution; if it is out of focus, it shows poor resolution. The line-pair test pattern has lead lines separated by equal size interspaces. Spatial resolution is measured by imaging this test pattern and expressing the number of line pairs per millimeter. The higher the number, the better the detail of the object to be imaged. The 800 to 1000 class image receptors can resolve approximately 6 lp/mm and 100 class image receptors can resolve 10 lp/mm. By contrast, the unaided eye can resolve about 10 lp/mm; direct-exposure film can resolve 50 lp/mm. (p. 194)
5. A description and illustration of the layers are found on p. 196.
6. The steps where major differences occur can be seen in Table 16-1. These are due to the interaction of x-rays with the screen phosphor and to the large number of visible-light photons produced by each of these interactions. (p. 197)
7. Pros and cons of each are discussed on p. 198.
8. Steps in preventing artifacts and degradation of the radiographic image when handling film are described on p. 201.

Across
1. kVp (p. 199)
2. quantum mottle (p. 198)

3. outer (p. 191)
4. ground state (p. 192)
5. felt (p. 196)
6. interact (p. 191)
7. high atomic (p. 190)
8. light (p. 192)
9. single (p. 195)
10. tungstate (p. 198)
11. decreases (p. 198)

Down

1. K-shell (p. 199)
2. intensifying (p. 192)
3. bent (p. 202)
4. yttrium tantalate (p. 198)
5. mA (p. 196)
6. greater (p. 195)
7. thermal (p. 191)
8. absorption (p. 190)
9. to-light (p. 193)
10. increased (p. 198)
11. spatial (p. 194)
12. line (p. 194)
13. heat (p. 196)
14. spec- (p. 197)

Chapter 17

1. d (p. 205)
2. a (p. 207)
3. d (p. 205)
4. b (p. 207)
5. b (p. 205)
6. b (pp. 211 and 212)
7. d (pp. 209–210)
8. a (pp. 210–211)
9. d (pp. 211–212)
10. c (p. 206)
11. The correct sequence is d, a, e. (p. 212)
12. Two kinds of x-rays are responsible for the optical density on a radiograph: (1) those that pass through the patient without interacting and (2) through Compton interaction. Together, these two types of x-rays are called remnant x-rays. (p. 205)
13. increased kVp; increased x-ray field size; increased anatomic part thickness (p. 205)
14. The image will be better in the film taken with the restricted x-ray beam because it results in less scatter radiation because of a smaller field size. (p. 207)
15. The x-ray beam is restricted to reduce patient dose and improve image contrast. (p. 209)
16. The key to improving spatial resolution in mammography is the use of a compression device because it reduces patient thickness, patient dose and tissue–image receptor distance. (p. 208)
17. image receptor (p. 213)
18. Carolyn may either increase mAs or kVp. Pros and cons of each are discussed in considerable detail on page 205.
19. 21%; 79% (p. 205)
20. a. 40%
    b. increased contrast at 60 kVp (Jeff's procedure)
    c. increased Compton interaction, which is scattered in the patient increasing patient dose. (Table 17-1)
21. Figure 17-1 on p. 205 demonstrates the two sources of remant radiation (those x-rays that are transmitted through the patient without interacting and those scattered in the patient).
22. At 50 kVp, Davis's procedure produces a photoelectric interaction of 79%; Jackie's, at 110 kVp, has a photoelectric interaction of 23%. As a result, Jackie's image will have greater contrast than Davis's. (p. 205)
23. About 59% of the x-ray beam is scattered through Compton interaction. (p. 205)
24. Davis's last procedure required 50 kVp; this one requires 70 kVp. As kVP is increased, the level of scatter radiation also increases. An increase in scatter radiation causes the radiographic contrast to decrease. Contrast will be reduced, although perhaps not by much. (p. 205)
25. An aperture diaphragm is the simplest of all beam-restricting devices. It is basically a lead or lead-lined metal plate attached to the x-ray tube head. The opening in the plate is design to cover just less than the size of the image receptor used. A properly designed aperture diaphragm is meant to project an image 1 centimeter smaller on all sides than the size of the image receptor. (p. 209)
26. See Figure 17-1.
27. This helps to reduce patient dose and improve image quality. (p. 209)
28. Cone cutting occurs when the x-ray tube, the extension cone, and the image receptor are

not aligned on the same axis. When this happens, the cone may interfere with the x-ray beam and one side of the image will be cut off. Hence the name cone cutting. (p. 210)

29. (a) The problem is most likely catter of the useful beam in the cone tip. (b) Many dental radiography units now use lead=lined cones for less distortion and lower patient dose. (p. 211)

30. Off-focus radiation refers to x-rays produced when projectile electrons stray and do not intersect with the focal spot. Control of off-focus radiation, through the use of first-stage entrance shutters and second-stage collimator shutters, is described on page 211.

31. The roles that key components in the collimator play in light localization are described on pages 211 and 212; the two chief components involved are a lamp and a mirror. The mirror must be far enough on the tube side of the collimator to project a sufficiently sharp light pattern through the collimator when the lamp is on. All three—the lamp, mirror, and collimator—must be adjusted so that the projected light field coincides with the x-ray beam.

32. Extension cones use an extended metal structure to restrict the useful beam to a required size; this beam is usually circular. One difficulty with cones is alignment. If the x-ray tube, extension cone, and image receptor are not aligned on the same axis, the cone may interfere with the x-ray beam and once side of the image will be cut off (cone cutting). In addition, their openings, like those of aperture diaphragms, are fixed so that they are appropriate for only specific types of exams. Extension cones are reserved primarily for examinations of the head, sinuses, and coned-down views of the spine. (pp. 210–211)

33. Uses of PBL devices are described at some length on page 212.

34. Tim should adjust the mirror or lamp. (pp. 211–212)

Challenge Questions

1. Eliot's reason is the easiest to start with. He knows that scatter radiation is controlled by keeping kVp at low levels; he is not wrong. Dennis and Molly need two different arguments against keeping kVp at low levels. Therefore, one might argue that as kVp is lowered, photoelectric interaction increases, resulting in a considerable increase in patient dose. This would still leave either Dennis or Molly to argue that fewer x-rays reach the film at low kVp, and thus the technical factors must be compensated for by increasing the mAs. The end result of this will also be a higher patient dose, but from a different source than the other argument. (p. 205)

2. A detailed discussion of extension cones and cylinders appears on pp. 210 and 211. Basically, (a) their limitations lie in alignment difficulties and the subsequent possibility of cone-cutting interference. In addition, like aperture diaphragms, their openings are fixed, making them appropriate for only specific types of exams. (b) While they were once used extensively in diagnostic radiology, today they are reserved primarily for examinations of the head, sinuses, and coned-down views of the spine. In modern radiography, the light-localizing variable-aperture collimator has replaced the extension cone and aperture diaphragms in most exams. (c) Extension cones can improve image contrast, and beam-defining cones are frequently used in dental radiography, in particular lead-lined extension cones. (pp. 210 and 211)

3. A full discussion and illustration of how the variable-aperture collimator is both constructed and operates is given on pages 211 and 212.

Chapter 18

1. d (p. 215)
2. c (p. 216)
3. b (p. 217)
4. b (p. 216)
5. d (p. 217)
6. d (p. 218)

7. c (p. 218)
8. b (p. 218)
9. a (p. 218)
10. c (p. 218)
11. c (p. 218)
12. d (p. 217)
13. d (p. 218)
14. c (p. 217)
15. F (pp. 223–224)
16. T (pp. 223-224)
17. F (p. 223)
18. T (p. 220)
19. T (p. 220)
20. F (p. 220)
21. F (p. 219)
22. T (p. 219)
23. 55 / (375 + 55) = 55 / 430 = .1279 = 12.8% of incident x-rays will be absorbed by this grid. (p. 216)
24. k = 3.5 / 1.6 = 2.19 is the contrast improvement factor. (p. 218)
25. The grid's line pair = 240 + 60 = 300 μm. So 1 cm (10,000 μm) divided by 300 μm = 33.3 lines/cm. 33.3 lines/cm x 2.54 cm/in = 64.6 lines/in. (p. 217)
26. (a) h/D = 1.5 millimeters/300 μm
    = 1500 um/300 μm
    = 5:1 is the grid ratio
    (b) This grid is not appropriate for Mike to use for a high-kVp procedure. Such procedures require higher ratio grids. (p. 217)
27. Distance to cutoff = 200 / 18 = 11.1 cm (p. 220)
28. Distance to cutoff = 180 / 14 = 12.9 cm (p. 220)
29. A grid is a carefully fabricated series of sections of radiopaque material, which are usually made of lead, alternating with sections of radiolucent material (interspace material), which are usually made of aluminum or plastic. The grid is designed to transmit only those x-rays whose direction is straight from the source to the image receptor. Gustave Bucky invented the first grid in 1913. The ideal grid would allow all primary x-rays to be transmitted and all scatter x-rays to be absorbed. (pp. 216, 218-219)
30. See Figure 18-4.
31. See Table 18-2.
32. See Figure 18-7 and 18-11.

33. The three interrelated factors that must be examined when selecting a grid with the proper ratio include kVp, degree of cleanup, and patient dose. When using high kVp, high-ratio grids are needed. The size and shape of the body part being radiographed also plays a part. As grid ratio increases, the amount of cleanup also increases. As a general rule, grid ratios up to 8:1 are satisfactory at tube potentials below 90 kVp. Grid ratios above that are used when kVp exceeds 90. (p. 225)
34. See the yellow box on page 225.
35. See page 226.
36. No doubt Hillary feels justified in calling the air-gap technique air filtration—after all, this is a commonly used name for this technique since you are using an air gap instead of a grid to reduce scatter radiation. However, Freddie is right. The term air filtration is a misnomer. In the air-gap technique, the air does not act as a filter of low-energy scattered x-rays; rather the distance between the patient and the film is what permits the scattered x-rays to escape before they reach the film. (p. 227)
37. The intensity of scatter is a function of kVp level, beam or field size, and thickness of irradiated tissue. (p. 215)
38. While linear grids clean up scatter radiation in only one direction, crossed grids are much more efficient, to the point that a crossed grid has a higher contrast improvement factor than a linear grid of twice the grid ratio. This advantage increases as the kVp of operation is increased. This advantage is accomplished in the manufacturing: Crossed grids have lead grid strips running parallel to both the long and short axes of the grid; they are usually made by sandwiching two linear grids together with the grid strips perpendicular to one another. Two serious disadvantages of the crossed grid is the care that must be taken to coincide the central ray with the center of the grid and the limitations it has in tilt-table operations. (p. 220)
39. The disadvantage of increased patient dose with high-frequency grids is compensated for by using high-speed intensifying screens to reduce patient dose significantly. (p. 217)

40. Answers should come from pages 219–223 and will vary greatly, depending on which grids the student writes about.
41. (a) The higher ratio grid, with a ratio of 14:1, would be more appropriate for high-kVp radiography. (b) The 8:1 grid is compatible with general-purpose equipment. (p. 217)
42. See Table 18-7.

Challenge Questions

1. Carolyn is right on both counts. Ron and Steve have forgotten to figure in the line pair measurement. While the interspace width is 300 μm, the line pair total would be 300 plus the 60-μm width of the grid strips, for a total of 360 μm. This must be the number in the calculation's denominator:
60 / (300 + 60) = 60 / 360 = .166 = 16.6 % (p. 216)
2. No, Robin and Eliot should not make such a prediction. Selectivity is related to grid ratio, but the total lead content in the grid has the primary influence on selectiity. Two grids can have the same grid ratio yet greatly differ in lead content. The more lead a grid contains, the higher its selectivity. (p. 219)
3. Advantages and disadvantages to both aluminum and plastic fiber grids' interspace materials are discussed on p. 217.
4. The information needed to prepare this demonstration is given in detail on pp. 219–223.

Chapter 19

1. F (p. 235)
2. F (p. 235)
3. T (p. 235)
4. F (p. 235)
5. F (p. 235)
6. T (p. 236)
7. T (p. 236)
8. F (p. 237)
9. F (p. 237)
10. F (p. 237)
11. F (p. 237)
12. F (p. 237)
13. F (p. 237)
14. F (p. 237)
15. T (p. 237)
16. F (pp. 235, 238)
17. T (pp. 235, 238)
18. T (pp. 235, 238)
19. F (p. 238)
20. F (p. 238)
21. An optical density of 3 means that only 1 in 1000 (103) light photons is capable of penetrating the x-ray film. (p. 233)
22. Speed = 1/23 mR = 1/0.023 R = 43.5 R (p. 237)
23. Speed = 1/Exposure
Exposure = 1/Speed = 1/500 = 0.002 R = 2 mR = 500 speed (pp. 237-238)
24. New mAs = (7 mAs) x 100/200 = 3.5 mAs
Therefore, the new technique is 140 kVp at 3.5 mAs. (p. 238)
25. New mAs = (9 mAs) x 150/250 = 5.4 mAs
The new technique is 120 kVp at 5.4 mAs. (p. 238)
26. MF = 14.1 cm / 10.7 cm = 1.32 is the approximate MF. (p. 239)
27. Focal spot blur = (1.6 mm) x (6 + 5 / 180 - (6 + 5) = 1.6 mm x (11 / 169) = 1.6 mm x 0.065 = 0.104 mm (p. 244)
28. (4.1)(4.3) = 17.63 (p. 245)
29. See preface on page 230.
30. Radiographic quality is the exactness of representation of the anatomic structure on the radiograph within the useful density range. Resolution is the ability to visually detect separate objects on a radiograph. Noise is the undesirable fluctuation in the optical density of the image. Speed is a measurement of the ability of an x-ray film to respond to an x-ray exposure. (p. 230)
31. See the discussion of quality control programs on page 230.
32. See Figure 19-1 on page 231.
33. See the discussion of characteristic curve on pages 231 and 232.
34. See Figure 19-2 on page 231.
35. See yellow box on page 233.
36. See yellow box on page 233.
37. The slope of the straight-line portion of the curve indicates film contrast. (p. 234)
38. Two radiographic factors are film contrast, which is inherent in the film and influenced by processing, and subject contrast, which is

determined by the size, shape, and x-ray–attenuating characteristics of the anatomic part. (p. 234)

39. 0.5 to 2.5 OD. (p. 234)

40. Film contrast and subject contrast are the two main factors affecting radiographic contrast. Film contrast is inherent in the film and is influenced by processing. Subject contrast is determined by the size, shape, and x-ray–attenuating characteristics of the anatomic part. In the clinical setting, it is usually best to standardize the film contrast and alter the subject contrast according to the needs of the exam. (p. 234)

41. average gradient (p. 235)

42. The average gradient is the slope of a straight line drawn between two points on the characteristic curve at optical densities 0.23 and 20 above base and fog densities. It is a method used to numerically specify film contrast. (p. 235)

43. See box on page 236.

44. See Figure 19-11 on page 236.

45. See formula on page 237.

46. See Figure 19-14 on page 238.

47. Short SIDs for mammograms are necessary, considering the low kVp and low radiation intensity of mammography units. Such units have a device for compression of the breast to reduce OID magnification and spread breast tissue. (p. 240)

48. Mark's image will show greater distortion because thick objects result in unequal magnification and therefore more distortion than thin objects. In addition, when these objects are positioned laterally to the central axis, the thicker object is even more dramatically distorted, especially given the many irregular shapes found in the chest. (pp. 240–241)

49. (a) The bullet has been x-rayed on end. A lateral radiograph can be taken to approximate position and further indicate dimension of the bullet. (b) By performing a cross-table lateral of the anatomy of interest. (p. 242)

50. See yellow box on page 243.

51. (a) The three main causes of focal-spot blur include large effective focal spot, short SID, and long OID. These are described on p. 243. (b) The heel effect, the varying intensity across an x-ray field that is caused by attenuation of x-rays in the heel of the anode,

affects focal-spot blur. The size of the effective focal spot is not constant across the radiograph, and this is what can cause a variation in focal-spot blur—namely, the focal-spot blur will be small on the anode side (where higher blur and poorer spatial resolution will occur) and large on the cathode side. (c) The most common method of minimizing focal-spot blur is to use a small focal spot when applicable and to position the patient so that the anatomy under examination is as close as possible to the image receptor. (pp. 243–244)

52. See Table 19-2 on page 244.

53. Low kVp results in high subject contrast, called short-scale contrast, since the radiographic image will appear either black or white with few shades of gray. On the other hand, high kVp results in low subject contrast, or long-scale contrast, since the radiographic image will display many shades of gray. It would be easy to assume that low-kVp techniques are always more desirable than high-kVp techniques. However, as kVp is lowered, the x-ray beam becomes less penetrating, in turn requiring a higher mAs to produce an acceptable optical density. The result, of course, is higher patient dose. (p. 246)

54. See page 238 under "latitude" and page 246.

55. See box on page 247.

Challenge Questions

1. (1) Use of rare-earth intensifying screens decreases patient dose by a factor of at least 20 times compared with direct-exposure film; (2) As the speed of the image receptor increases, spatial resolution is decreased and radiographic noise increases, which results in reduced radiographic quality; (3) Direct exposure x-ray film always results in lower contrast than screen-film combinations but is rarely used in modern departments, except for studies of arthritic pathology; (4) Low-contrast imaging procedures allow for a wider margin of error in producing an acceptable radiograph. (p. 247)

2. Image quality is improved with short exposure times. (p. 248)

3. The principle advantages to the use of high kVp are the great reduction in patient dose

and the wide latitude of exposures allowed in the production of a diagnostic radiograph. (p. 248)

4. An effective summary of key points one might expect to see are covered on pages 247–248.

5. As the kVp is increased, the penetrability of the x-ray beam and the total number of x-rays emitted at any x-ray energy are also increased. As mAs increases, the quantity of radiation is increased proportionately. As kVp is increased, more x-rays are transmitted through the patient so that a higher portion of the primary beam reaches the film. Thus optical density is affected. Of those x-rays that interact with the patient, the relative number of Compton interactions increases with increasing kVp, resulting in less differential absorption and reduced subject contrast. As for fog density, this is increased with increased kVp because of an increase in the percentage of scatter radiation. Finally, though, the primary control of optical density is mAs, not kVp. As mAs increases, the number of x-rays arriving at the image receptor increases, which results in higher optical density and lower radiographic noise. (p. 248)

6. A change in SID results in a change in optical density because x-ray intensity varies with distance. Adding filtration to the x-ray tube head reduces the intensity but increases the quality. (p. 249)

7. See Table 19-3 on page 249.

8. .32% = 0.0032
$OD = \log_{10}(I_o/I_t) = \log_{10}(1/0.0032)$
Using Table 19-1, $I_t/I_o \times 100 =$
.0032 / 1 x 100 = 0.32, therefore, optical density = 2.5 (pp. 232-233)

9. $OD = \log_{10}(I_o/I_t) = \log_{10}(1500/375)$
Using Table 19-1, $I_t/I_o \times 100 =$
375 / 1500 x 100 = 25, therefore, optical density = 0.6 (p. 233)

10. See Figure 19-4 on page 232.

Chapter 20

1. c (p. 252)
2. c (p. 252)
3. a (p. 252)
4. b (p. 252)
5. b (p. 253)
6. c (p. 253-254)
7. b (p. 254)
8. b (pp. 254–255)
9. d (p. 254)
10. a (p. 255)
11. 2.84×10^{18} electrons per second (p. 252)
$1 A = 6.3 \times 10^{18}$ electrons per second =
450 mA = 0.45 A =
$(0.45)(6.3 \times 10^{18}$ electrons/sec/A) =
2.84×10^{18} electrons per second (p. 252)

12. Freddie's best station selection option is that of 600 mA because the resultant 2256 mR is the highest possible without exceeding the 2300 mR ESE limit set for this particular projection. (p. 252)
At 800 mA, ESE = 752 mR x 800/200 = 3008 mR
At 700 mA, ESE = 752 mR x 700/200 = 2632 mR
At 600 mA, ESE = 752 mR x 600/200 = 2256 mR (p. 252)

13. 4/5:　　0.8 s and 800 ms
1/2:　　0.5 s and 500 ms
1/5:　　0.2 s and 200 ms
1/20:　　0.05 s and 50 ms
1/120: 0.008 s and 8 ms (p. 253)

14. 500 mA x 75 milliseconds = 500 mAs x .075 seconds = 37.5 mAs (p. 253)

15. Michelle's technique will require a higher mAs of 180 mAs. (p. 253)
600 mA x 300 milliseconds = 600 x .3 seconds = 180 mAs
200 mA x 500 milliseconds = 200 x .5 seconds = 100 mAs

16. 400 mA (p. 253)

Time (1st exposure)	mA (2nd exposure)
Time (2nd exposure)	mA (1st exposure)

$$\frac{x}{200\ mA} = \frac{400}{200}$$
(200 milliseconds)x =
(400 milliseconds) (200 mA)
(0.2 seconds)x = (.4 seconds)(200 mA)
0.2x = 80 mAs
x = 80 mAs/0.2 second
x = 400 mA

17. Ellie's technique will use the shorter exposure time of 375 milliseconds, as compared to Bill's 667 milliseconds. (p. 254)
Ellie: 300 mAs/800 mA = .375 second = 375 milliseconds

Bill: 400 mAs/600 mA = .6666 second = 667 milliseconds

18. 30 mAs/35 mAs = .857 = (.86)(120 mR) = 103 mR (p. 254)

19. 50 mAs is the new factor for 150 cm. (p. 254)

$$\frac{\text{mAs (2nd exposure)}}{\text{mAs (1st exposure)}} = \frac{(\text{SID})^2(\text{2nd exposure})}{(\text{SID})^2(\text{1st exposure})}$$

$$\frac{x}{200 \text{ mA}} = \frac{150^2}{300^2}$$

$x = 200(150/300)^2$

$x = 200(1/2)^2$

$x = 200/4 = 50 \text{ mAs}$

20. $\dfrac{x}{140} = \dfrac{120^2}{200^2}$

$x = 140(3/5)^2$

$x = 50\text{mAs}$ (p. 254)

21. $\dfrac{x}{120} = \dfrac{90^2}{180^2}$

$x = 120(1/2)^2$

$x = 30\text{mAs}$ (p. 254)

22. $\dfrac{x}{100} = \dfrac{100^2}{160^2}$

$x = 100(5/8)^2$

$x = 39\text{mAs}$ (p. 254)

23. a (p. 255)
24. c (p. 256)
25. d (p. 256)
26. d (p. 256)
27. b (p. 256)
28. c (p. 256)
29. kilovolt peak (kVp) and milliampere second (mAs) (p. 252)
30. With increasing kVp, more x-rays are produced, and they have a greater penetrebility. (p. 252)
31. 1 A = 1 C/s = 6.3×10^{18} electrons per second (p. 252)
32. See the discussion on page 254.
33. Small focal spots are designed for imaging very small microcalcifications at relatively short SIDs; they are reserved for fine-detail radiography in which the quantity of x-rays is relatively unimportant; they are normally used in imaging extremeties or other thin body parts. (pp. 254-255)
34. Most mammography tubes have 0.1-mm/0.4-mm focal spots. (p. 254)
35. See Table 20-3.
36. See Table 20-4.

Challenge Questions

1. Answers should resemble those in Table 20-2 on page 253.
2. Charts should contain highlights of the information found on pages 255–256.
3. Answers will vary from site to site.

Chapter 21

1. a. sthenic
   b. hyposthenic
   c. hypersthenic
   d. asthenic
2. d (p. 260)
3. d (p. 270)
4. b (p. 270)
5. d (p. 259)
6. b (p. 268)
7. a (pp. 266 and 269)
8. a (p. 261)
9. a (p. 266)
10. The fifteen-percent rule increases the kVp by 15% while reducing the mAs by one-half (p. 268). Thus:
    58 kVp x 0.15 = 9.7 kVp
    58 + 10 = 68 kVp
    14 mAs x 0.5 = 7 mAs
    Therefore, Daryl's repeat technique should be 68 kVp/7 mAs.
11. The five-percent technique calls for an increase of 5% in kVp accompanied by a 30% reduction in mAs (p. 268).
    58 kVp x 0.05 = 2.9
    58 + 3 = 61 kVp
    14 mAs x 0.3 = 4.2 mAs
    14 - 4 = 10 mAs
    The repeat technique should be 61 kVp/10 mAs.
12. 20 x 2 = 40
    40 + 30 = 70 kVp
    Begin with 70 kVp on a single-phase generator.
    40 + 25 = 75 kVp is the starting kVp on a three-phase generator.
    40 + 23 = 73 kVp is the starting kVp on a high-frequency generator. (p. 271)
13. High-contrast radiographs do produce shorter scales of contrast because there are fewer shades of gray between black and white.

Low-contrast radiographs, by comparison, produce many more shades of gray, making a longer scale of contrast. (p. 266)

14. See Table 21-3. (p. 260)

15. Answers may be somewhat lengthy and should be based on the discussion on pages 270 through 272.

16. Wendy is no doubt trying to remind Dennis that it is not appropriate to use a radiographic technique chart straight from a book or pamphlet. Each radiographic unit is unique in its radiation characteristics, so a specific chart should be prepared and tested for each exam room. (p. 271)

17. Phyllis is giving Bernie sound advice. The fixed-kVp radiographic technique chart selects exposures that produce radiographs with longer scales of contrast that are consistent within anatomic regions. Fixed-kVp charts also tend to result in somewhat higher kVp values and lower patient doses. (p. 272)

18. See Table 21-7. (p. 270)

19. See Table 21-10. (p. 274)

20. The phototimer records the amount of radiation falling on the image receptor. Radiation exposure is automatically terminated when a sufficient number of x-rays have reached the image receptor. Jack will select the appropriate kVp, and the phototimer will do the rest. In addition to selecting the exposure cells, Jack may have to adjust the optical density, depending on body habitus. (p. 274)

21. (a) A microprocessor would allow Jack to digitally select any kVp or mAs, for which the microprocessor will then automatically activate the appropriate mA station and exposure time. (b) To reduce motion blur, the microprocessor minimizes exposure time in a falling-load generator by beginning the exposure at a maximum value and then reducing the current during exposure. (p. 274)

Challenge Questions

1. Finished checklists will vary but should take into consideration each of the following image quality factors: optical density, contrast, image detail, and distortion. (p. 260)

2. (a) The blackening on the radiograph is a result of the development of the silver-bromide crystals in the film emulsion. (b) Black

is numerically equivalent to an optical density of 3 or greater, whereas clear is less than 0.2. (c) Optical density is the logarithm to the base 10 of the ratio of light incident on a film to the light transmitted through the film. The amount of light transmitted through the radiograph is determined by the optical density of the film. (d) Underexposure (too light) is a result of the radiograph being exposed to too little radiation. Overexposure is a too-dark radiograph with a high optical density, caused by too much radiation being converted to light in the intensifying screen and reaching the film. (p. 261)

3. All answers should be based on the discussion concerning Figure 21-11.

4. All answers should be based on the discussion on p. 272.

Across

1. part thickness (p. 272)
2. attenuation (p. 266)
3. increase (p. 268)
4. shorter (p. 268)
5. hypersthenic (p. 259)
6. contrast (p. 259)
7. align (p. 269)
8. bromide (p. 261)
9. mAs (p. s65)
10. low degree (p. 266)
11. range (p. 266)
12. anatomic regions (p. 272)

Down

1. motion (p. 269)
2. chart (p. 270)
3. ratio (p. 261)
4. adjacent (p. 265)
5. elongation (p. 269)
6. development (p. 261)
7. automatic (p. 273)
8. sharpness (p. 269)
9. intermediate (p. 259)
10. density (p. 259)
11. five percent (p. 268)
12. black (p. 261)
13. shorter (p. 266)
14. photo (p. 273)
15. light (p. 269)

Chapter 22

1. a (p. 282)
2. b (p. 291)
3. c (pp. 283–284; 286)
4. d (p. 286)
5. d (p. 282)
6. b (p. 282)
7. b (p. 286)
8. b (p. 286)
9. c (p. 285)
10. in order: c, d, a, b, e (pp. 287–289)
11. Tube shift = 0.1 x 200 centimeters = 20 centimeters (p. 288)
12. MF = Image size/Object size
    Object size = Image size/MF (pp. 290–91)
    MF = 120/(120 – 30) = 120/90 = 1.33
    Object size = Image size/MF
    20/1.33 = 15 mm
13. The tomographic x-ray equipment appears similar to conventional radiographic equipment except for a vertical rod that fixes the x-ray tube head to the table Bucky device. This rod attachment is the feature unique to tomography. (pp. 282 and 291)
14. Tomography avoids superimposition by bringing into focus only that anatomy lying in the plane of interest, while blurring structures on either side of the plane. (p. 282)
15. These can be viewed through a stereoscope or through crossed eyes. Both techniques are fully described on page 289.
16. Presentations will vary but should point out that book cassettes often prevented repeat exposures, thus helping to reduce patient dose. (p. 282)
17. Panoramic tomography. (p. 286)
18. Linear anatomic structures will be imaged better if they are positioned with their length parallel to the x-ray tube motion. Linear structures that lie perpendicular to the x-ray tube motion are more easily blurred. (p. 284)
19. The streaking may be due to part of the long bone lying outside the object plane and being oriented in the direction of x-ray tube and image-receptor movement. The uneven blurring Patrick gets in his second image is probably due to the changes in distance between x-ray tube and patient and in the angulation of the x-ray beam during exposure. These

can result in a lack of uniform optical density. The solution? Multidirectional motion. (p. 285)
20. Claire is right. When the tomographic angle is very small, the section thickness is the entire anatomic structure, and it becomes a conventional radiograph. (p. 284)
21. Comptued tomography (CT) and magnetic resonance imaging (MRI) have largely replaced tomography because of their superior contrast resolution. The three-dimensional images made using CT and MRI provide a volume of data and can be viewed from any direction, making them examples of virtual reality in use. (p. 289)
22. The tomographic angle determines the thickness of tissue that will not be blurred (section thickness). The larger a tomographic angle, the thinner the imaged section will be. The smaller the angle, the thicker the section. (pp. 282 and 284)
23. It has been largely replaced by three-dimensional computed tomography and magnetic resonance imaging. These can provide three-dimensional images but without the doubled patient exposure or the need for quite the same extensive practice and patient cooperation. (p. 287)

Challenge Questions

1. Demonstrations should be based on the discussion on pages 282–285.
2. Follow instructions given with such items to practice stereoscopy viewing.
3. See discussion on pages 282–284.
4. Time lines will vary depending on the procedures researched.
5. Image A: The long axis of the foot is parallel with the tube motion; Image B: The long axis of the foot is perpendicular to the tube motion (p. 285).

Across
1. stereoradiography
2. blurring
3. superimposition
4. thinner
5. hypocycloidal
6. small
7. linear

8. nephrotomography

Down

1. position
2. vascular
3. grids
4. fixed
5. virtual
6. stereoscopy
7. uniform
8. tomography
9. dominant

Chapter 23

1. b, d, c, a, g, f, h, e (p. 295)
2. e (p. 295)
3. a (p. 295)
4. e (p. 295)
5. c (p. 295)
6. e (p. 295)
7. d (p. 296)
8. b (p. 297)
9. b (p. 297)
10. a (p. 297)
11. b (p. 298)
12. d (p. 300)
13. b (p. 300)
14. e (p. 300)
15. e (p. 300)
16. c (p. 300)
17. a (p. 301)
18. d (p. 301)
19. Target x-ray tube material; Preferred filter; Rationale
    Tungsten; Molybdenum or rhodium; To reduce higher bremsstrahlung x-rays
    Molybdenum; Molybdenum or rhodium; Provides the molybdenum characteristic x-rays for imaging along with the shaped bremsstrahlung x-ray emission spectrum
    Rhodium; Rhodium; Provides a slightly higher quality x-ray beam of greater penetrability. Preferred for thicker, more dense breasts. (p. 299)
20. Diagnostic mammography is performed on patients with symptoms or elevated risk factors. Two or three views of each breast may be required. Screening mammography is performed on asymptomatic women using one

view, the medial lateral oblique (MLO). (p. 294)

21. The first exam of a patient's breasts serves as the baseline mammographic exam. It is saved in the file and never discarded. Radiologists may use this baseline mammogram for comparison with all future mammograms. (p. 295)
22. Answers may be somewhat lengthy but should reflect the information given in column 2 on page 295.
23. The three types of image receptors that have been used for mammography include direct-exposure film, xerox, and screen-film. Screen-film is used at the present time. Xero-mammography is of historical interest only, and direct exposure mammography is associated with excessively high patient dose. (p. 300)

Challenge Questions

1. Advantages noted on the diagram should include the following: Compression immobilizes the breast for better spatial resolution and less blur, minimizes scatter for better contrast resolution, and irradiates less tissue for more uniform optical density and lower patient dose. (p. 296)
2. It sounds like Helen had screening mammography. This is performed on asymptomatic women and it requires only one view, the medial lateral oblique. Elaine probably had diagnostic mammography, which is performed on patients with symptoms or elevated risk factors. Two or three views of each breast may be required. (p. 294)
3. See the discussion on page 298
4. See Table 23-3 on page 302.

Chapter 24

1. Q (p. 307)
2. S (p. 307)
3. D (p. 307)
4. S (p. 307)
5. M (p. 307)
6. D (p. 307)
7. Q (p. 307)
8. W (p. 307)

9. S (p. 307)
10. W (p. 307)
11. M (p. 307)
12. c (p. 306)
13. d (p. 306)
14. d (p. 307)
15. b (p. 307)
16. e (p. 307)
17. b (p. 307)
18. e (p. 307)
19. a (p. 307)
20. e (p. 308)
21. d (p. 310)
22. c (p. 310)
23. a (p. 311)
24. c (p. 311)
25. a (p. 311)
26. c (p. 313)
27. b (p. 314)
28. b (p. 316)
29. d (p. 317)
30. 7, 2, 1, 4, 6, 5, 3 (pp. 309–310)
31. 3, 5, 2, 1, 6, 4 (pp. 316–317)
32. MD; DD (p. 308)
33. +0.15; +0.1 (p. 308)
34. fog; +0.03 (p. 310)
35. 0.5; four; three; three (p. 311)
36. Steps in darkroom cleanliness are covered on page 307.
37. (a) Chris should be careful to adhere to the film manufacturer's recommendations regarding the proper combination of film, processor, chemistry, developer temperature, immersion time, and replenishment rate. (b) She should be made aware that the use of strips exposed more than an hour or two before processing is unacceptable since the strips may be less sensitive to changes in the processor (p. 310)
38. (a) An archival quality check is a quarterly task done to determine the amount of residual fixer in the processed film. The result is used to indicate the film's storage quality. (b) One sheet of unexposed film is processed. Next, one drop of residual hypo test solution is placed on the emulsion side of the film and allowed to stand for 2 minutes. The excess solution is blotted off and the stain compared with a hypo estimator, using a white sheet of paper as background. The matching number from the hypo estimator is recorded. (p. 314)

39. She may not have made the comparison immediately after blotting. It must be done at that time to prevent the spot from darkening. (p. 314)
40. Checklists should cover key points discussed on page 316.

Challenge Questions

1. See page 306.
2. Yes! Janet must investigate the cause for such a wide variation. This needs to be remedied—merely adjusting the control values is not enough. (p. 310)
3. The chart should reveal the following data: (a) A fiber may be given the following scores—provided each occurs at the correct location and with the correct orientation: Count it as 1 if its entire length is visible. Give it a score of 0.5 if more than half its length is visible, and a score of 0 if less than half is visible. (b) A speck group may be given a score of 1 if four or more of the six specks are visible, a score of 0.5 if at least two are visible, and a score of 0 for fewer than two. Count a mass as 1 if a density difference is seen at the correct location with a circular border. A score of 0.5 may be given to a mass if a density difference is seen at the correct location but the shape is not circular. If there is only a hint of a density difference, the score is 0. (p. 311)
4. (a) The repeat analysis determines the number and cause of repeated mammograms. It also identifies ways to improve efficiency, reduce costs, and reduce unnecessary patient exposure. (b) Approximately 250 patients are needed for this evaluation to be valid. (c) All rejected films are collected for a quarter or until 250 patients have been examined. The rejected films are sorted into different categories such as poor positioning, patient motion, too light, and other categories. Next, the total number of films repeated and the total number of films exposed are counted. The repeat rate is computed by dividing the number of repeated films by the total number exposed and multiplying this by 100 to get a percentage. (p. 313)

5. 24/640 x 100 = 15/4 = 3.75% = the repeat rate

This is considered too high for an overall repeat rate. The overall repeat rate for each category should be less than or equal to 2%, and the rates for each category should be from 2% to 5%. (pp. 313–314)

6. 14/851 x 100 = 1400/851 = 1.645% = 1.6%

This is an acceptable rate. (pp. 313–314)

Chapter 25

1. g, e, a, h, c, f, d, b (p. 322)
2. a (p. 323)
3. c (p. 323)
4. d (p. 324)
5. e (pp. 324–325)
6. d (p. 325)
7. a (p. 325)
8. b (p. 325)
9. b (p. 325)
10. b (p. 327)
11. a (p. 331)
12. lamberts; millilamberts (p. 323)
13. cornea; lens; retina; iris (p. 323)
14. intense; fovea centralis; low light; periphery of the retina. (p. 323)
15. 2.5 or 5; 10 to 35 (p. 325)
16. output phosphor; milliroentgen per second (mR/sec). (p. 325)
17. 50 to 300; 5000 to 30,000. (p. 325)
18. direct; ratio of the diameters (p. 326)
19. high; low (p. 326)
20. higher (p. 326)
21. vertical; horizontal; electron beam; modulated; higher (p. 330)
22. Brightness gain = $17^2/2.5^2$ x 140 = 46 x 140 = 6440 (p. 325)
23. MF = 23/10 = 2.3 (p. 326)
24. $25^2/12^2$ = 635/144 = 4.34 times as high. (p. 326)
25. The input phosphor is cesium iodide (CsI). These CsI crystals are grown as tiny needles and are tightly packed, resulting in microlight pipes with little dispersion and excellent spatial resolution. When an x-ray interacts with the input phosphor, its energy is converted into visible light—an effect similar to that of radiographic intensifying screens. (p. 324)

26. This difference is maintained so that the electrons of photoemission will be accelerated to the anode. (p. 324)
27. It is inherently unfocused and suffers from vignetting, which is a reduction in brightness at the periphery. (p. 326)
28. Spatial resolution tends to be better because only the central region of the input phosphor is used in the magnification mode. (p. 326)
29. These are discussed on page 327.
30. It is absolutely essential that the lenses and mirror remain precisely adjusted. The alignment of the camera lenses is the most critical part of the optical chain. Malpositioning results in a blurred image. (p. 328)
31. Bandpass is expressed in frequency (Hz) to describe the number of times per second that the electron beam can be modulated or changed. A 1-MHz bandpass would indicate that the electron beam intensity could be changed a million times each second. The higher the bandpass, the better the horizontal resolution. (p. 330)
32. When a cassette spot-film exposure is desired, Jesse must actuate a control that properly positions the cassette in the x-ray beam and changes the operation of the x-ray tube from low fluoroscopic mA to high radiographic mA. The spot film is masked by a series of lead diaphragms to allow several image formats. When the entire film is exposed, that is called one-on-one. When only half of the film is exposed at a time, two images result, which is called two-on-one. (pp. 330–331)
33. See Table 25-1.

Challenge Questions

1. Answers will vary slightly but should certainly include functions of the glass envelope, the electron gun, the electrostatic grids and the target assembly. Discussion and properly labeled illustration are found on page 327 and in Figure 25-11.
2. Answers should reflect the lengthy description of this process on page 326.
3. Answers should reflect the discussion on page 326.
4. Discussion of both methods appears on page 328.

5. Answers should reflect the discussion on pages 329–330.

Across

1. plumbicon
2. phototopic
3. Chamberlain
4. thermionic
5. scotopic
6. Edison
7. contrast

Down

1. bandpass
2. visual
3. photocathode
4. brightness
5. vignetting
6. minification
7. cesium
8. active

Chapter 26

1. c, e, a, f, d, b (p. 334)
2. d (p. 337)
3. a (p. 337)
4. b (p. 338)
5. c (p. 338)
6. c (p. 338)
7. low osmolality (p. 335)
8. bleeding at puncture site; hypersensitivity reaction to contrast media; kidney failure (p. 335)
9. small; large-diameter massive; magnification (p. 336)
10. anode heat capacity (p. 337)
11. two to three; 20 to 40 (p. 339)
12. $MF = SID/SOD = 100/70 = 1.4285 = 1.43$

    Focal-spot blur = $(EFS) OID/SID = (0.3)30/100 = .09$ mm

    Approximate spatial resolution = $2 \times$ focal-spot blur = .18 millimeters (p. 337)
13. It requires a suite of rooms. The procedure room itself should not be less than 20 feet along any wall and not less than 500 square feet. Such a size is required to accommodate the amount of equipment required and the large number of people involved in most procedures. The control room should be large and connect directly with processing and viewing areas. (pp. 335–336)
14. There may be two or three radiographers setting up runs, as well as the interventional radiologist who performs the procedure, and a radiology nurse. When the patient must be highly medicated, there must also be an anesthesiologist present. (p. 336)
15. Two ceiling track-mounted radiographic x-ray tubes are generally required with an image-intensified fluoroscope mounted on a C or an L arm. (p. 336)
16. Answers should reflect Table 26-2.
17. The 35-millimeter film format requires more patient exposure than the 16-millimeter film format, but the image quality is also better. (p. 338)
18. The x-ray tube is energized only during the time when the cine film is in position for exposure. The x-ray tube is not energized during the time between frames when the film is advancing because this would result in considerably excessive and unnecessary patient exposure. (p. 338)
19. See page 334.

Challenge Questions

1. Christa has selected the wrong frame rate. High frame rates are necessary for cardiac studies; 7.5 frames per second may be adequate for other examinations, but not this one. (p. 338)
2. a. Rapid flow requires two or three frames per second (p. 339)
   b. During exposure the screens are pressed against the film. This is to ensure good screen-film contact. Precise mechanical and electrical synchronization are essential. (p. 338)
   c. This test is to check that the catheter tip is not wedged and is in the correct vessel. Injection rates of the automatic power injector are gauged by the test flow speed. A scout film will be obtained to check positioning and exposure factors. (p. 339)
   d. After catheter placement and the injection have helped in checking catheter tip

location and after the gauging of injection rates and the obtaining of a scout film, the catheter is attached to the unit that injects the contrast media. If subtraction films are needed, then the film and injection parameters include one exposure before injection of the contrast material. Exposures are made at the frame rate and injection sequence specific for the procedure. (p. 339)

Chapter 27

1. b (p. 342)
2. a (p. 342)
3. b (p. 343)
4. d (p. 344)
5. c (p. 344)
6. c (p. 344)
7. b (p. 344)
8. d (p. 344)
9. e (p. 345)
10. b (p. 348)
11. a (p. 348)
12. a (p. 349)
13. c (p. 350)
14. 2, 9, 5, 7, 4, 3, 8, 1, 6 (pp. 342–344)
15. a. bootstrap
    b. application programs
    c. memory manager
    d. file manager/scheduler
    e. assemblers, compilers, interpreters
    f. primary memory
    g. i/o manager
    h. device driver
    i. terminal
    j. printer
    k. modem
    l. disk storage
    (p. 350)
16. logic functions (p. 343)
17. direct memory access (DMA) controllers (p. 345)
18. read-write memory; static RAM (SCRAM); dynamic RAM (DRAM); computer instructions; system programs (p. 346)
19. alphanumeric; letters and numbers; character generator; graphic output; intelligent; nonintelligent (p. 347)
20. random access; fixed-length blocks; 1 Gbyte;

CD-ROMs; read-only (p. 347)
21. binary digit (0 or 1); 8, 16, 32; 8; bytes; encode; 16; 32; megabytes (p. 349)
22. 214 falls between 2^7 and 2^8.

Yes	2^7	= 1	=	128
Yes	2^6	= 1	=	64
No	2^5	= 0		
Yes	2^4	= 1	=	16
No	2^3	= 0		
Yes	2^2	= 1	=	4
Yes	2^1	= 1	=	2
No	2^0	= 0		

11010110 = 214

23. 630 falls between 2^9 and 2^{10}.

Yes	2^9	= 1	=	512
No	2^8	= 0		
No	2^7	= 0		
Yes	2^6	= 1	=	64
Yes	2^5	= 1	=	32
Yes	2^4	= 1	=	16
No	2^3	= 0		
Yes	2^2	= 1	=	4
Yes	2^1	= 1	=	2
No	2^0	= 0		

1001110110 = 630

24. 4; 0100; 4
    11; 1011; B
    23; 10111; F8
    See Table 27-3. (p. 352)
25. The computer can make decisions based on conditions previously known, currently known, and expected. Besides, computing manipulating, and making decisions, it is also capable of interacting with the user by accepting data from the user and providing results to the user. (p. 342)
26. In the mid-1970s, the magnetic core memory was changed to semiconductor memory. The magnetic core consisted of small magnetic dipoles that existed in one of two states, depending on the direction of the electric current passing through them. Semiconductor memory consists of extremely small storage circuits etched on a silicon chip. These chips are arranged in groups to form a memory module complete with all interconnections to

plug into the computer. Semiconductor memory was cheaper and faster, but the word core survived and is used to refer to primary memory even though primary memory now is based on semi-conductors rather than magnetic loops. (p. 345)

27. Semiconductor storage operates on the principle of a flip-flop. A switch is set in one of two states variously described as one or zero, A or B, "yes" or "no," "true" or "false," "set or reset," and "plus" or "minus." Each individual flip-flop stores one bit (binary digit) of information. (p. 345)

28. Answers should be based on the extensive discussion on pages 345–346.

29. Each memory location has a unique label identifying its position. Memory operates much like a person's home address, where mail received is uniquely his or hers. This allows the computer's CPU access to the data at specific spots in memory without disturbing the rest of memory. The CPU keeps track of the address in memory where the current program instructions are stored so that it can hop to other memory locations to read or write data and then return to the proper place in the program. (p. 346)

30. Secondary memory devices are described on pages 347–348.

31. The decimal system is a number system to the base ten; in other words, it has 10 digits. The duodecimal system has 12 digits, and the binary system has two: 0 and 1. The computer performs all operations by converting alphabetic characters, decimal values, and logic functions to binary values. Even the computer's instructions are stored in binary form. (p. 350)

32. Margie is using a remote job-entry (RJE) system. (p. 353)

33. Margie is using a time-sharing system. (pp. 353–354)

34. Pipeline processors work like an assembly line. Different parts of the data are processed by different parts of the processor at the same time. The data move through the processor and are fully processed by the time they reach the output. Array processors perform the same computations in parallel on many items of data at once. (p. 354)

Challenge Questions

1. Time lines should reflect material covered on pages 342–348. Key features that have been particularly revolutionary include the transistor, the computer chip, the semiconductor, and the optical disk.

2. Hank is developing an applications program, not a systems software. Systems software consists of programs that make it easy for the user to operate the computer to its best advantage. Application programs are those written in a higher-level language expressly to carry out some user function. (p. 349)

3. Answers should reflect Table 27-4. (p.352)

Across

1. scram
2. Hollerith
3. integrated circuit
4. Atansoff
5. VDT
6. chip
7. software
8. Pascal
9. batch
10. Mauchly
11. central processing
12. electronic

Down

1. Shockley
2. random access
3. microprocessor
4. control unit
5. input
6. semiconductor
7. output
8. optical disk
9. Babbage
10. hardware
11. hard disk

Chapter 28

1. e (p. 358)
2. a (p. 358)
3. c (p. 359)
4. c (p. 360)
5. e (p. 366)

6. b (p. 366)

7. c (p. 366)

8. d (p. 366)

9. a (p. 366)

10. b (p. 368)

11. d (p. 368)

12. e (p. 369)

13. a (p. 370)

14. e (p. 370)

15. d (p. 370)

16. receptor; radiation detector; computer; matrix of intensities; dynamic range (p. 359)

17. pixel; pixel brightness; subtraction images; image contrast; Hounsfield unit; composition (p. 359)

18. larger (p. 360)

19. dynamic range; numerical range; greater (p. 360)

20. mask; energy subtraction (p. 369)

21. pulsed; intermittent (p. 370)

22. imaging time; detector efficiency (p. 370)

23. a gas-filled detector assembly; scintillation detectors coupled to solid-state photo-diodes (p. 370)

24. $10^{24} \times 10^{24}$ = 1,048,576 pixels (p. 360)

25. 5 inches = 127 mm. Therefore, the size of each pixel is 127 mm/512 (image matrix) = 0.248 mm. (p. 360)

26. The two principal advantages are (a) speed of image acquisition and (b) the post-processing image enhancement. (p. 358)

27. These three are summarized concisely on pages 358–359.

28. One screen is for patient data, one for current image display, and one for subtracted image display. (p. 362)

29. (a) There are two limitations: First, the interlaced mode of reading the target of the television camera can significantly degrade a digital image, and second, the conventional television camera tubes are relatively noisy, with a signal-to-noise ratio of about 200:1. In DF, an SNR ratio of 1000:1 is necessary. A tube with a 1000:1 SNR ratio contains five times the useful information and is more compatible with computer-assisted image enhancement. (b) Progressive mode is preferred because there is no interlace of one field with another, and this produces a sharper image with less flicker. (p. 365)

30. It will drop by a factor of about 4 (about 8 images per second) because of the time required to conduct such enormous quantities of data from one segment of memory to another. (p. 366)

31. Micah is using temporal subtraction; Carla is using energy subtraction. Advantages and disadvantages of each are found in Table 28-2. (p. 366)

32. In temporal subtraction using the mask mode (as Micah is), because the video system is relatively slow to respond and the video noise may be high, several video frames may be added to the memory to make each image. This is image integration. Although it improves contrast resolution, it also increases patient dose because more image frames are acquired. (p. 367)

33. Micah may use a later image as the mask image. He can even integrate several images and use that composite image as the mask. Other causes for unacceptable mask images include noise and technical factors. (p. 367)

34. TID stands for time interval difference mode. This calls for each subtracted image to be made from a different mask and follow-up frame, using a constant image-acquisition rate. The principal application of this mode is in cardiac studies. The procedure is described in more detail on page 367. Its main advantage over mask mode is that it is relatively free of motion artifacts, but it has less contrast than mask-mode imaging. (p. 367)

35. If patient motion occurs between the mask image and a subsequent image, the subtracted image will contain misregistration artifacts. The same anatomy is not registered in the same pixel of the image matrix. This type of artifact can frequently be eliminated by reregistration of the mask; that is, by shifting the mask by one or more pixels so that superimposition of images is again obtained. (p. 368)

36. Answers should reflect the information in column 1 on page 372.

37. The PACS display sytem uses a CRT montior in a video workstation. Subtraction of one image from another emphasizes vascular structures. Edge enhancement is effective for fractures and small, high-contrast objects. Windowing is useful for amplifying soft tis-

sue differences. Highlighting can be effective in identifying diffuse nonfocal disease. Pan, scroll, and zoom allow for careful visualization of precise regions of an image. (p. 373)

38. Teleradiology involves remote transmission and viewing of images. The network enables many computers to be connected and to interact with one another. Further details on the network's function are on pages 373–374. With PACS, a film room is replaced by a magnetic or optical memory device. (p. 374)

Challenge Questions

1. Producing a film image from the CRT that will have proper density and contrast is done by using the computer to postprocess the image through windowing. This is used to allow one to see only a window of the computer's much greater dynamic range. The two characteristics of the window are window level and window width. Window level identifies the type of tissue to be imaged; window width determines the gray-scale representation of that tissue. The wider the window width, the longer the gray scale will be. Narrow window widths produce high contrast. (p. 361)

2. Dennis is correct about the wide discrepancy in tube currents used in these two fluoroscopic procedures, but the high mA used in DF is not a concern because the tube is not energized continuously. (p. 362)

3. The time required for the x-ray tube to be switched on and reach the selected level of kVp and mA is called the interrogation time. The time required for the x-ray tube to be switched off is the extinction time. A time of a little less than 2 seconds is unacceptable for either of them. To avoid unnecessary patient dose, it is required that DF systems show interrogation and extinction times of approximately 1 millisecond. (p. 365)

4. Answers will be lengthy but should reflect the discussion on pages 366–367.

Chapter 29

1. See Figure 29-14. (p. 383)
2. c (p. 378)
3. a (p. 378)
4. c (p. 379)
5. b (p. 380)
6. c (p. 380)
7. d (pp. 380–81)
8. c (p. 381)
9. a (p. 381)
10. b (p. 388)
11. b (p. 389)
12. d (p. 390)
13. rotate-only; concentrically (p. 381)
14. linear detector; curvilinear (p. 381)
15. third-generation; annulus (p. 381)
16. patient dose (p. 382)
17. rotates; nutates (p. 382)
18. x-ray tube failure (p. 383)
19. continuous; pulsed (p. 383)
20. 2400; scintillation detectors; gas detectors (p. 383)
21. cadminum tungstate ($CdWO_4$) (p. 384)
22. area of the patient that intercepts the useful beam; slice thickness; patient dose; x-ray field viewed by the detector array (p. 384)
23. pixel size; thickness of the CT scan slice; field of view (FOV). (p. 386)
24. brightness; optical density (p. 387)
25. spatial resolution; contrast resolution; linearity; noise (p. 388)
26. artifact generation; contrast resolution; spatial resolution (p. 390)
27. T (p. 385)
28. F (p. 385)
29. T (p. 386)
30. T (p. 386)
31. F (p. 388)
32. T (p. 389)
33. F (p. 390)
34. T (p. 390)
35. a. 240 mm/120 pixels = 2 mm/pixel
    b. 320 mm/512 pixels = 0.62 mm/pixel
    c. 270 mm/512 pixels = 0.53 mm/pixel
    (p. 387)
36. The reciprocal of 2 lp/cm = $(2\ lp/cm)^{-1}$
    = 1/2 lp/cm
    = 1 cm / 2 lp
    = 10 mm / 2 lp
    = 5 mm/lp (p. 390)
37. See discussion on page 384.
38. The detector signal during each translation is registered in increments with values as high

as 1000. The value for each increment is related to the x-ray attenuation coefficient of the total path through the tissue. Through the use of simultaneous equations, a matrix of values is obtained that represents the cross section of the anatomy scanned. (p. 379)

39. See pages 385–386.

40. CT number $= k \times (\mu_o - \mu_w)/\mu_w$
In the equation, μ_o is the x-ray attenuation coefficient of the pixel, μ_w is the x-ray attenuation coefficient of water, and k is a constant that determines the scale factor for the range of CT numbers. (p. 387)

41. a. CT number $= 1000$; Linear attenuation coefficient $= 0.528$
    b. CT number $= 40$; Linear attenuation coefficient $= 0.163$
    c. CT number $= 20$; Linear attenuation coefficient $= 0.182$ (p. 387)

42. See page 389.

Challenge Questions

1. Current software includes programs to generate CT number historgrams along any preselected axis, computation of mean and standard deviation of CT values within an ROI, subtraction techniques, and planar and volumetric quantitative analysis. Reconstruction of images along coronal, sagittal, and oblique planes is also possible.

2. Answers will be lengthy but should reflect the discussion on page 391.

3. See page 391 under "Spatial Uniformity."

Chapter 30

1. d (pp. 397–98)
2. d (p. 401)
3. a (p. 401)
4. c (Table 30-4)
5. b (Table 30-4)
6. interpolation; exterpolation; interpolation; transverse (p. 397)
7. 360; Z-interpolation (p. 398)
8. spiral scan pitch ratio (p. 398)
9. pitch; 360; 180 (p. 399)
10. slip-ring; continuously (p. 400)
11. one breathhold (p. 401)
12. 9 mm / 6 mm $= 1.5{:}1$ (p. 398)

13. Tissue imaged
    $= 9$ mm $\times 27 \times 1.5$
    $= 365$ mm
    $= 36.5$ cm (p. 398)

14. Tissue imaged
    $= \dfrac{4 \text{ mm} \times 1.6 \times 16 \text{ s}}{2 \text{ s}}$
    $= 111$ mm
    $= 11$ cm (p. 399)

15. The two slip-ring designs are the disk and the cylinder. The disk design incorporates concentric conductive rings in the plane of rotation. The cylindrical design has the conductive rings lying parallel to the axis of rotation forming a cylinder. (p. 400)

16. One provides high-voltage power to the x-ray tube and high-voltage generator. A second provides low-voltage power to control systems on the rotating gantry. The third slip ring transfers digital data from the rotating detector array in the case of a third-generation scanner.

17. One approach generates the high voltage off the gantry. In this design the slip ring must be sealed to insulate the transfer of up to 150 kVp. Another approach transfers a low voltage to the rotating gantry, where it is increased to the desired kVp. This requires that invertors and transformers be designed to produce that high power but also compact enough to fit on the rotating gantry. In between these two approaches are hybrid designs. (p. 400)

18. Volume of tissue imaged is determined by examination time, couch travel, pitch, and collimation. Also, gantry rotation time, reconstruction algorithm, reconstruction interval, and skip scan delay must be selected. (p. 401)

19. It may be necessary for Mike to skip scan with a 10-second interscan delay to allow the patient to breathe. (p. 401)

20. Kate may choose from shaded volume display, shaded surface display, or CT angiography. (p. 402)

21. MIP reconstructs an image by selecting the highest value pixels along any arbitrary line through the data set and exhibiting only those pixels. MIP images can be reconstructed very fast. Only approximately 10% of the three-dimensional data points are used. (p. 402)

22. See page 404.

Challenge Questions

1. This procedure requires high Z-axis resolution. Other representative technique factors are shown in Table 30-3. To be sure to cover the required anatomy, Mike's department should contruct a table similar to the one in Table 30-3. (pp. 401–402)

2. a. In general, image quality in CT is measured by spatial resolution and contrast resolution, which is comparable with conventional CT. Since the number of detectors, detector spacing, and the number of projections in the scan plane are generally the same as that in conventional CT, inplane resolution is the same.

   b. Although the SSP is worse in spiral CT, there can be notable improvement in the Z-axis spatial resolution because there are no gaps in the data and image reconstruction can be made at any position along the Z-axis. Reconstructed images can even overlap.

   c. In conventional CT, the nodule may be missed if it lies at a section interface. With spiral CT a 50% overlap can be performed in reconstruction to improve the contrast resolution.

   d. Spiral CT excels in three-dimensional multiplanar reformation (MPR). Transverse images are stacked to form a three-dimensional data set that can be rendered as an image in several ways. The following three-dimensional MPR algorithms are most frequently used: (1) maximum intensity projection (MIP), (2) shaded surface display (SSD) and (3) shaded volume display (SVD). (p. 402)

Chapter 31

1. a (p. 408)
2. d (p. 408)
3. c (p. 409)
4. a (p. 410)
5. b (p. 410)
6. c (p. 410)
7. d (p. 411)

8. b (p. 412)
9. d (p. 414)
10. d (p. 414)
11. acceptance testing; routine performance evaluation; error correction (p. 408)
12. ± 2% (p. 409)
13. focal-spot size of the x-ray tube (p. 410)
14. ±4 kVp of the actual kVp. (p. 411)
15. ±5%; ±20% (p. 411)
16. 3 to 5 rad (30 to 50 mGy); 10 rad (p. 412)
17. 10 R (100 mGy); 20 R (200 mGy) (p. 412)
18. 10 to 40 µR (or 0.1 to 0.4 µGy) (p. 413)
19. ±5; ±2; ±1 (p. 413)
20. ±10 HU; ±10 HU; ±10 HU (p. 414)
21. $x / 60 = 15 / 30$
    $x = 60 (15 / 30)$
    $x = 30$ mrad (p. 413)
22. $x / 55 = 20 / 25$
    $x = 55 (20 / 25)$
    $= 55 (4 / 5)$ mrad
    $= 11 (4)$ mrad
    $= 44$ mrad (p. 413)
23. See page 408.
24. See Table 31-1. (p. 409)
25. Both methods rely on a precision radiation dosimeter. First, one can make a series of at least three exposures at the same technique factors, changing the technique controls between each exposure. If the result is not reproducible, it is usually so because of error in the kVp control. Second, one can select a combination of technique factors and hold them constant for a series of 10 exposures. There are mathematical formulas that allow the determination of reproducibility in both instances. They basically require that the output radiation intensity not vary by more than ±5%. (pp. 411–412)
26. The use of photo-fluorospot images is fairly routine. These images use less film, require less personnel interaction, and are produced with a lower patient dose. (p. 413)
27. See page 416.
28. See page 417.
29. See page 417.

Challenge Questions

1. The fabrication of an x-ray tube is an exceptionally complex process. Specification of focal-spot size depends not only on the

geometry of the tube but also on the focusing of the electron beam. The consequent permitted variations in advertised focal-spot size are shown in Table 31-3. (p. 410)

2. See page 413.
3. See pages 415 and 416.
4. See Table 31-9. (p. 416)

Chapter 32

1. during handling and storage; during exposure; during film processing (p. 420)
2. obscure (p. 420)
3. geometric (p. 420)
4. gelatin; emulsion; sharp (p. 420)
5. curtain; two colors; yellow; green; blue; purple (p. 420)
6. turn-around; sprung (p. 420)
7. white-light (p. 422)
8. hypo; thiosulfate (p. 423)
9. Artifacts interfere with the radiologist's diagnosis by limiting the entire view of the image. (p. 420)
10. Pi lines occur at 3.1416-inch (π) intervals because of dirt or a chemical stain on a roller. Since the rollers are 1 inch in diameter, 3.1416 inches represent one revolution of a roller. (p. 422)
11. Chemical fog is produced with improper or inadequate processing chemistry and appears as a dichroic stain, a curtain effect. Chemical fog is usually a uniform, dull gray. Dichroic stains can appear yellow, green, blue or purple. When chemistry is not properly squeezed from the film, it either runs down the leading edge of the film or up the trailing edge, producing the curtain effect. White-light leaks from a safelight that is used improperly can cause streak-like densities on the film. This is light fog. Films left in the x-ray room during an exposure can become fogged by radiation exposure. Radiation fog and light fog look alike. (pp. 420 and 422)
12. a.   Exposure artifacts are associated with the manner in which the radiographer conducts the exam. Patient motion produces unsharp or blurred images; lack of centering produces cut-off artifacts; improper screen-film contact produces smoothness; and warped cassettes cause geometric artifacts. Finally, of course, failing to remove articles like jewelry and eyeglasses produces still other artifacts.

   b.   Processing artifacts include the following: Dirty or warped rollers can cause emulsion pickoff and gelatin buildup, which result in sludge deposits on the film. These artifacts appear as sharp areas of altered optical density. Chemical fog, dichroic stain, and curtain effect are the result of improper processing chemistry. Guide-shoe marks occur when the guide shoes on the turn-around assembly are either sprung or out of position. Pi lines occur because of dirt or a chemical stain on the roller. Finally, wet-pressure sensitization occurs because of irregular or dirty rollers. It shows up as circular patterns of increased optical density.

   c.   Handling and storage artifacts occur as a result of radiation fog (excess exposure) or light fog (due to white-light leaks). Kink marks and scratches occur as a result of rough handling, showing fingernail marks when the film is kinked or abruptly bent. Static is caused by a buildup of electrons in the emulsion. The most common versions are crown, tree, and smudge. Finally, hypo retention causes a yellowish stain during storage. (pp. 420–423)

Challenge Questions

1.   Charts and quizzes will be based on information found throughout this chapter.

Across
   1. chemical
   2. geometric
   3. pi lines
   4. radiation
   5. curtain
   6. mammography
   7. double exposures

Down
   1. warped
   2. optical density
   3. smoothness

4. wet-pressure
5. dichroic
6. static
7. cut-off
8. fingernail
9. unsharp
10. sludge

Chapter 33

1. The diagram on the left shows (a) mitosis; the one on the right is (b) meiosis. Mitosis is the phase of the cell cycle during which the chromosomes become visible, divide, and migrate to daughter cells. The letters in the diagram indicate each of the following: A, interphase; B, prophase; C, metaphase; D, anaphase; E, telophase; and F, interphase. In the diagram on the right we see meiosis. Meiosis is the process of reduction and division, and it occurs only in germ cells. The letter n in the diagram is the number of similar chromosomes. The topmost arrow shows the shift from interphase to DNA replication, where the number of chromosomes doubles. The second arrow shows a mitosis-like division of the germ cell into two copies of the original. The bottom two arrows show these two new cells each splitting into yet two more daughter cells, with no DNA replication to produce four daughter cells with half the chromosome number of the original cell in interphase. (p. 437)
2. E, F, E, F, E, L, L, E, L, L, E, L (p. 430)
3. a (p. 430)
4. b (p. 431)
5. c (p. 431)
6. d (p. 431)
7. d (p. 432)
8. d (p. 435)
9. c (p. 435)
10. b (p. 435)
11. early (or immediate); late (or delayed) (p. 430)
12. ionizing radiation; biologic (p. 431)
13. proteins; lipids (or fats); carbohydrates (or sugars and starches); nucleic acids (p. 431)
14. life; carbon (p. 432)
15. proteins; lipids; carbohydrates (pp. 431–432)
16. 2; hydrogen; 1; oxygen (p. 432)

17. provide fuel for cell metabolism (p. 433)
18. nucleus; cytoplasm; messenger RNA (mRNA); transfer RNA (tRNA) (p. 433)
19. nucleus; cytoplasm; DNA; RNA; protein; water (p. 435)
20. 1 Mrad (10 kGy); 100 rad (1 Gy) (p. 435)
21. two-chromatid; four-chromatid (p. 437)
22. become visible; divide; migrate to daughter cells (p. 437)
23. reduction; division; germ cells (p. 437)
24. 60% hydrogen
    25.7% oxygen
    10.7% carbon
    2.4% nitrogen
    0.2% calcium
    0.1% phosphorus
    0.1% sulfur
    0.8% trace elements (p. 431)
25. 80% water
    15% protein
    2% lipids
    1% carbohydrates
    1% nucleic acid
    1% other   (p. 432)
26. c, h, i, b, f, a, g, d, e (p. 432)
27. a.   mitochondria
    b.   secretory channel
    c.   cell membrane
    d.   lysosomes
    e.   ribosomes
    f.   endoplasmic reticulum
    g.   nucleus
    h.   nuclear membrane
    i.   nucleoli (p. 435)
28. Its chemical-binding properties change. If the atom is a constituent of a large molecule, the ionization may result in breakage of the molecule or relocation of the atom within the molecule. The abnormal molecule may in time function improperly or cease to function, which can result in serious impairment or death of the cell. (p. 430)
29. The basis of the cell theory is Schneider and Schwann's proof that all plants and animals contain cells as their basic functional units. (p. 431)
30. The formula for a protein is $C_nH_nO_nN_nT_n$. The formula for a lipid is $C_nH_nO_n$. (p. 432)
31. DNA consists of a backbone composed of alternating segments of deoxyribose (a sugar)

and phosphate. For each deoxyribose-phosphate conjugate formed, a molecule of water is removed. Attached to each deoxyribose molecule is one of four different nitrogen-containing or nitrogenous organic bases: adenine, guanine, thymine, or cytosine. Adenine and guanine are purines. Thymine and cytosine are pyrimidines. For a discussion of how nucleotides (the base sugar-phosphate combinations) are strung together and attached in ladder fashion, see page 433. The completed ladder is twisted on an imaginary axis to form a molecule in a double-helix configuration. (p. 435)

32. RNA resembles DNA structurally. The sugar component is ribose rather than deoxyribose, and uracil replaces thymine as a base component. In contrast, RNA forms a single spiral, not a double helix. (p. 435)

33. Cell proliferation is the act of a single cell or group of cells reproducing and multiplying in number. This increase in number of cells by reproduction is a result of the process of cell division, a mechanism that results in twice the number of cells. (p. 436)

34. Basically, when somatic cells undergo proliferation, they undergo mitosis. Genetic cells undergo meiosis. More extensive differences are described on pages 436–437.

35. Each cycle includes the various states of cell growth, development, and division. The geneticist considers only two phases of the cell cycle: mitosis (M) and interphase. Mitosis, the division phase, is characterized by four subphases: prophase, metaphase, anaphase, and telophase. The portion of the cell cycle between mitotic events is termed interphase. Interphase is the period of growth of the cell between divisions. The cell biologist usually identifies four phases of the cell cycle: M, G_1, S, and G_2. These phases of the cell cycle are characterized by the structure of the chromosomes, which contain the genetic material DNA. The gap in cell growth between M and S is G_1. It is termed the pre-DNA synthesis phase, while the DNA synthesis phase is S. More detailed descriptions of all these phases are found on pages 436–437.

36. Changes in genetic material occur during meiosis, the division process of genetic cells.

The primary genetic cells, the germ cells, begin with the same number of chromosomes as somatic cells, 23 pairs (46 chromosomes), but for a germ cell to be capable of marriage with another germ cell, its complement of chromosomes must be reduced by half to 23 so that, following the conception and union of two germ cells, the daughter cells will contain 46 chromosomes. This process of reduction division of germ cells is meiosis. It is more thoroughly described on page 437. "Crossing over" is a process by which, during the second division, there is some exchange of chromosomal material among chromatids. Crossing over results in changes in genetic constitution and changes in inheritable traits. (p. 437)

37. Basically, these types can be broken down into epithelium, connective and supporting tissues, muscle, and nervous tissue. (p. 438)

38. The parenchymal part contains tissues that are representative of that particular organ, whereas the stromal part is composed of connective tissue and vasculature that provides structure to the organ. (p. 438)

Challenge Questions

1. Tables will vary, of course, but should be accurately based on the information provided on pages 432–433.

2. Diagrams will use the discussion on page 438 as their bases.

Chapter 34

1. The illustration demonstrates the various shapes that nonlinear dose-response relationships can assume on a graph. (p. 445)
2. c (p. 442)
3. a (p. 442)
4. c (p. 442)
5. b (p. 443)
6. d (p. 443)
7. ionizing radiation; soft tissue (p. 442)
8. 3 keV/μm (p. 442)
9. 200 to 250 kVp; 1 (p. 442)
10. 5% to 10% (p. 444)
11. radiosensitizers; halogenated pyrimidine; methotrexate; actinomycin D; hydroxyurea; vitamin K (p. 444)

12. radioprotectors (p. 444)
13. Radiosensitivity is a function of metabolic state of the tissue being irradiated. Basically, this law states that the radiosensitivity of living tissue varies as follows:
    a. Stems cells are radiosensitive. The more mature a cell is, the more resistant to radiation it is.
    b. The younger the tissues and organs are, the more radiosensitive they are.
    c. When the level of metabolic activity is high, radiosensitivity is also high.
    d. As the proliferation rate for cells and the growth rate for tissues increase, the radiosensitivity increases also. (p. 442)
14. If the time of irradiation is lengthened, a higher dose is requried to produce the same effect. This lengthening of time can be accomplished in two ways. Dose protraction causes less effect because of the lower dose rate and the longer irradiation time. Dose fractionation causes less effect because tissue repair and recovery occur between doses. (p. 442)
15. Aerobic means oxygenated, anoxic means without oxygen, and hypoxic refers to a low-oxygen condition. (p. 443)
16. Biologic tissue is more senstive to radiation when irradiated in an oxygenated (aerobic) state than when in an anoxic or hypoxic state. This characteristic of biologic tissue is called the oxygen effect. It is described numerically by the oxygen enhancement ratio (OER). The OER is calcuated as follows:

$$OER = \frac{\text{Dose necessary under anoxic conditions to produce a great effect}}{\text{Dose necessary under aerobic conditions to produce a great effect}}$$

(p. 443)
17. Tissue is generally irradiated under full oxygenation (aerobic state). (p. 443)
18. (a) If the radiation dose is not sufficient to kill the cell before its next division (interphase death), then given sufficient time, the cell will recover from sublethal radiation damage. (b) This intracellular recovery is due to a repair mechanism inherent in the biochemistry of the cell. Some types of cells have greater capacity for repair of sublethal

damage than others. (c) At the whole-body level this recovery from radiation damage is assisted through repopulation by the surviving cells. (p. 444)
19. These two types of agents are radiosensitizers, which have an effectiveness ratio up to 2, and radioprotectors, which have an effectiveness ratio that is also approximately 2. (p. 444)
20. Radioprotective agents have not found human application because, to be effective, they must be administered in toxic levels. Thus, the protective agent can be worse than the radiation. (p. 444)
21. A dose-response relationship is a mathematical relationship between different radiation doses and the magnitude of the observed response. Radiation dose-response relationships have two important applications in radiology. First, these experimentally determined relationships are used to design therapeutic treatment routines for patients with cancer. Second, radiobiologic studies have been designed to provide information on the effects of low-dose irradiation. (p. 444)
22. See lengthy discussion on page 445.
23. See discussion on page 446.

Challenge Questions

1. See pages 443–444.

Chapter 35

1. A. main-chain scission
   B. cross-linking
   C. point lesions
   D. transcription
   E. transfer
   F. translation
   Explanations of each of these processes are found on pages 450–451.
2. e, g, a, c, f, b, h, d (pp. 450–453)
   a. outside the body or cell
   b. within the body or cell
   c. breakage of the thread or backbone of the long-chain macromolecule
   d. thick fluidity
   e. process in which small, spurlike molecules extend off the main chain and

attach to a neighboring macromolecule or to another segment of the same molecule

f. disruptions of single chemical bonds in a molecule that can result in minor modifications of the molecule

g. uncharged molecules containing a single unpaired electron in the valence or outermost shell

h. molecular lesions of the DNA that cause genetic mutations occurring as a result of radiation damage

3. d (p. 450)
4. b (p. 450)
5. a (p. 453)
6. b (p. 453)
7. c (p. 454)
8. a (p. 454)
9. c (p. 459)
10. d (p. 459)
11. b (p. 459)
12. molecular; macromolecules; water (p. 450)
13. water; water (p. 450)
14. in vitro (p. 450)
15. translation; transferred; transcribed (p. 450)
16. deoxyribonucleic acid; genetic; chromosomes (p. 450)
17. cell death; malignant disease; genetic damage; linear, nonthreshold dose-response (p. 452)
18. dissociates; radiolysis (p. 452)
19. direct; indirect; free radicals (p. 453)
20. hit; larger; free radicals (p. 454)
21. maximal (p. 459)
22. See discussion on page 451.
23. These include the following categories:
    1. main-chain scission with only one side rail severed
    2. main-chain scission with both side rails severed
    3. main-chain scission and subsequent cross-linking
    4. rung breakage causing a separation of bases
    5. a change or loss of a base (p. 452)
24. (a) The equation for radiolysis of water is shown on page 453, along with a discussion. Basically, what happens is that the atom dissociates into two ions, or an ion pair. (b) See page 453 for the formulas. When an atom of water is irradiated and ionized, it dissociates

into two ions (an ion pair). After initial ionization, a number of reactions can happen. First, the ion pair may rejoin into a stable water molecule, and no damage occurs. Second, if these ions do not rejoin, it is then possible for the negative ion (the electron) to attach to another water molecule and produce yet a third molecule. (pp. 452–453)

25. See page 453.
26. During radiolysis of water, the OH* free radical can join with a similar molecule and form hydrogen peroxide. The H* free radical can interact with molecular oxygen if it is present to form the hydroperoxyl radical. The hydroperoxyl radical, along with hydrogen peroxide, is considered to be the principal damaging product after the radiolysis of water. Hydrogen peroxide can also be formed by interaction of two hydroperoxyl radicals. See page 453 for equations.

27. According to target theory, for a cell to die after radiation exposure, its target molecule must be inactivated. There is considerable experimental evidence in support of the target theory that suggests overwhelmingly that the key molecular target is the DNA. Originally, target theory was used to represent cell lethality. It can be used equally well, however, to describe nonlethal radiation-induced cell abnormalities. (p. 454)

28. The interaction between radiation and cellular components is random. When an interaction does occur between radiation and the target, a "hit" is said to have occurred. (p. 454)

29. See the raindrop analogy on pages 456–457.

30. When this type of experiment was first conducted with human cells, the observed extrapolation number was 2. That result agreed with the hypothesis that similar regions on two homologous chromosomes (an identical pair) had to be inactivated to produce cell death. Since chromosomes come in pairs, the experimental results confirmed the hypothesis. Subsequent experiments, however, have resulted in extrapolation numbers ranging from 2 to 12, and therefore the precise meaning of n in the model's equation is unknown. The D_Q is called the threshold dose. It is a measure of the width of the shoulder of the multitarget, single-hit model

and is related to the capacity of the cell to recover from sublethal damage. A large D_Q indicates that the cell can readily recover. (p. 457)

31. The split-dose technique is designed to describe the capacity of a cell to recover from sublethal damage. Related experiments show that cells that survive an initial radiation insult exhibit precisely the same characteristics as nonirradiated cells, and therefore they have fully recovered from the sublethal damage produced by the initial irradiation. Consequently, D_Q is not only a measure of the capacity to accumulate sublethal damage but also a measure of the ability of the cell to recover from sublethal damage. (p. 458)

32. Age-response function is the pattern of change in radiosensitivity as a function of phase in the cello cycle. (p. 458)

33. RBE =

$$\frac{D_O \text{ (standard radiation)}}{D_O \text{ (test radiation)}}$$ to produce the same effect (p. 459)

Challenge Questions

1. See Figure 35-3. (p. 451)
2. See page 454.
3. The single-target, single-hit model applies to biologic targets such as enzymes, viruses, and simple cells like bacteria. The multitarget, single-hit model applies to more complicated biologic systems such as human cells. The equations for each are found and interpreted on pages 455–457.

Chapter 36

1. b (p. 464)
2. a (p. 464)
3. d (pp. 464–465)
4. d (p. 467)
5. a (p. 467)
6. c (p. 468)
7. a (p. 468)
8. c (p. 470)
9. b (p. 470)
10. d (p. 472)
11. d (p. 475)
12. 100 rad (p. 464)
13. 200 to 1000 rad (p. 465)

14. 100 rad (1 Gy); 600 rad (6 Gy); 1000 rad (10 Gy) (p. 466)
15. $LD_{50/30}$; 30 days; 300 rad (3 Gy) (p. 466)
16. nonlinear, threshold (p. 466)
17. hematologic; CNS; GI effects (p. 467)
18. fractionated; 200 rad (2 Gy); five (p. 468)
19. lymphocytes; spermatogonia; direct; lymphocytes; precursor (p. 471)
20. ring; dicentric; chromatid (p. 474)
21. SED50; 600; 200 rad; 500 rad (p. 475)
22. Draw a horizontal line from the 75% level on the y-axis until it intersects the S curve. Now drop a vertical line from this point to the x-axis. This intersection with the x-axis occurs at approximately 325 rad (3.25 Gy). (p. 466)
23. Draw a horizontal line from the 8% level on the y-axis until it intersects the S curve. Now drop a vertical line from this point to the x-axis. This intersection with the x-axis occurs at approximately 200 rad (2 Gy). (p. 466)
24. Draw a horizontal line from the 91% level on the y-axis until it intersects the S curve. Now drop a vertical line from this point to the x-axis. This intersection with the x-axis occurs at approximately 420 rad (4.2 Gy). (p. 466)
25. See page 465.
26. (a) After a single dose of 300 to 1000 rad (3 to 10 Gy), an initial mild erythema may occur within the first or second day. This first wave of erythema then subsides, only to be followed by a second wave that reaches maximum intensity in about 2 weeks. At higher doses, this second wave of erythema is followed by a moist desquamation. Moist desquamation is known as clinical tolerance for radiation therapy. (p. 468)
27. See Figure 36-4. (p. 469)
28. Information on how radiation effects on the ovaries are somewhat age-dependent is found on page 469. The ovaries are especially radiosensitive at the fetal stage and in early childhood.
29. See page 469.
30. Radiation doses as low as 10 rad (100 mGy) can result in a reduction in the number of spermatozoa. With increasing doses, the depletion of spermatozoa becomes greater and extends over a longer period of time. A dose of 200 rad (2 Gy) produces temporary infertility, which will commence approximately 2 months after irradiation and persist

for up to 12 months. A dose of 500 rad (5 G7) to the testes produces permanent sterility. (p. 469)

31. The first cells to become affected are the lymphocytes. The lymphocytes and spermatogonia are considered the most radiosensitive cells in the body. (p. 471)
32. These responses are covered on page 471.
33. See pages 473–474.
34. Single-hit aberrations are produced with a linear, nonthreshold dose-response relationship. Multihit aberrations are produced after a nonlinear, nonthreshold relationship. The approximate equations for each of these relationships are as follows:

single hit: $Y = a + bD$

multihit: $Y = a + bD + cD^2$

Y is the number of single- or multihit chromosome aberrations, a is the naturally occurring frequency of chromosome aberrations, and b and c are coefficients of damage for single- and multihit aberrations. the variable, radiation dose is represented by D. (pp. 474–475)

Challenge Questions

1. For a full discussion of the hematologic syndrome, see page 465.
2. See Table 36-2.
3. Answers will be gleaned from the entire chapter.
4. Since male gametogenesis is a self-renewing system, there is some evidence to suggest that genetic mutations induced in surviving post-spermatogonial cells represent the most hazardous mutations. Consequently, after testicular irradiation of doses above approximately 10 rad (100 mGy), the male should refrain from procreation for 2 to 4 months until all cells in the spermatogonial and postspermatogonial stages at the time of irradiation have matured and disappeared. This will reduce but probably not eliminate any increase in genetic mutations because of the persistence of the stem cell. (pp. 469–470)

Across
1. thrombocytes
2. gastrointestinal
3. prodromal
4. lymphopenia
5. dermis
6. erythrocytes
7. epilation
8. granulocytosis
9. atrophy
10. oogonia
11. erythrocytes
12. granulocytes

Down
1. erythema
2. acute
3. basal
4. desquamation
5. graunlocytopenia
6. gametogenesis
7. cytogenetics
8. manifest
9. epidermis
10. leukocytes
11. thrombocytes
12. leukopenia
13. grenz
14. oocytes
15. latent

Chapter 37

1. a. exposure
   b. latent period
   c. excess incidence
   d. spontaneous incidence
   e. exposure
   f. latent period
   g. excess incidence
   h. spontaneous incidence
   i. In the absolute age-response relationship, the increased incidence of cancer is a constant number of cases after a minimal latent period. The relative age-response relationship suggests that the increased incidence of cancer is proportional to the natural incidence. This second model is the one most subscribe to. (p. 488)
2. a (p. 478)
3. d (p. 478)
4. c (p. 480)
5. d (p. 480)
6. b (p. 481)

7. a (p. 482)
8. b (p. 483)
9. d (p. 489)
10. d (p. 490)
11. dose; LET (p. 478)
12. 300,000; 100,000; 100,000; 10 rad; 100; linear, nonthreshold (p. 483)
13. prenatal death; spontaneous abortion (pp. 489–490)
14. linear, nonthreshold; quality; frequency (p. 491)
15. T (p. 480)
16. T (p. 481)
17. F (p. 486)
18. F (p. 486)
19. T (p. 488)
20. F (p. 488)
21. T (p. 492)
22. F (p. 492)
23. Relative risk = Observed / Expected = 00.00300 / 00.00150 = 2 (p. 481)
24. Relative risk = Observed / Expected = 00.00250 / 00.00150 = 5 / 3 = 1.67 (p. 481)
25. Excess cases = observed – expected = 30 – 0.005 = ~ 30 (p. 482)
26. (Six cases / 10^6 persons/rad/yr) (10^5 persons) (0.15 rad) (20 years) = 1.8 (p. 482)
27. (10 cases / 10^6 persons/rad/yr) (0.3 x 10^6) (0.01 rad) = 10 / 0.003 = 0.03 cases per year. (p. 482)
28. These studies are difficult because (a) the dose is usually not known but is presumed to be low, and (b) the frequency of response is very low. Consequently, the results of radiation epidemiologic studies do not carry the statistical accuracy that observations of early radiation effects do. (p. 478)
29. (a) The radiosensitivity of the lens of the eye is age-dependent. The older the individual, the greater the radiation effect and the shorter the latent period. (b) Latent periods varying from 5 to 30 years have been observed in humans, and the average latent period is approximately 15 years. High-LET radiation, such as neurons, has a high RBE for the production of cataracts. The dose-response relationship for radiation-induced cataracts is apparently threshold, nonlinear.
30. Occupational exposures to the lens of the eyes are too low to require protective lens shields for radiographers or radiologists. It is nearly impossible for a medical radiation worker to reach the threshold dose. However, the radiation administered to patients undergoing head and neck examinations by either fluoroscopy or CT can be significant. In CT, the lens dose can be 5 rad per slice. In either case, protective lens shields are not normally required. (p. 479)
31. Unlike the relative risk, which is a dimensionless ratio, the absolute risk has units of number of cases/10^6 persons/rad/year. Absolute risk values range from approximately one to ten cases/10^6 persons/rad/year. Ten cases is the approximate absolute risk of death from all malignant disease. To determine the absolute risk factor, one must assume a linear dose-response relationship. (p. 482)
32. Some suggest that the reason British radiologists did not show the same elevated risk of leukemia as their American counterparts did from the turn of the century to 1960 could be the fact that radiation therapy activities in Great Britain have always been attended by medical physicists, who presumably were more radiation safety-conscious. (p. 484)
33. Results suggested a linear, nonthreshold dose-response relationship. (p. 485)
34. It is difficult to ascribe any case of cancer to a previous radiation exposure, regardless of its magnitude because cancer is so common. Approximately 20% of all deaths are caused by cancer; therefore, any radiation-induced cancers are obscured. Leukemia, on the other hand, is a rare disease. That makes analysis of radiation-induced leukemia easier. (p. 485)
35. See page 486.
36. The radiation exposure in the uranium mines occurs because the high concentration of uranium ore, which is radioactive with a very long half-life, decays through a series of radioactive nuclides by successive alpha and beta emissions, each accompanied by gamma radiation. The relative risk to uranium minors is approximately 8:1. Interestingly, uranium miners who smoke have a relative risk of approximately 20:1. (p. 487)
37. First, they estimated the excess mortality from malignant disease after a one-time acci-

dental exposure to 10 rad that is highly unlikely in diagnostic imaging. Second, they considered the response to a dose of 1 rad/year for life. This situation is possible in diagnostic imaging but is certainly rare. Finally, they considered excess radiation-induced cancer mortality after a continuous dose of 100 mrad/year. This is considerably higher than that found for radiographers. (p. 488)

Challenge Questions

1. See page 485.
2. See pages 486–487.
3. In addition to drawing from research, answers should reflect the text by asserting the following: (a) Responses of concern to diagnostic imaging include spontaneous abortion, congenital abnormalities, mental retardation, and childhood malignancy. (b) Radioiodine is known to concentrate principally in the thyroid gland. The thyroid gland begins to function at approximately 10 weeks of gestation, and since the radioiodine readily crosses the placental barrier from the mother's blood to the fetal circulation, radioiodine should be administered during pregnancy only in trace doses and before the 10-week gestation period. At any time thereafter, the hazard of such an administration increases. See also Table 37-8 and the discussion on page 491.

Chapter 38

1. b (p. 496)
2. a (p. 499)
3. d (pp. 499–500)
4. b (p. 501)
5. c (p. 502)
6. c (p. 502)
7. a (p. 502)
8. c (p. 502)
9. d (p. 502)
10. d (p. 502)
11. time; distance; shielding (p. 496)
12. motion blur; patient and personnel exposure (p. 496)
13. decreases; inverse square law (p. 497)

14. reduce; one-tenth (p. 497)
15. 10^{-4}/year; NCRP Dose Limits (p. 499)
16. occupational; 100 mrem (1 mSv); downward (p. 499)
17. one-tenth (p. 501)
18. as low as reasonably achievable (p. 502)
19. Occupational exposure =
    (300 mR/hr) (40 min / 60 min/hr) =
    200 mR. (p. 496)
20. Time = exposure / exposure rate =
    40 mR / 500 mR/hr =
    2 / 25 hour = 4.8 minutes (p. 496)
21. Patient exposure =
    (5 R/mA-minute) (2.2 mA) (3 minutes) =
    33 R (p. 496)
22. (2.4 mR/mAs) $(100 / 400)^2$ =
    (2.4 mR/mAs) (0.0625) =
    0.15 mR/mAs (p. 496)
23. 500 mR/hr at patient's head
    500 mR / 60 min = x mR / 3 min
    x = 25 mR
24. (400,000) (10-4) = 40 (p. 499)
25. 1 TVL = 3.3 HVL (p. 497)
26. See Table 38-3. (p. 500)
27. Jackie should wear an extremity personnel monitor. This device is worn on the wrist or finger.
28. The effective DL is 50 mSv per year; environmental background radiation is approximately 1 mSv per year. Finally, occupational exposures are closer to the latter (environmental background radiation) than to the former (effective DL). (p. 504)
29. Elective booking is the most direct way to ensure against the irradiation of an unsuspected pregnancy. This requires that the clinician or radiologist determine the time of the patient's previous menstrual cycle. X-ray exams in which the fetus is not in or near the primary beam may be allowed, but should be accompanied by pelvic shielding.
30. (a) The first step is to estimate fetal dose. If it exceeds 1 rad, a more complete dosimetric evaluation should be conducted. (b) In the case of a KUB exam, fetal dose is approximately 70 mrad. (c) Once this is known, the physician and radiologist should determine the stage of gestation at which the x-ray exposure occurred. They can then advise the patient accordingly. (p. 507)

Challenge Questions

1. Answers are found on pages 499–501.
2. (a) Since essentially all exposure to occupational workers occurs during fluoroscopy and the trunk is shielded by a lead apron, the response of the monitor on the collar overestimates the effective dose (E). (b) A conversion factor of 0.3 is applied to the monitor reported value to estimate E. (c) For a radiographer who does no fluoroscopy, the monitor response may be considered the effective dose. (p. 501)
3. You should agree with this student. The fetus protected by the mother's lead apron, and the dose at waist level under a protective apron would be less than 10% of the collar dose. In addition, because of attenuation by maternal tissues overlying the fetus, the dose to the fetus is approximately 30% of the abdominal skin dose. (p. 503)
4. Steps that Pete should incorporate into the radiation protection program include (1) new employee training, (2) periodic in-service training, and (3) counseling during pregnancy. Issues to be covered in each category are discussed on pp. 502–505.
5. Problems suggested here would be based on the box on page 504.

Chapter 39

1. d (p. 511)
2. a (p. 512)
3. d (pp. 514–515)
4. d (p. 515)
5. b (p. 515)
6. c (p. 515)
7. b (p. 515)
8. a. 2.5
   b. 1.5
   c. 0.5 (p. 510)
9. 0.25-millimeter; 0.25-millimeter (p. 512)
10. 5 (p. 512)
11. 2.1 R; 10 R; 20 R (p. 512)
12. 4 lb/ft^2; 4 inches (p. 512)
13. a secondary barrier (p. 513)
14. fluoroscopy (p. 514)
15. controlled area; less than 100 mR; uncontrolled; 2 mR per week; two tenth-value layers (TVL) (p. 514)
16. thicker; workload (W); milliampere-minutes; mA-min/wk (p. 515)
17. use factor (A); 1/4; 1 (p. 515)
18. central collecting; electrons; increases; increases (p. 516)
19. photon; light; photoelectron; electron; energy absorbed by the crystal from the incident photon (p. 519)
20. F (p. 510)
21. T (p. 510)
22. F (p. 511)
23. T (p. 511)
24. F (p. 511)
25. F (p. 511)
26. F (p. 513)
27. F (p. 513)
28. T (p. 515)
29. T (p. 515)
30. T (p. 515)
31. T (p. 515)
32. At 1 meter:
    250 mR x 0.1% = 250 mR x 0.001 = 0.25 mR
    At 3 meters:
    0.25 mR $(1/3)^2$ = 0.25 mR (1/9) = 0.028 mR = 28 μR (p. 513)
33. From scatter radiation the barrier will receive the following:
    Total primary beam =
    6 mR mAs x 100 mA x 4 m x 60 sec/meter = 144,000 mR
    Scatter radiation =
    144,000 mR x 1/1000 x $(1/3)^2$ = 16 mR (p. 513)
    From leakage radiation, the barrier will receive the following:
    Leakage radiation at 1 meter =
    100 mR/hr x 4/60 hr = 6.6 mR
    Leakage radiation = 6.6 mR $(1/3)^2$ = 0.73 mR
    Total secondary radiation =
    10 mR + 0.73 mR = 10.73 mR or 11% of the dose limit (p. 514)
34. Answers should summarize the information given on pages 511–512.
35. The nine features are as follows:
    Source-to-skin distance (not less than 38 cm on stationary fluoroscopes and not less than 30 cm on mobile fluoroscopes); Primary pro-

tective barrier (Image-intensifier assembly; 2-millimeter lead equivalent, coupled with tube and interlocked); Filtration (at least 2.5 millimeter aluminum equivalent); Collimation (unexposed border visible on monitor when input phosphor is 35 cm above table top and collimators fully open); Exposure switch (dead-man type); Bucky slot cover (moved to end of table, leaving an opening of about 5 cm at gonad level, covered by Bucky slot cover of at least 0.25-mm lead equivalent); Protective curtain (at least 0.25 mm lead equivalent); Cumulative timer (interrupts beam when time exceeds 5 min.); X-ray intensity (at tabletop, no more than 2.1 R per min for each mA at 80 kVp; for no high level control, not more than 10 R per min; with high level control, maximum of 20 R per min) (pp. 511–512)

36. He will need to consider (a) the useful beam, (b) leakage radiation, and (c) scatter radiation. (p. 513)

37. Lead is rarely required for secondary protective barriers because the computation usually results in less than 0.4 mm lead. In such cases, conventional gypsum board, glass, or lead acrylic is adequate. (p. 513)

38. Centering the x-ray machine in the middle of the room means that no single wall is subjected to especially intense radiation exposure. (p. 514)

39. (a) The three types of radiation detection devices other than film badges are (1) gas-filled radiation detectors; (2) thermoluminescence dosimeters (TLD) used for patient and personnel monitoring; and (3) scintillation detectors, the imaging device used in the gamma camera in nuclear medicine and in some CT scanners. (b) The three types of gas-filled detectors are the ionization chambers, proportional counters, and Geiger-Muller detectors. (pp. 515–516)

40. Components should be labeled as follows:
    a. aluminum seal
    b. photocathode
    c. dynodes
    d. collector
    e. base
    f. glass envelope
    g. window
    A description of the function of each of these

components is discussed on pages 518–519.

41. See pages 519–520.

42. See pages 519–520.

Challenge Questions

1. The use of the area being protected is of principal importance, because if it were rarely occupied (like a closet), the required shielding would be less than if it were an office or lab occupied 40 hours a week. This reflects the time of occupancy factor (T). Guidelines for levels of occupancy, as suggested by the NCRP, are found in Table 39-3 on page 514.

2. See page 516.

3. See pages 517–519.

4. See pages 520–521

Chapter 40

1. 50 mSv (5000 mrem) per year; 5 mSv (500 mrem) per year (p. 524)

2. radiologists; radiographers; radiologist (p. 524)

3. fluoroscopy; portable radiography (p. 524)

4. 4 R per minute (p. 529)

5. 20 mrad (200 µGy) (p. 529)

6. two times (p. 530)

7. 100 mrad; 300 mrad (p. 530)

8. individual glandular (p. 530)

9. 1.8 meters (p. 532)

10. one quarter (p. 532)

11. no (p. 532)

12. 0.25; 0.5; 1 (p. 535)

13. wrap-around (p. 536)

14. Exposure = Exposure rate x Time = 300 mR per hour x 1.5 minutes = 300 mR per hour x 0.025 hour = 7.5 mR (p. 524)

15. Occupational exposure = 0.1 mR per scan x 25 scans = 2.5 mR (p. 526)

16. Estimate the intersection between a vertical line rising from 3 millimeters aluminum and a horizontal line through 70 kVp. Extend the horizontal line to the y-axis and read 4 mR/mAs.
    4 mR/mAs x 20 mAs = 80 mR = 0.08 mrad (p. 527)

17. At 80 cm SSD, the intensity wll be greater by $(100 / 80)^2 = (1.25)^2 = 1.56$
    3.2 mR/mAs $\times$ 1.56 = 4.9 mR/mAs (p. 528)

18. $(80/72)^2 = (1.1)^2 = 1.21$
    7.1 mR/mAs $\times$ 1.21 = 8.6 mR/mAs (p. 528)

19. At 80-centimeters SSD:
    Dose =
    (5 mR/mAs) $(63 \text{ kVp}/70 \text{ kVp})^2$ (200 mAs) =
    810 mR = 810 mrad
    At 90-centimeters SSD:
    Dose =
    (810 mrad) $(80/90)^2$ = 720 mrad (p. 528)

20. ESE = (4 R/minute)(3 minutes) = 12 R
    (p. 529)

21. ESE = (4 R/minute)(1.5 minutes) = 6 R
    (p. 529)

22. Dose =
    (420 mR)(45 mAs/90 mAs)
       $(74 \text{ kVp}/70 \text{ kVp})^2$ =
    (420 mR)(0.5)$(1.06)^2$ =
    (420 mR)(0.5)(1.1) =
    231 mR (p. 538)

23. Both are right. When protective barriers are not available, such as during portable examinations, the portable x-ray machine should be equipped with an exposure cord long enough to allow the radiographer to leave the immediate exam area. The radiographer should wear a protective apron for each portable examination. During fluoroscopy, both radiologist and radigorapher are exposed to relatively high levels of radiation. Personnel exposure, however, is directly related to the x-ray beam-on time. (p. 524)

24. Personnel engaged in angiointerventional procedures often receive higher exposures than do those in general imaging practice because of longer fluoroscopic exposure times. The frequent absence of an intensifier tower protective curtain and the extensive use of cineradiography also contribute to higher personnel exposure. (p. 524)

25. Personnel exposures associated with both types of exams are low. Exposures in mammography are low because the low kVp of operation results in reduced scatter radiation. Usually a long exposure cord and a conventional wall or window wall are sufficient to provide adequate protection. Rarely does a room used strictly for mammography require protective lead shielding. Exposures in CT are low too. Since the CT x-ray beam is finely collimated and only secondary radiation is present in the scan room, the radiation levels are low compared with those experienced in fluoroscopy. (p. 525)

26. There are two reasons for this. First, the frequency of x-ray exams is increasing among all age groups at a rate of between 6% and 10% per year in the United States. Second, there is increasing concern among public health officials and radiation scientists regarding the risk associated with medical x-ray exposure. (p. 526)

27. The three ways this is estimated and reported are via the (a) entrance skin exposure (ESE), the gonadal dose, and the dose to the bone marrow. (p. 526)

28. The first method is the use of a nomogram, in particular one that a medical physicist contstructs specifically for the unit. Another method requires that one know the output intensity for at least one operating condition. With this calibration value available, one would first make adjustment for a different SSD, by using the inverse square law. Knowing the ESE, the kVp, and mAs of the exam can be calculated. The final step in estimating ESE is to multiply the output intensity in mR/mAs by the examination mAs, since they are proportional. (p. 528)

29. The genetically significant dose (GSD) is the population gonad dose of importance since it is the radiation dose for the population gene pool. See page 529 for more information.

30. The technique to be used has an ESE of 10 mrad, 2 mrad mean marrow dose, and a gonad dose of less than 1. (Table 40-1)

31. See page 529.

32. See page 530.

33. See discussion on page 530, second column.

34. Patient dose = $k \times \text{IE} / \sigma^2 \times w^3 \times h$
    In this equation, k is a conversion factor, I is beam intensity in mAs, E is average beam energy in keV (approximately 0.45 kVp), σ is system noise, w is pixel size, and h is slice thickness. (p. 531)

35. See pages 532–533.

36. See pages 533–534.

37. See pages 534–535.

38. See page 535.

39. See page 537.
40. See page 537.
41. See page 539.

Challenge Questions

1. See page 535.
2. See applicable sections throughout this chapter.

Across
1. millirem
2. milliroentgen
3. quarter
4. effective dose
5. exposure
6. genetically

Down
1. millirad
2. control
3. gender
4. fluoroscopy
5. patient dose
6. dose
7. weighted

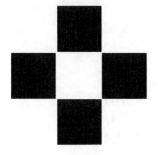

Math Tutor Answers

Working with Decimal Timers
Exercise 1
1 5 mAs
2 6.4 mAs
3 1.9 mAs
4 12.5 mAs
5 80 mAs
6 4 mAs
7 10 mAs
8 12.8 mAs
9 3 mAs
10 0.3 mAs
11 25 mAs
12 60 mAs
13 80 mAs
14 1.6 mAs
15 0.6 mAs
16 7 mAs
17 9 mAs
18 21 mAs
19 210 mAs
20 30 mAs
21 150 mAs
22 480 mAs
23 3.6 mAs
24 4.8 mAs
25 30 mAs
26 90 mAs
27 12 mAs
28 4.5 mAs
29 75 mAs
30 7.5 mAs
31 45 mAs
32 1.8 mAs
33 1.2 mAs
34 4 mAs
35 16 mAs
36 32 mAs
37 64 mAs
38 6.4 mAs
39 132 mAs
40 320 mAs
41 280 mAs
42 2.8 mAs

43 40 mAs
44 15 mAs
45 100 mAs
46 350 mAs
47 3.5 mAs
48 62.5 mAs

Working with Fractional Timers
Exercise 2
1 50 mAs
2 5 mAs
3 2 mAs
4 20 mAs
5 approx. 12 mAs
6 approx. 1.2 mAs
7 approx. 8 mAs
8 approx. 0.8 mAs
9 approx. 15 mAs
10 approx. 7 mAs
11 2.5 mAs
12 approx. 33 mAs
13 approx. 3.3 mAs
14 approx. 16 or 17 mAs
15 approx. 1.6 or 1.7 mAs
16 approx. 66 or 67 mAs

Exercise 3
1 approx. 24 or 25 mAs
2 2.5 mAs
3 40 mAs
4 4 mAs
5 approx. 6 mAs
6 approx. 2.4 or 2.5 mAs
7 approx. 16 or 17 mAs
8 approx. 1.6 or 1.7 mAs
9 approx. 4 mAs
10 approx. 0.4 mAs
11 approx. 7 to 8 mAs
12 approx. 14 mAs
13 5 mAs
14 approx. 16 or 17 mAs
15 approx. 1.6 or 1.7 mAs
16 approx. 66 or 67 mAs
17 approx. 6.6 or 6.7 mAs

18 approx. 32 to 34 mAs
19 approx. 3.2 to 3.4 mAs
20 approx. 132 to 134 mAs
21 approx. 8 to 9 mAs
22 approx. 0.8 to 0.9 mAs
23 approx. 0.6 to 0.7 mAs
24 approx. 30 mAs

Exercise 4
1 60 mAs
2 50 mAs
3 6 mAs
4 5 mAs
5 15 mAs
6 150 mAs
7 20 mAs
8 25 mAs
9 2.5 mAs
10 12 mAs
11 75 mAs
12 7.5 mAs
13 approx. 36 mAs
14 approx. 3.6 mAs
15 approx. 45 mAs
16 10 mAs

Exercise 5
1 20 mAs (4 sets of 5)
2 25 mAs (5 sets of 5)
3 30 mAs (6 sets of 5)
4 80 mAs (4 sets of 20)
5 120 mAs (6 sets of 20)
6 8 mAs (4 sets of 2)
7 12 mAs (6 sets of 2)
8 125 mAs (5 sets of 25)
9 150 mAs (6 sets of 25)
10 12.5 mAs (5 sets of 2.5)
11 15 mAs (6 sets of 2.5)
12 20 mAs (1/3 of 60, or 6 sets of 3.3)
13 approx. 13 mAs (4 sets of 3.3)
14 approx. 6.4 mAs (4 sets of 1.6)
15 approx. 60 mAs (4 sets of 15)
16 approx. 48-50 mAs (4 sets of 12 or 12.5)
17 approx. 4.8-5 mAs (4 sets of 1.25)
18 approx. 60 mAs (5 sets of 12)
19 approx. 48-50 mAs (6 sets of 8)
20 approx. 5 mAs (6 sets of .8)
21 approx. 40 mAs (5 sets of 8)
22 approx. 3.2-3.3 mAs (4 sets of 0.8)
23 approx. 28 mAs (4 sets of 7)
24 approx. 35 mAs (5 sets of 7)

25 approx. 16 mAs (4 sets of 4)
26 approx. 20 mAs (5 sets of 4)
27 approx. 24 mAs (6 sets of 4)
28 approx. 120-132 mAs (4 sets of 33)

Exercise 6
1 40 mAs
2 approx. 14 mAs (2 sets of 7)
3 approx. 21 mAs
4 15 mAs (3 sets of 5)
5 35 mAs
6 150 mAs
7 80 mAs (2 sets of 40)
8 120 mAs
9 160 mAs
10 60 mAs
11 140 mAs
12 approx. 28-30 mAs (2 x 7 x 2)
13 approx. 42 mAs (2 x 7 x 3)
14 30 mAs (3 sets of 10)
15 70 mAs
16 160 mAs (2 sets of 80)
17 240 mAs
18 320 mAs
19 120 mAs (3 x 40)
20 280 mAs
21 200 mAs
22 120 mAs (2 x 60)
23 180 mAs
24 240 mAs
25 90 mAs
26 210 mAs (7 x 30)
27 40 mAs (2 x 20)
28 60 mAs
29 45 mAs (3 x 15)
30 60 mAs
31 140 mAs
32 200 mAs
33 150 mAs
34 350 mAs (7 x 50)
35 75 mAs (3 x 25)
36 240 mAs (2 x 120)
37 360 mAs
38 180 mAs (3 x 60)
39 90 mAs (3 x 30)
40 120 mAs*

* Note that on question 40 you may simply take double the answer you would get at the 300 mA station. If you have memorized that 15s and 20s go together at the 300 mA station, then a 15th at 600 would be double 20 or 40. Then take 3 sets

of 40. Many problems at the 600 mA station can be solved this way, just doubling the answer you would get at 300 mA. Also, many mAs values can be figured at the 400 mA station in a similar manner by doubling numbers you are familiar with using at the 200 mA station.

Timers: Converting Fractions into Decimals and Vice Versa

Exercise 7

1 0.75
2 0.667
3 0.25
4 0.2
5 0.167
6 0.142
7 0.125
8 0.083
9 0.0667
10 0.05
11 0.04
12 0.033
13 0.025
14 0.02
15 0.0167
16 0.0125
17 0.01
18 0.0083
19 0.7
20 0.133
21 0.15
22 0.4
23 0.6
24 0.8
25 0.33
26 0.2
27 0.35
28 0.0067
29 0.375
30 0.3125

Exercise 8

1 1/20
2 1/30 (common denominator is 333)
3 1/5
4 3/4
5 1/40
6 2/3
7 1/7 (common denominator is 143)
8 1/500

9 4/5
10 1/6 (common denominator is 167)
11 1/8
12 3/5
13 1/16
14 1/12 (common denominator is 833)

Finding mA and Time Combinations for a Desired mAs

Exercise 9

1 2 sets of 40
2 3 sets of 15
3 2 sets of 33
4 3 sets of 25
5 3 sets of 60
6 3 sets of 40 *or* 2 sets of 60
7 2 sets of 80 *or* 4 sets of 40
8 3 sets of 80 *or* 4 sets of 60
9 3 sets of 30
10 4 sets of 80

Exercise 10

1 1/50
2 1/40
3 2/3 (2 sets of 33)
4 1/15
5 1/6
6 1/12
7 1/30
8 1/60
9 1/80
10 1/120
11 2/5 (2 sets of 20)
12 1/30
13 1/20
14 1/40
15 1/8
16 1/5
17 3/5 (3 sets of 40)
18 1/40
19 1/40
20 2/15 (2 sets of 7)
21 1/6
22 1/50
23 1/15
24 1/120
25 3/20 (3 sets of 15)
26 3/5 (3 sets of 60)
27 4/5 (4 sets of 60)
28 1/4 (cut in half twice)

29 1/5
30 3/5 (3 sets of 80)

Exercise 11

1 0.04
2 0.025
3 0.67
4 0.07
5 0.16
6 0.08
7 0.033
8 0.017
9 0.4
10 0.05
11 0.025
12 0.125
13 0.2
14 0.6
15 0.025
16 0.0125
17 0.7
18 0.17
19 0.02
20 0.07
21 0.6
22 0.25
23 0.2
24 0.6

Technique Adjustments

Exercise 12

1 6
2 4.5
3 4
4 2.5
5 3
6 10.5
7 6
8 9
9 16.5
10 3
11 approx. 5
12 6
13 approx. 4
14 approx. 7
15 9
16 102 kVp
17 46 kVp
18 64-65 kVp
19 74 kVp

Exercise 13

1 approx. 75
2 approx. 30
3 approx. 30
4 approx. 36
5 15
6 10
7 15
8 25
9 68-70
10 four times
11 two times
12 1/4
13 1/2
14 62.5
15 3.47
16 0.77
17 0.28
18 70
19 12-in
20 30-in
21 40-in
22 60-in
23 1.17
24 4.34
25 8.1
26 0.31
27 0.69
28 1.93
29 0.56